PRAISE FOR GOOD HEALTH FOR
AFRICAN AMERICANS

"A valuable resource for both African Americans and health professionals who need to better understand the situation faced by contemporary black America."

—*Oakland Tribune*

"*Good Health for African Americans,* an expansive, yet concisely written work . . . is a winner of a book."

—*Quarterly Black Review of Books*

"Dixon supplies a fascinating historical explanation as to why disease and mortality rates differ between blacks and other Americans. . . . These are potentially political issues, and Dixon handles them with grace and sensitivity while mapping lifestyle changes needed for improved health."

—*Publishers Weekly*

"An intriguing mix of historical perspective and informative, valuable information."

—*Detroit Free Press*

"The most comprehensive self-help book of its kind."

—*Cleveland Plain-Dealer*

"Good, solid health information."

—*The Sunday Denver Post*

"An important new book."

—*Orange County Register*

Also by Barbara M. Dixon, R.D., L.D.N., with Josleen Wilson

Good Health for African Americans

This Book Recommends Reg. milk for Black folks so Read everything else with caution

GOOD HEALTH
FOR AFRICAN-
AMERICAN
KIDS

Barbara M. Dixon, R.D., L.D.N.,

with Josleen Wilson

Foreword by Melvin E. Jenkins, M.D.

Preface by Keith C. Ferdinand, M.D., F.A.C.C.

Crown Trade Paperbacks
New York

For my Aunt Mateal and Uncle Oliver Douglas,
my second parents, for all the years of love, support,
and being there always. I wish all children could
experience the same kind of caring.

Copyright © 1996 by Barbara M. Dixon and Josleen Wilson
Foreword copyright © 1996 by Melvin E. Jenkins, M.D.
Preface copyright © 1996 by Keith C. Ferdinand, M.D.

Published by Crown Trade Paperbacks, 201 East 50th Street, New York, New York
10022. Member of the Crown Publishing Group.

Random House, Inc. New York, Toronto, London, Sydney, Auckland

CROWN TRADE PAPERBACKS and colophon are trademarks of Crown Publishers, Inc.

Printed in the United States of America

Design by Lenny Henderson

Library of Congress Cataloging-in-Publication Data
Dixon, Barbara M.
   Good health for African-American kids/Barbara M. Dixon, with Josleen Wilson.—1st pbk. ed.
   Includes bibliographical references and index.
   1. Afro-American children—Health and hygiene.   2. Pediatrics—Popular
works.   3. Afro-American children—Nutrition.   I. Wilson, Josleen.   II. Title.
RJ61.D612   1996
649'.4'08996073—dc20   95-34601
                                                                    CIP

ISBN 0-517-88269-8

10 9 8 7 6 5 4 3 2 1

First Edition

CONTENTS

ACKNOWLEDGMENTS

I am especially grateful for the love, patience, and invaluable medical advice I received from my husband, Henry C. Dixon, M.D., who reminded me always about the importance of encouraging good health and disease prevention for prospective mothers, children, and families. I also wish to thank all of those friends and readers I have met over the last two years who showed so much interest in our first book, *Good Health for African Americans,* and asked time and again that we expand that work into a book for parents and children.

Josleen Wilson and I wish to thank our agent, Barbara Lowenstein, whose insight into the wide reading audience among African Americans was accurate and timely; and our editor, Carol Taylor, for her strong support, steady hand, and belief in this work. We are also grateful to Steve Magnuson and all of our friends at Crown Publishers who have been so supportive to us over the last two years.

We gratefully acknowledge the contributions of Donald Biglands, who illustrated the Kids' Food Pyramid, and the four outstanding researchers and editors who helped gather and analyze the vast amount of information that underlies this work. Roslyn Tolson of Southern University Library (Baton Rouge, Louisiana)—thank you again for helping us get started with an important collection of research. Jeffrey Felshman (Chicago) and Lee Seifman (New York) provided both research and editorial support for the major chapters on lifestyle and various diseases, and Sheila Gaffney (New York) provided editorial support throughout.

My special thanks to Tom Ketterer, food service director, and Debbie Budd of the Baton Rouge General Medical Center for their invaluable assistance in computing the nutrient content of the recipes in Chapter 18.

I am indebted to Melvin M. Murrill, M.D., and Karen Williams, M.D., for their advice and thorough medical review of the manuscript. I am especially grateful to Irene Jackson-Townsend, M.D., for her guidance and encouragement, as well as for her friendship over the years.

FOREWORD

Good physical and mental health in childhood leads to good health during adulthood. In African Americans, this positive relationship is not necessarily a given. Our child health statistics are totally unacceptable, just as comparable adult health parameters are far below desired levels. For African Americans a vicious health circle is created: Unmet health needs at any point on the circle augment unfulfilled health needs at every other point. Poor child health and poor adult health complement each other, and perpetuate the endless circle. By the same token, interventions to break the circle have far-reaching effects—particularly if they begin in childhood.

Barbara M. Dixon's sequel to her earlier book, *Good Health for African Americans,* published in 1994, completes a unique literary unit of two volumes. This second book, *Good Health for African-American Kids,* also written with Josleen Wilson, is presented in that similar refreshing and personable writing style, which facilitated the easy reading and comprehension of the first book.

As a pediatrician for almost fifty years and also a pediatric endocrinologist for most of that time, I am very aware that two of the core philosophies that buffer the strength of this book are ones that took me many years to fully appreciate. First, at least one-third of this second work analyzes, emphasizes, and utilizes childhood nutrition and places it at the core of child health. This encompasses the broad expanse of growth and development, mental health, disease prevention and treatment, as well as the interplay of poverty and environment that impacts so profoundly on the health of African-American children.

In most European countries, as reported at the 1990 conference on "Cross National Comparisons of Child Health," poor child health statistics correlate most consistently with geographic pockets of poverty. Poverty begets poor health everywhere. Among African Americans, racism adds another deleterious dimension that augments their health discrepancies. Barbara Dixon uses her expertise in nutrition to pursue logical and forceful arguments, which place into a practical perspective the critical position of major and minor nutrients in the health of African-American infants, children, and adolescents. The influence of good nutrition during the pregnancy and prenatal periods is also appropriately covered.

Second, this book also addresses the interaction between emotional stress and physical disease, both from a causative as well as a responsive perspective. Stress is a major cause of health problems, but, on the other hand, illness causes stress. Hans Selye, the long-time director of the Institute of Experimental Medicine and Surgery in Montreal, Canada, spent a lifetime developing theoretical constructs that explain the impact of stress on disease. Most of his thirty-four books, including *The Stress of Life* (2nd Ed., 1976), attempted to develop a unifying concept for all disease reactions and outcomes. The common denominator in his hypotheses was stress, which produces chemical changes that are mediated through a chain reaction triggered by an increase in hydrocortisone from the adrenal gland.

Barbara Dixon's emphasis on stress as a part of poor health in African-American children, particularly the stress of racism, gives considerable credence to a holistic approach to child health care. Folk practices, like chicken soup for colds, are not to be scoffed at if used within a framework of accepted medical practice. Actually, Tom Lambo, a Nigerian psychiatrist who was deputy director of the World Health Organization for many years, advocated the use of traditional healers alongside modern physicians to treat Nigerian patients. His system has been successfully incorporated into the curricula of many African medical schools.

This book properly places considerable priority on disease prevention and health maintenance. Major diseases in African-American children such as AIDS, diabetes, high blood pressure, sickle-cell disease, asthma, and lead exposure are singled out for special emphasis, and conflict-resolution strategies are presented as violence preventives.

Barbara Dixon and Josleen Wilson have written a book that should be considered valuable reading not only for African-American families but also for health-care professionals who care for children. Our individual and collective responsibilities to African-American children are especially large. It is with the execution of tenets such as those presented in this book that good child health will improve health parameters in African-American adults.

Melvin E. Jenkins, M.D.
Professor Emeritus and Past Chairman
Department of Pediatrics and Child Health
Howard University College of Medicine
Washington, D.C.

PREFACE

As a parent of four children, I know that raising a child can be complicated. With *Good Health for African-American Kids*, Barbara M. Dixon offers an excellent addition to our base knowledge about our children's nutrition and health, starting with early childhood and continuing all the way through adolescence. Through these years, she appropriately looks at the whole child, and includes in the total picture dental health, common childhood ailments, and lifestyle habits, as well as serious diseases such as childhood HIV and AIDS, asthma, and sickle-cell anemia that are known to disproportionately affect African-American children.

Ms. Dixon shows how parents and children can alter or improve nutrition and lifestyle practices that have significant impact on health issues in the African-American community. This is crucial information for African-American families.

With increasing urbanization and poor health habits, cardiovascular disease (heart attack and stroke) has quickly become the most common cause of death in the African-American community and among all Americans. Each year there are 1.5 million new heart attacks, with 500,000 deaths. One-half million people suffer strokes each year, and nearly 150,000 die from them.

Most of these events occur in the over-forty age group. But we know that the process of atherosclerosis (hardening of the arteries) leading up to heart attack and stroke begins early in life. The history of that process goes from a normal artery, through which blood and oxygen freely flow, to the initial appearance of a fatty streak, to a fibrous plaque, and finally to a complicated lesion that may rupture, causing heart attacks, strokes, gangrene, and aortic aneurysms.

In an autopsy study of 110 children and young adults (mean age 17.9 years) in the recent Bogalusa Heart Trial, almost all subjects were found to have deposits of fatty streaks in coronary arteries, and 6 had more advanced plaques.

In the past twenty years, researchers have increasingly recognized that certain risk factors—hypertension, obesity, smoking, lack of exercise—promote this process. All of these risk factors occur more frequently among African Americans, and all are affected by lifestyle habits that begin during childhood.

It's true that heart transplants and artificial hearts are exciting developments in modern medical technology. However, expensive and complicated surgeries and interventions do not decrease the chance of developing a heart attack or sudden death. Clearly, from every vantage point—individual well-being, long life, and economics—preventing these episodes is by far the most productive path to the future. As a researcher and practicing cardiologist, especially treating African-American patients, I have been increasingly convinced that the leading causes for death and disability in black Americans are largely preventable.

In the Heartbeats Life Center, our cardiovascular clinic in New Orleans, we help patients understand the workings of bodies and help prevent disease before it happens. For many years, I have personally known of the work of nutritionist and dietitian Barbara Dixon in neighboring Baton Rouge. She has led the charge in getting the message out to the African-American community that premature death and disability can be avoided. I consider her book on the health of African-American children essential in that struggle.

Modifying risk factors in childhood and shaping a child's perception of health and well-being remain the most important aspects of addressing cardiovascular diseases. After all the headlines and front-page stories about new medical technologies are forgotten, our children will benefit most from knowing how to take care of their own bodies and avoid disease. Our children are our future and our most important resource. *Good Health for African-American Kids* goes a long way toward helping us raise our children in an environment with the best circumstances possible.

Keith C. Ferdinand, M.D., F.A.C.C.
Medical Director, Heartbeats Life Center, New Orleans, LA
Associate Professor, Clinical Pharmacology, College of Pharmacy, Xavier University of New Orleans
Editor in Chief, *Urban Cardiology*
Past Chairman, Association of Black Cardiologists

INTRODUCTION

African-American kids are bubbling over with vitality. When I think of my own childhood, I remember being constantly busy, listening to music, dancing, and never tiring of playing games with my friends. I also remember the closeness I felt within my family, my sweetest bond. Most of my friends felt the same way about their own families. In general, African-American families tend to create a warm and joyous environment for kids. In some ways, black families are stricter than those of other cultural and ethnic groups; in other ways, they are looser and more accepting of differences among children.

Despite the horrifying images we see on the nightly news, most African-American kids are not violent, uneducated street thugs—far from it. Most are encouraged to do well in school and to prepare themselves for college, where they can receive the education needed to fulfill their dreams.

The health of African-American kids, like that of all children, depends largely on their environment, the foods they eat, their access to regular medical checkups and health care, and the stability of their families. And like children from all ethnic groups, African-American children have biological strengths and vulnerabilities that are passed along within families.

Yet, there's an increasing health gap between black Americans and the rest of American society, even when you compare similar levels of income. It's a gap that begins widening very early in life. Today, black children are the single most vulnerable group in our nation, as indicated by the following statistics from the U.S. Department of Health and Human Services and other health agencies.

Black infants are twice as likely as white infants to die at birth.

They are twice as likely to be born prematurely and underweight, which increases their risk of birth defects, autism, physical and mental handicaps, and respiratory and infectious diseases.

They are four times as likely to be born HIV-positive, making them the fastest-growing group of patients with AIDS.

If they survive their first twenty-eight days, black infants are three times more likely to die from sudden infant death syndrome (SIDS).

As they grow up, health problems increase. African-American children are more likely to be victims of accidents; they are more likely to suffer infections such as whooping cough and measles; they are three times as likely to die of asthma; and they are four times as likely to contract and die of tuberculosis. Black children are twice as likely to suffer from lead poisoning as white children living in identical environments.

Most researchers believe that in one way or another, poverty causes most of their health problems. Poor children everywhere are much more likely to live in toxic environments, to suffer from malnutrition, and to have little or no access to health care. Poverty tends to perpetuate itself; it's hard to break the cycle when you are the product of a broken family, when you lack education and training, and when you suffer from poor health.

The question is, If family income were equal for blacks and whites, would health status be equal, too? Perhaps not. Startling differences in birth weight and the incidence of infant mortality, asthma and other respiratory ailments, and lead poisoning persist even when environments are similar. Something larger appears to be involved.

Rich or poor, African-American children appear to suffer different health problems from those of other children because of certain accumulating risk factors. Although scant, new research points to a complex web of history, culture, environment, genetics, and racism.

Several researchers have suggested that it's not inherited genes that cause health problems, but inherited stress. At an early age and even *in the womb*, black children suffer great stress. Like African-American adults, they suffer from racism, which is incredibly stressful.

Health professionals are only beginning to understand how significant stress is to a child's health; for example, stress can initiate or exacerbate many illnesses that begin in childhood, including heart disease and high blood pressure. By adolescence, stress may be expressed as free-floating anger, which has been linked to violent and risky behavior and deadly accidents—leading causes of mortality in this age group. In Baton Rouge where I live, black-on-black crime, mostly involving teenagers and young adults, is responsible for over 70 percent of homicides yearly.

Health problems are compounded by lack of good health information in our communities. African-American parents and children at all income levels lack access to good prevention programs, including nutrition education, exercise, and reinforcement of positive health practices. Such programs are vital in helping families learn how to take care of their own health.

Where such programs are available, black families tend *not* to participate in them. Basically, we view these programs as white-oriented and fail to recognize that they are beneficial for everyone.

Culture affects our nutritional status as well as the foods we choose. Early reports released from the ongoing Bogalusa Children's Heart Study in Louisiana show that the high-fat, high-salt, high-sugar diet many black children eat may be setting them up for early health problems.

Culture also determines the ways in which we do (or do not) seek health care. Our past experiences in the United States created a distrust of the medical establishment, which may partially explain why African-American kids often do not see a doctor or dentist yearly, or receive timely immunizations, even when cost is not a factor.

Our family culture influences our lifestyle practices. The use of cigarettes, alcohol, and drugs starts early in the black community, where youngsters are often targeted by advertisers. Smoking cigarettes and drinking alcohol, destructive in themselves, can also trigger a hidden genetic predisposition toward certain diseases, as well as aggravate many others.

The wide range of possible health dangers seems frightening. But whether our children are babies or teenagers, we don't have to wait for all medical mysteries to be solved. Nor do we have to wait for federal and state health initiatives that may never happen.

My goal is to bring the diverse elements that impact on the health of African-American children into focus so we can start to reverse the statistics. This book is designed to address the specific issues that disproportionately affect African-American children. It's not, however, an encyclopedia of child health.

I have tried to identify economic and environmental issues that affect the health of all children, then separate these from cultural and genetic issues that primarily affect African-American children.

The theme of this book is prevention. It concentrates on changes in lifestyle, fitness, and nutrition that your whole family can make happen today, and offers information to help you protect the health of your children, beginning with your own health before pregnancy. Finally, the book tackles certain critical ailments that affect African-American children disproportionately in comparison with other groups.

Good health is a gift we can give our children now, whether they are babies, children, or adolescents. Promoting good health in childhood is the primary and most effective way to close the health gap and improve life expectancy for all African Americans.

A NOTE ABOUT HEALTH AND RACIAL STATISTICS

In this book, "racial" groups are identified by broad regional divisions: The word *African* or *black* means a population that originated in Africa. Similarly, the word *white* denotes a population that originated on the continent of Europe.

Most scientists agree that biologically speaking there is no such thing as race. "Races," as we think of them, share characteristics that arose when spontaneous mutations proved to be protective in a particular environment. Beneficial mutations survived and were genetically passed on because they were life-giving. Over the course of human history, as different groups of *Homo sapiens* moved and merged, individual genes traveled and were assimilated by thousands of generations living in many different environments.

For convenience, anthropologists later separated humans into three arbitrary groups—Caucasoid, Mongoloid, and Negroid—based on hair color and texture, eye color and shape, stature and shape of the head, and skin color. However, every individual carries millions of inherited genes, and there are often greater biological differences among individuals in the same group than between groups.

Many modern scientists prefer to identify population groups by geographic or cultural origin—hence the current use of terms like *Asian* and *Hispanic*—although, carried to its logical end, we would then have hundreds, or perhaps even thousands, of racial groups.

For thousands of years human beings have been migrating all over the globe, and they continue to do so today. Few groups remain isolated from the rest of the world. Certainly, few Americans today are purely one thing or another, regardless of their skin color.

For all of these reasons, most geneticists study inherited genes within families but not within races. Like everyone else, African Americans inherit genetic traits from their parents, and our parents may have had African, European, Asian, Hispanic, and Native American ancestors.

If that's the case, what do health statistics reported by race tell us? Often, they don't tell us much at all. One glaring example concerns the way birth certificates and death certificates are reported.

Less than ten years ago, the race of each baby born in the United States was classified by the Center of Health Statistics according to the racial identity of one parent or the other. Which parent was chosen depended on which race was involved. If both parents were white, a newborn was classified as white. If both parents were other than white, the child was assigned its father's race. But if one parent was white and the other nonwhite, no matter which, the child was assigned the race of its nonwhite parent.

The guidelines were changed in 1987, although the new classifications are only beginning to be reflected in current statistics. Now every American baby is classified according to its mother's race. Although the system is uniform, it still tells us very little about a child's racial makeup.

Statistics become even more unreliable if an infant dies. African-American infant mortality has always been known to be high, but now we know that the numbers are higher than previously reported. Dr. Robert Hahn, an epidemiologist at the federal Centers for Disease Control and Prevention, examined the records of 117,188 infants born from 1983 through 1985 who died within a year. He found that infant mortality was slightly overreported for whites, but underreported for all other groups, *because on their death certificates, some babies were incorrectly reported as white.* How is that possible?

Funeral directors or municipal officials who prepare death certificates fill in a race classification based on the infant's *appearance.* Many newborns categorized as "nonwhite" according to federal guidelines actually looked white. If an infant died, funeral directors often unwittingly recorded a different racial classification. As a result, infant mortality among all nonwhite groups was vastly underestimated.

After Dr. Hahn's discovery, death and birth certificates began to be matched through computer linkups. When future data are recorded, both documents should at least record the same race. But as long as American babies are classified only by the mother's race, health statistics reported along racial lines can never be depended upon to provide quality information.

There are even more problems with racial designation and health statistics. It's not unusual to find "black children" and "low-income children" grouped together, then compared with "white children," as if economics and skin color were somehow the same. This kind of reporting is bound to be misleading. To yield useful facts, health statistics of low-income black children would have to be compared with low-income white children, and so on up the economic ladder.

Moreover, research studies involving African-American children are still fairly few and far between. All of these factors contribute to contradictory and often unreliable information regarding the health of African-American kids, which makes it extremely difficult to discover the root causes of particular health problems.

In this book I have tried to use only those research statistics which were objectively analyzed. I wish that we could provide absolute answers, but that is impossible at this stage. However, every effort has been made to present conflicting evidence fairly, and to draw fair-minded conclusions based on the available evidence.

Many factors make good health harder for black children to achieve. But it's not impossible. Historically, the ability of African Americans to overcome adversity has been miraculous. We are a determined and vigorous people, and I believe we can overcome our most desperate health statistics by drawing on our past for strength and knowledge. We can—indeed, we must—become more actively involved in teaching our children about the importance of a healthy diet and living habits. Taking charge of your children's health and teaching them how to maintain it is important for their personal happiness and productivity, and also for the strength of our community as a whole.

My hope is that this information will also motivate the health-care professionals working in our communities to seek imaginative ways to help solve the health crisis. As I traveled across the country last year promoting our first book, *Good Health for African Americans*, I saw many examples of community empowerment that convinced me that we can do this job. The Free Health Clinic in Kansas City, Missouri, is one good example. This clinic provides free, quality health care and mental-health counseling to pregnant women, infants, children, adolescents, and people with a variety of health problems. Clinic volunteers—blacks, Hispanics, and whites—go into the community to provide vital health information. This is the kind of outreach we can accomplish, even with humble beginnings.

Part One

___

AFRICAN-AMERICAN CHILDREN— OUR MOST PRECIOUS RESOURCE

1

YOUR CHILD'S FAMILY TREE

Because many serious health problems may be inherited, including hypertension, diabetes, and heart disease, knowing the health status of a child's immediate ancestors can help identify, and often prevent, potential problems.

The tradition of keeping the extended family close has been a long-standing practice among African Americans. Our heritage, like the heritage of many ethnic cultures in the United States, holds that all adults are responsible for nurturing all children. The tradition continues today, even though many more adult children are moving away from the towns and communities where their families have lived for generations. Still, holiday gatherings and family reunions remain popular traditions. These events when your family is together are good opportunities to gather health information about various family members. At just such a family get-together, I learned more about my own family health tree, including the fact that on my mother's side, high blood pressure and stroke were common, and on my father's side, heart disease and renal (kidney) failure were common.

Because of the widespread custom of informal adoption in our communities, it may not be easy to assess all of your child's antecedents. The practice of informal adoption has its roots in the period of enslavement, when children could be sold away from their parents and husbands and wives were sold away from each other. At the same time, slaveholders also encouraged new marriages, knowing that family ties would reduce rebellion and escape. Those who were enslaved never forgot their own lost children and loved ones, and yet they also accepted other children brought into their care.

Our African heritage and our experiences in the period of enslavement continue to shape our families today. Modern black families have many faces—urban and rural, wealthy and poor, and everything in between—but the tradition of extended family is shared by all. A family may include aunts, uncles, cousins, in-laws, grandparents, informally adopted children, and single moms and dads. If you're unable to determine the health status of your child's immediate relatives, you can begin a new family tree now, which will later benefit his or her children.

TEN RISK FACTORS THAT AFFECT AFRICAN-AMERICAN KIDS

When the American Heart Association speaks of "risk factors," they mean conditions that lead to heart disease. For example, people with high blood pressure or diabetes are more likely than others to develop heart disease. So are people who smoke. But when it comes to African-American children, we need to think about risk factors in a new way.

Most health research is carried out on adults. However, the persistent decline in the health status of children in the United States has caused researchers to realize that we could learn a great deal about the development of adult diseases by discovering when and how these diseases *begin*.

Identifying and eliminating risk factors in young children may help them avoid life-threatening diseases in adulthood. At the very least, identifying risk factors will put them in the best possible position to receive early treatment and management if health problems arise later.

Here are ten risk factors that sooner or later are most likely to cause health problems for African-American kids:

> *Cultural/Social*
>> *Fatty diet*
>> *Lack of physical exercise*
>> *Childhood stress*
>> *Too much salt (sodium) in the diet*

> > *Smoking, alcohol, drugs*
> >
> > *Poverty, which can contribute to all of the above, plus increase the risk of:*
> >
> > > *Exposure to lead in paint*
> > >
> > > *Exposure to accidents*
> > >
> > > *Poor nutrition*
> >
> > *Genetic risk factors*
> >
> > > *Parents who carry the sickle-cell gene*
> > >
> > > *Parent(s) with diabetes*
> > >
> > > *Parent(s) with hypertension*
> > >
> > > *Parent(s) with high blood cholesterol (familial hyper-cholesterolemia)*

Each risk factor can lead to a range of devastating health problems; two or more together compounds the risk. Only 10 percent of risk factors fall into the genetics category. You don't have much control over genetic risk factors, since you cannot change your child's genetic blueprint. However, knowing that a child may have a genetic tendency toward a particular disease can help you prepare for and better manage the disease should it develop. Fully 80 percent of risk factors fall into the cultural/social category, meaning that these are risks you can change.

To a great extent, cultural/social risk factors are also passed along within families. One excellent way to identify in advance risk factors to which your child is vulnerable is to make a family tree.

MAKING YOUR FAMILY TREE

When a doctor asks you whether you have a "family" history of certain diseases, he's talking about diseases that are known to run in your immediate family, such as heart disease, diabetes, hypertension, sickle-cell anemia, or others.

Your child's family tree is a graphic depiction of all known family members, beginning with your child at the base. Right above are you and your child's other parent, along with the siblings of both parents. Then come both sets of grandparents, and so on, until the tree is as tall and full as possible. You can go back as far as your research takes you. For each person, write in health information, including diseases that person suffered from and the cause of death. Leave room to include lifestyle/environmental influences that affect health, such as smoking, alcohol, type of diet, and exercise.

Here is a sample outline:

Grandmother	Grandfather	Grandmother	Grandfather
_____	_____	_____	_____
a _____	a _____	a _____	a _____
b _____	b _____	b _____	b _____
c _____	c _____	c _____	c _____
c _____	c _____	c _____	c _____

Aunt/Uncle	Aunt/Uncle	Aunt/Uncle	Aunt/Uncle
_____	_____	_____	_____
a _____	a _____	a _____	a _____
b _____	b _____	b _____	b _____
c _____	c _____	c _____	c _____
c _____	c _____	c _____	c _____

Mother	Father
_____	_____
a _____	a _____
b _____	b _____
c _____	c _____
c _____	c _____

Sibling	Sibling	Child	Sibling	Sibling
_____	_____	_____	_____	_____
aa _____	aa _____	aa _____	aa _____	aa _____
aa _____	aa _____	aa _____	aa _____	aa _____
aa _____	aa _____	aa _____	aa _____	aa _____

Family Health Tree

a – Disease(s) b – Cause of Death c – Lifestyle Practices
aa – Childhood Diseases or Health Problems

2

PREPARING FOR PREGNANCY

Every child's health begins in the womb, where the mother's body supplies all of its needs. Your own health plays an essential part in getting your child off to a good start. This is a particularly vital issue for African-American women. In 1994, almost 13.6 percent of African-American babies were of low birth weight—more than double the rate for whites. Low-birth-weight babies are more likely to be born with physical and mental handicaps, as well as respiratory and infectious diseases; if they survive, they may also suffer from behavioral problems in childhood.

The term *low birth weight* is confusing. All babies born under five and a half pounds are classified as low-birth-weight babies. However, low-birth-weight infants are of two different types: those who are born too small because they are born too soon; those who are born on time but are too small for their gestational age.

This differentiation is extremely important when it comes to pregnancy in African-American women. It is well known that African-American infants are somewhat smaller than others at birth, and most of the medical attention has been directed toward increasing birth size. However, the results of new studies released in 1995 by the National Institute of Environmental Health Sciences indicate that *prematurity* is the main underlying cause of stillbirth and early infant death. Ninety percent of very low-birth-weight babies (under 3.3 pounds) are born too soon. And African-American women are much more likely than other women to go into premature labor (see chapter 4).

Over the past ten years, preterm deliveries among all pregnant women have been gradually, and steadily, rising, even among women who received early prenatal care. This suggests that those who provide prenatal care are failing to recognize some of the causes of prematurity or failing to intervene to correct them. We desperately need new strategies for preventing premature delivery.

CAUSES OF PREMATURITY

The four common complications that account for most preterm deliveries are:

> *Infection or premature rupture of the amniotic membranes*
> *Premature labor for no apparent reason*
> *High blood pressure*
> *Hemorrhaging (blood loss)*

These conditions cause premature birth and dangerously under-sized babies among all women, regardless of race or ethnicity. But black women are three times as likely to experience these problems during pregnancy.

Moreover, African-American women are three times more likely than white women to die from complications of pregnancy. The difference seems to be due to a greater incidence of ectopic pregnancies and toxemia, conditions that often can be diagnosed early or prevented with early and continued prenatal care. (An ectopic pregnancy means the fertilized egg has implanted outside the uterus. This embryo cannot survive; it must be surgically removed immediately to protect the mother's life. Toxemia is caused by poisons circulating in the blood, often associated with high blood pressure, inadequate kidney function, and convulsions. The underlying cause must be discovered and treated immediately, before the fetus is damaged.)

A MOTHER'S RISK FACTORS

Prematurity and/or low birth weight appear to be caused by a complex interplay of risk factors. Most studies show that preventing or treating the following maternal risk factors can help lower the rate of infant mortality and also preserve a mother's life.

- Little or no prenatal care
- Being too heavy or too thin going into pregnancy
- Smoking during pregnancy
- Using alcohol and/or drugs
- Anemia or inadequate nutrition
- Being younger than age twenty
- Preexisting medical conditions
- Too much or too little weight gain during pregnancy
- Having several previous children, particularly if they were born underweight

All of these risks, or contributors, disproportionately affect African-American women, especially the first. Reducing risk factors vastly improves any woman's chance of giving birth to a healthy baby. Yet African-American women *without* apparent risk factors are still twice as likely as other low-risk women to give birth to a low-birth-weight baby. The reasons are unclear.

From earliest records, African-American infants have been smaller at birth than other American babies. The difference in size was presumed to be genetic, but it has become clear that genetic studies based on race are unreliable. A few current researchers have explored, with limited results, a possible correlation between low birth weight and environmental factors such as prenatal care.

As research continues to rock back and forth between genetic and environmental causes, new studies are probing more deeply into income, health care, and stress to try to uncover the root cause of low birth weight and infant mortality among African Americans. Although we don't yet know the truth, every day we are discovering variables that may be involved in the outcome of pregnancy.

One intriguing possibility is being examined in an ongoing study at Meharry Medical College, in Nashville, Tennessee. In most modern pregnancy studies, low-, middle-, and high-income black women are compared with their white economic counterparts. It sounds fair, but this method assumes that their economic environments have remained the same for several generations. However, the first poor woman to make it into a higher income group may carry emotional, nutritional, and physical residuals of generations of poverty. If she is compared with a woman who grew up relatively well-off, and whose immediate ancestors were all relatively well-off, we would expect her pregnancy outcome to fare worse.

The Meharry researchers decided to include a new variable in their study: how *long* a woman's family had sustained poverty or wealth. Early results from this study suggest that when the generational income variable is factored into the analysis, the birth weight and mortality rate of black infants may correlate with other American infants.

Another new study, from Illinois, has raised a different possibility. Here the offspring of biracial couples were compared with babies born to two white parents. Babies born to white mothers and black fathers had birth weights similar to all-white babies. But babies born to black mothers and white fathers were one and a half times more likely to be born small.

The researchers say that it is unlikely the difference could be accounted for by genetics. Instead, they believe the stress imposed by racism may account for the difference in birth weight. No matter whom she is married to, a pregnant black woman is more vulnerable to stress than a pregnant white woman married to a black man. From childhood on, black women experience chronic emotional and physical stress, and their health often begins deteriorating in early adulthood.

While the Meharry and Illinois studies are inconclusive, they offer new ways to look at seemingly intractable health problems. Whenever the complete answer is determined, it will not be simple. What seems clear is that black women must pay attention to *all* known risk factors for *all* pregnant women. And more than other women, they must look for ways to reduce stress in their lives. Stress can affect every pregnancy, but stress imposed by racism is difficult to assess, difficult to admit, and difficult to cope with.

HOW STRESS AFFECTS THE FETUS

Emotional stress produces biological responses in a mother that may have a lasting effect on an unborn baby. The mother's thoughts and feelings affect muscle tension and hormone output. Increased levels of stress hormones in her bloodstream cross the placental barrier and enter the bloodstream of the unborn baby. Her emotional state also affects her heart, respiratory, and metabolic rates. Years ago, researchers discovered that when a mother experiences emotional stress, fetal movements increase several hundred percent and a residual effect lingers for several hours. Stress and anxiety also decrease a pregnant woman's ability to absorb nitrogen, phosphorus, and calcium, all of which the baby needs. Newborn infants of stressed mothers are often irritable and hyperactive.

These are just some of the ways a mother's feelings, experiences, and perceptions biologically affect her baby's development.

A crucial stress factor in a pregnant woman's life is her relationship with the baby's father. A baby's health is vastly improved when both mother and father are prepared for and feeling positive about parenting. A father's attitude toward the mother has a direct effect on her emotional well-being. Both parents need to lower their stress levels and reduce any tension between them. The most important role a father can play throughout the pregnancy is to support the mother emotionally. A pregnant woman cannot always put personal problems in perspective. The flood of increased hormones in her body makes her feelings run up and down the emotional scale. These are the times when the father's reassurance and support are invaluable.

Unfortunately, many African-American mothers do not have the baby's father in the picture. Teen mothers especially are often very much alone. In these situations, it's doubly important for the immediate family to contribute emotional support and to help reduce a pregnant woman's stress.

Unintended pregnancies are much more likely to be stressful and to produce small, weak babies. Studies have proved this: Of the babies born to 8,823 married pregnant women enrolled in the Child Health and Development Studies from 1959 to 1966, those born to women who said the pregnancy was unwanted were 2.4 times more likely to die in the first twenty-eight days of life.

PREPARE YOUR BODY

GET A PHYSICAL CHECKUP

A baby's good health begins in its mother's healthy body—even before she becomes pregnant. It makes sense for both parents to have a prepregnancy medical checkup to make sure you are both in good health. A prepregnancy checkup is similar to a first prenatal exam, which is described on page 19.

Both partners can be tested for sickle-cell disease, a severe form of anemia. If both carry the sickle-cell trait, there is a one in four chance of having a baby with sickle-cell disease. If this is the case, the doctor will probably advise genetic counseling before pregnancy (see chapter 29).

A prepregnancy exam also gives the prospective mother an opportunity to discover whether she has any preexisting diseases (such as diabetes or high blood pressure) and to get them under control *before* conception. Sexually transmitted diseases or other infections can also be diagnosed and successfully treated prior to conception.

A woman who has never had rubella (German measles) or mumps, or has never been immunized against them, can be vaccinated now. She will have to wait at least three months following the vaccination before she tries to conceive.

In addition, the doctor can check her nutritional status, and if her eating habits or nutrition is poor, the physician may recommend early start-up supplements of vitamins and minerals.

LOWER YOUR RISK PROFILE

It's important to assess all of your risk factors *before* you conceive. Your baby is at its most vulnerable during the first eight to twelve weeks following conception—a time when you may not even know that you're pregnant. Since it takes time to give up risky lifestyle practices such as smoking, drinking, and drug use, you don't want to wait until you're pregnant to stop.

Smoking. From the moment of conception to the moment of birth (and afterward), a baby is threatened by repeated, cumulative assaults of cigarette smoke. This is true whether the mother smokes herself or whether she breathes in secondhand smoke. Chemicals in smoke reduce the amount of oxygen available to the baby, constrict the blood vessels feeding the placenta, and strip away nutrients. The baby's heart beats faster and breathing is abnormal.

Pregnant women who smoke have an increased risk of spontaneous abortion, early separation of the placenta from the uterus, misplaced placenta, and bleeding during pregnancy. Their babies also have a higher risk for brain damage and sudden infant death syndrome (see chapter 4).

Smokers are also more likely to weigh less before pregnancy and tend to gain less weight during pregnancy, which can seriously affect the growth of the fetus.

After being born, the baby can continue to suffer from parental smoking by receiving nicotine in breast milk or by inhaling secondhand smoke. Breathing secondhand smoke makes a child more vulnerable to a host of ailments, including ear, nose, and throat infections, bronchitis, pneumonia, asthmatic attacks, and decreased lung efficiency.

Before you conceive, you want to make sure that you and the people you live with and work with are not smoking. Once you are pregnant, you want to stay off cigarettes and away from smoky environments.

If you need help giving up cigarettes, check out stop-smoking programs in your community or ask your doctor's advice about antismoking aids.

Alcohol. We have known for a long time that women who drink heavily during pregnancy run a significant risk of giving birth to a baby with fetal alcohol syndrome, a cluster of severe physical and mental defects. These include growth retardation, facial abnormalities, brain damage, abnormal development of various organs (including heart defects), poor muscle coordination, learning disabilities, and hyperactivity. Babies of mothers who drink heavily (five to six drinks a day), especially early in pregnancy, are likely to suffer the most severe abnormalities. Binges or sporadic drinking are particularly dangerous, since the pregnant body is unable to detoxify sudden large amounts of alcohol.

Even women who drink as few as two drinks a week have a higher rate of miscarriage than those who don't drink at all.

Most doctors advise giving up drinking altogether—before becoming pregnant. If you find you are unable to stop, get help immediately.

Drugs. A mother's drug use during pregnancy is associated with spontaneous abortion, premature birth, low birth weight, and SIDS.

Drug-addicted mothers give birth to drug-addicted babies; those babies who survive may have developmental problems and brain damage, severe learning disabilities, and behavioral problems.

Let's be straight. I know that many alcohol- or drug-using pregnant women stay away from prenatal clinics because they feel ashamed—and also because they fear their babies may be taken away from them. In certain parts of the country, these fears are real. But these are the very women who most need quality prenatal care.

A pregnant woman hooked on drugs or alcohol *can* get help without fear that her children will be permanently taken away. Discussing her addiction with someone she can trust—a doctor, mother, sister, minister, or friend—is beneficial. But she also needs help from a treatment center. If you or someone you know is in this position, take steps to find safe and fair treatment.

Caffeine. Caffeine interferes with the body's ability to absorb and use certain nutrients, specifically iron and some forms of protein. Caffeine also crosses the placental barrier and is distributed to all fetal tissues. Your baby is drinking that cup of coffee, too.

Although harmful effects to the fetus have not been proved, I recommend that a pregnant woman stop consuming caffeine or at least limit herself to one or two cups of coffee or other caffeine-containing beverages or foods daily (unless her doctor advises less). Unfortunately, those who are hooked on caffeine usually consume much greater quantities than this. Eliminating caffeine definitely causes withdrawal symptoms. If you suddenly stop consuming beverages/foods with caffeine, you'll probably have headaches and feel nauseated. However, after a few days, these symptoms disappear. You can reduce the withdrawal effects considerably by cutting back gradually. Eliminate by one serving a day until you've reached safe amounts or have quit altogether.

GETTING TO YOUR BEST WEIGHT

Once you become pregnant, it's too late to start changing your basic body weight. Therefore, if you are very thin or extremely overweight before pregnancy, it's important to achieve a healthy weight and also to make sure you're eating nourishing foods. In this way, during the first weeks following conception—when most women can't stand food—your good nutritional stores will carry you and the baby through.

If you are overweight. If you are thirty or more pounds overweight before pregnancy, complications in pregnancy and delivery could jeopardize both you and your baby. You need to lose weight— gradually—before becoming pregnant.

Do not go on a crash diet. Precipitous weight loss depletes essential nutrients that you'll need during pregnancy. A nutritionist can advise you on specific ways to reduce your calories, fat, sugar, and cholesterol without compromising good nutrition.

If you're underweight. Due to such adverse factors as smoking or poor eating habits, your baby is more likely to be born prematurely or dangerously small. The best way to gain weight before you conceive is simply to eat more at meals and add snacks in the form of protein and carbohydrates. Choose *nutritious* high-calorie foods. Whole nuts and seeds, dried fruits, sweet potatoes, and avocados are examples. You can add a daily drink made from well-balanced high-protein powder. These are particularly good if you are a vegetarian and don't eat meat, fish, or eggs. If you are still underweight when you conceive, you can afford to gain a little more weight than usual during pregnancy, but don't go overboard. Unless you're very underweight or are carrying twins or triplets, gaining more than forty pounds will not do you or your baby any good. Your doctor will advise you along the way if your weight gains are unhealthy.

BUILDING UP YOUR NUTRITIONAL LEVEL

The most important nutrients for pregnancy are protein, calcium, magnesium, vitamins C and E, iron, folic acid, and the B complex vitamins. These are the very nutrients many black women are short on.

A preliminary trial of six hundred black women is under way in Washington, D.C., designed to find out if poor maternal nutrition is responsible for the high incidence of low-birth-weight babies. So far, the study analyses show that about 35 percent of these pregnant women are getting less than 70 percent of the recommended daily allowance (RDA) for vitamins A, B_6, B_{12}, calcium, and iron; 25 percent are getting less than 70 percent of the RDA for protein, vitamin C, and thiamine, riboflavin, and niacin (all B complex vitamins).

Protein. (Recommended: 75 gm per day.) High-quality protein helps form healthy new body tissue for you and the baby. "High-quality" means a complete protein that contains all eight essential amino acids (found in eggs, meat, chicken, and fish). Beans, legumes, and grains contain protein, too, but they must be combined or eaten in the same day to provide the complete set of essential amino acids.

Calcium. Extra stores of calcium during pregnancy are essential for the baby's bones and tooth buds to develop. If you don't consume extra calcium, the fetus will drain it from your bones and teeth. Refined sugar (and also alcohol and caffeine) can also rob the body of calcium.

It's a good idea to start increasing calcium before conception. You want to add at least 400 mg of calcium to your daily diet, for a total of 1,200 to 2,000 mg each day. Calcium is best found in low-fat and nonfat dairy products, dark green vegetables, tofu, canned sardines and salmon (eat the soft bones), and dried beans and peas.

Calcium should be in a state of equilibrium with phosphorus in the body; therefore, a pregnant woman also needs 50 percent more phosphorus each day. However, phosphorus is prevalent in common foods and this extra need is easily met by almost every diet.

Vitamin D is essential for calcium absorption and balance, and if vitamin D levels are adequate, calcium/phosphorus will be in balance. Some doctors recommend 10 mcg (400 IU) of vitamin D per day during pregnancy.

Folic acid and the B complex vitamins. When you are pregnant, you need to double your usual intake of folic acid, and add 50 percent more of the B complex vitamins, which promote healthy red blood cells in the mother and the fetus. More importantly, these vitamins work together to prevent certain birth defects (such as spina bifida) that develop in the very early weeks of pregnancy. Start now to increase your B complex vitamins and folic acid, then continue at that higher level all the way through your pregnancy.

Good food sources: dark green vegetables, asparagus, legumes (especially lima beans), whole grains, nuts, salmon, and lean meats. Vitamin B_{12} is found in fish, organ meats, egg yolks, and cheese.

Iron. Iron-deficiency anemia has been associated with a higher risk of preterm delivery. Your blood volume will double during pregnancy, and few women have enough iron stored in their bodies to meet this increased need. The usual 15–18 mg RDA increases to 30–36 mg daily.

It's difficult to get enough iron from any source—only 10 percent of the iron consumed in food or taken in supplements is actually absorbed by the body. Iron from red meat is absorbed better than iron from vegetables. Therefore, adding food fortified with iron, such as iron-fortified breads and cereals, is a good idea. Increasing foods high in vitamin C will help improve iron absorption.

Good food sources: lean meats, dark green vegetables (especially parsley and kale), beets and beet greens, dried fruits, egg yolks, shellfish, molasses, and whole grains. Organ meats, such as liver, heart, and kidney, are also iron-rich, but make sure these come from organic sources free from chemicals. Dried beans and peas also provide some iron.

Vitamin E. A pregnant woman needs twice as much vitamin E as usual (10–11 mg), particularly during the second trimester.

Good food sources: meat, fish, grains, liver, yeast, nuts, and oils of wheat germ, soybeans, cottonseed, and corn.

Vitamin C. The recommended daily allowance of vitamin C, or ascorbic acid, increases by about 10 mg during pregnancy, for a total of 70 mg (additional supplements are usually recommended by physicians, see page 18).

Good food sources: Vitamin C is found naturally in a wide variety of fruits and vegetables, including all citrus fruits, papaya, mango, guava, cantaloupe, broccoli, brussels sprouts, green and red peppers, parsley, and strawberries.

Zinc. The usual RDA of 15 mg a day increases to 20 mg during pregnancy. Too little zinc in a mother's diet is associated with retarded fetal growth, abnormal fetal development, and prolonged labor. To help your body absorb zinc, you need adequate amounts of iron, vitamin B_6, and tryptophan (an amino acid found in lean meats, fish, eggs, and dairy products).

The best food source is oysters, but eating one serving of raw oysters every day is not a good idea because of the possibility of contamination. You can get zinc from a variety of other foods, including herring, whole grains, liver, lamb, beef, poultry, nuts, brown rice, peas, peanuts, milk, and eggs.

DO YOU NEED VITAMIN/MINERAL SUPPLEMENTS?

A woman's body needs so many extra vitamins and minerals to support a healthy pregnancy that it's almost impossible to get them all from food sources alone. Most doctors recommend taking a multivitamin/mineral supplement, which you can start even before you conceive and then continue throughout pregnancy. But you should take supplements only in the amounts prescribed by your doctor or nutritionist, since getting too much can be just as damaging as getting too little. Your doctor will recommend a combination that's right for you—*but it's up to you to take them.*

The most common pregnancy supplements—and their average recommended dosages—are:

Calcium—1,200 mg/day
Folic acid—400 mg/day
Vitamin E—16 mg/day
Vitamin C—500 mg/day

If you are used to taking large quantities of vitamin C supplements and would like to continue throughout your pregnancy, discuss the dosage with your doctor. Megadoses of vitamin C are not recommended for pregnant women, because they are thought to create a transient vitamin dependency in the fetus. It's usually safe to continue vitamin C in low to moderate levels—up to 1,000 mg daily.

Many doctors also recommend iron and/or zinc supplements during pregnancy. However, it's important that you follow your doctor's recommendation carefully and do not add additional amounts yourself.

PRENATAL VISITS

If you are planning to become pregnant, you should have your first prenatal visit *before* you conceive, in which case it is called a prepregnancy checkup. As soon as you suspect or know you are pregnant, you should have another one.

The initial prenatal visit is usually a long one, in which the doctor (preferably an OB/GYN—a specialist in obstetrics and gynecology) or midwife takes a complete history, draws blood and urine samples for lab tests, and carries out a physical examination. You and your partner will also have a chance to ask questions and see if the doctor's approach to labor and delivery agrees with your own.

Subsequent visits take less time and usually include some routine lab tests and an opportunity to ask questions. The heartbeat and position of the baby will be checked during each visit; you will have a urinalysis, and your blood pressure and weight will be recorded.

For the first six months, you'll want to see the doctor once a month. (If you have any health problems that put your pregnancy in a high-risk category, you will probably see the doctor more often.) Checkups increase in frequency as your pregnancy progresses. In the seventh and eighth month, you'll probably see your doctor every two weeks. And during the ninth month, you'll see the doctor every week until labor begins.

If you experience any problems in between visits, don't hesitate to call your doctor. Your doctor may also ask you to keep a diary to record how you feel, which helps you keep track of how things are going. You can also use the diary to jot down any questions you have for your next checkup.

Most prenatal visits are routine. At the same time, the purpose of regular visits is to detect potential problems. For example, diabetes and high blood pressure—two causes of life-threatening complications in pregnancy—are common among African Americans. A pregnant woman may not even know when she has one of these diseases, and sometimes the disease actually develops during pregnancy. Regular prenatal care can help bring these conditions under control. During the course of your pregnancy, the doctor can also discover if the baby is too small for its gestational age, if you're carrying twins, or if the baby is in a breech presentation.

Prenatal visits also allow you and your doctor and/or midwife to get to know each other. At each visit, you will have the chance to talk about how you are faring emotionally and about other issues that may be affecting your family life. Prenatal visits are also a good opportunity to ask questions about advice you may have received from well-meaning friends and relatives.

THE INITIAL EXAM

Because lack of prenatal care is a serious problem for African-American mothers and babies, I'm going to take some time to describe the first prenatal exam and the many benefits it can yield.

Your doctor will want to know about any past history of serious illness in you and your family, which inoculations you have had, and whether you take any medications. The doctor or midwife should specifically ask:

- Are there any twins in your family? Twins are more common among black women than among other groups, and if it turns out you are pregnant with twins, you will need special prenatal care.

- Do you have any history of sickle-cell disease in your family? If so, your doctor is likely to refer you to a genetic counselor to assess the chances of passing along the disease to your baby.

- If you have been pregnant before, did you encounter any complications? Previous miscarriage, premature birth, or toxemia are a few of the conditions that may have a bearing on the outcome of your next pregnancy.

- Can you describe your menstrual pattern? Problems related to menstruation—endometriosis, erratic ovulation, unbalanced hormonal cycles, or premature menopause—can interfere with conception and pregnancy.

The doctor will estimate the baby's due date, counting forty weeks from the first day of your last period. (The average pregnancy lasts thirty-eight weeks from the date of conception. However, it is impossible to know the precise moment conception occurred, since sperm is viable for several days after intercourse. Nor does every normal pregnancy last exactly the same number of days. Labor may start a week early or late and still be perfectly normal.)

The physical exam and lab tests come next. Your height and weight are measured to assess your posture and provide a baseline for weight gain through pregnancy.

The internal pelvic exam. This will detect any structural abnormalities of the pelvis, vagina, and cervix. During the exam, the physician can take cervical swabs for a Pap smear and test for any sexually transmitted diseases (STDs).

Urinalysis. This lab test can detect excess protein, which may indicate kidney disease; glucose, which would indicate the presence of diabetes; ketones, which may indicate that you're not eating enough; pus or blood, which could mean kidney infection.

Blood analysis. This identifies your blood group, in case you need an emergency transfusion, and tests for venereal diseases, anemia, and the rhesus (Rh) factor. (If your blood is Rh-negative and your partner's is Rh-positive, you may have a high-risk pregnancy. About 15 percent of the white population has Rh-negative blood, but the trait is less common among other groups.)

Your blood sample also can be tested for the sickle-cell trait, for rubella antibodies, and for toxoplasmosis, an infection that can severely affect fetal development.

Rubella vaccinations. Even if you think you have had rubella in the past, or were vaccinated against it, your doctor should check to make sure you are still immune. Rubella, or German measles, can have serious consequences for an unborn baby. Once you are pregnant, you cannot be vaccinated, because the live vaccine might harm the unborn child. If you are already pregnant, and not immune to rubella, you will have to stay away from young children who have not been vaccinated.

Other immunizations. During your pregnancy, circumstances may arise—travel to foreign countries, exposure to epidemics, animal bites—that require various shots or vaccinations.

Most vaccines used today have not been associated with untoward effects for the mother or fetus. However, a theoretical risk to the fetus exists. Live viral vaccines, in particular MMR (measles/mumps/rubella) and oral polio, are not given during pregnancy except under very special circumstances. *Therefore, do not have any shots or vaccines without first consulting your obstetrician.* If for any reason you are not receiving prenatal care, be sure to tell any other doctor or nurse you are pregnant before getting any shots.

At the end of every prenatal exam, you will have time to talk over anything that worries you. If you know you always forget your questions the minute you walk into a doctor's office (lots of people do), write them down beforehand and take them along with you.

SPECIAL PREGNANCY CONCERNS

Any preexisting disease can affect a pregnancy. For African-American women, the two most common, and most dangerous, illnesses are diabetes and hypertension. Both may preexist before pregnancy, or they may appear for the first time during pregnancy.

DIABETES

Uncontrolled diabetes increases the risk that the child will be stillborn or have congenital defects. The fetus may grow excessively large, which can contribute to difficulties at birth. However, if the diabetes is carefully controlled, the risks are greatly reduced. A diabetic woman will need regular monitoring of blood-glucose (or blood-sugar) levels, a careful diet, or possibly insulin injections or pills for hypoglycemia.

One kind of diabetes, called gestational diabetes, develops only during pregnancy. It carries the same risks to the fetus as regular diabetes. This kind of diabetes can often be controlled by diet alone, although in some cases, insulin injections are also required.

A woman with severe diabetes may be admitted to the hospital for the last days, or weeks, of her pregnancy so that the diabetes can be precisely controlled and the baby's condition can be monitored.

HIGH BLOOD PRESSURE

High blood pressure is one of the conditions you may have without knowing it, and it may be discovered for the first time during a routine prenatal visit. High blood pressure is sometimes caused by the pregnancy itself.

Extremely high blood pressure is associated with difficult childbirth and can harm the baby. Sudden elevations can also be a sign of toxemia, a potentially life-threatening complication.

With proper medical care, high blood pressure can be controlled, and the risk to mother and baby can be greatly lowered.

SEXUALLY TRANSMITTED DISEASES

STDs, which include herpes, chlamydia, gonorrhea, and syphilis, must be treated promptly for the health of both mother and fetus. Mothers infected with syphilis, for example, have a higher risk of miscarriage. If the baby is born with syphilis, it has an increased risk of low birth weight, mental retardation, chronic health problems, and premature death. When syphilis is detected early and treated in the mother, transmission to the baby can be prevented.

Gonorrhea can cause a buildup of scar tissue in and around a woman's reproductive organs. If a woman with gonorrhea becomes pregnant (often she cannot), she may have a higher risk of miscarriage or ectopic pregnancy. Gonorrhea is easily identified, usually by a slide test in the physician's office.

Dormant herpes does not ordinarily affect the developing fetus, but a flare-up during childbirth can expose the baby to the virus as the child passes through the birth canal. Herpes infection in a newborn is serious, and it may result in mental retardation, blindness, neurological problems, and even death. Since an episode of herpes

---

HIGH-RISK PREGNANCIES

Certain medical conditions automatically place a pregnant woman in a high-risk category, meaning that she requires closer observation and monitoring throughout the pregnancy. Pregnancy may have an adverse effect on an existing disease and, conversely, the disease may also affect the pregnancy and its outcome. Most high-risk pregnancies can be successfully handled with proper care. Any one of the following risk factors defines a high-risk pregnancy:

- *Being older than age thirty-five*
- *Diabetes*
- *Heart or lung disease*
- *High blood pressure*
- *Sexually transmitted disease*
- *Thyroid or neurological problems*

cannot be predicted, pregnant women with this disease should anticipate having a cesarean delivery.

AIDS also falls into the category of STDs, although there are other ways besides sex to contract the disease. Doctors often recommend that pregnant women be tested for HIV, the virus believed to cause AIDS, because of the likelihood of passing the virus to the fetus. New research suggests that taking the antiviral drug AZT may reduce this risk by two-thirds. Even if you are fairly certain you don't have HIV, it's still worth it to have the test, because you or your partner may have been exposed years earlier and unknowingly carry the virus. (See chapter 24 for more information on AIDS in children.)

ULTRASOUND AND AMNIOCENTESIS

Over the past twenty years, medical technology has made incredible progress in its ability to test for serious problems while the infant is still in the womb. All tests are not used on all mothers. However, two are now so common that we've included them here.

ULTRASOUND

Ultrasound can be used in the second and third trimesters of pregnancy to observe how well the fetus is developing in the womb. If the fetus is growth-retarded (growing too slowly), an effort can be made to improve growth before birth.

In this test, high-frequency sound waves are sent out by a scanning device and transmitted to a small crystal placed on the surface of the body. The sound waves enter the body and echo back when they strike the surface of an organ. The echoes are converted into electrical signals and transferred to a video screen, where internal structures, including the baby, are outlined in detail. The baby's size and position can be seen (so can its sex, but before disclosing that particular bit of news, the doctor will ask you whether you wish to know). Obvious birth defects may also show up, and a few of these can now be corrected while the baby is still in the mother's uterus.

Most pregnant women have ultrasound at around the twentieth

week; depending on the results, some women continue to have periodic ultrasound checks until the delivery.

Ultrasound is painless, and it takes only a few minutes. The bonus part is that the image of your baby on the screen can be photographed and you can take the picture home.

AMNIOCENTESIS

Amniocentesis is usually offered to older mothers, who have a higher risk of giving birth to a Down's syndrome baby. The test is also offered to parents who have a family history of sickle-cell anemia.

Amniocentesis does not reveal all birth defects, but it can discover about a hundred different ones—including Tay-Sachs disease and certain forms of muscular dystrophy. However, each test is separate and must be specifically ordered by the physician. If an abnormality is present, amniocentesis can help parents prepare for the birth. They also have the option of choosing abortion.

Amniocentesis is performed between the fourteenth and eighteenth week of pregnancy. The procedure begins with ultrasound, which is used to locate the fetus floating inside the amniotic sac. Then a thin needle is slipped into the surface of the abdomen. The procedure is painless, although occasionally a woman feels very slight contractions when the needle penetrates the uterus. The needle pierces the amniotic sac (the needle does not touch the baby) and about one ounce (30 ml) of fluid is withdrawn and transferred to a vial for delivery to a laboratory. When carried out by an experienced physician, as it always should be, amniocentesis is a safe and accurate procedure. Withdrawal of the fluid takes about three minutes.

Amniotic fluid contains cells that indicate the baby's genetic code. It takes between three and five weeks in the lab before these cells reproduce and grow large enough so that the chromosomes can be examined. Normal cells show forty-six matched chromosomes. If chromosome number twenty-one has three strands of DNA instead of two, the baby will be born with Down's syndrome. Amniocentesis is successful in establishing a genetic diagnosis in 95 percent of the cases, although there are rare instances when the laboratory analysis is in error. (For further information about sickle-cell disease, see chapter 29.)

WEIGHT GAIN DURING PREGNANCY

A baby's birth weight is directly related to its mother's weight gain during pregnancy. Your goal is to gain enough weight to give birth to a healthy child who weighs at least six and a half pounds.

Although bigger babies do better, extremely large babies do not. Babies weighing more than ten pounds at birth tend to have more problems during labor and delivery. (Excessive size is most frequently caused by a mother's obesity before pregnancy, poorly controlled diabetes, or a pregnancy that lasts longer than forty-two weeks. Mothers who have a family history of large newborns are also more likely to give birth to large babies.)

The American College of Obstetricians and Gynecologists recommends that women entering pregnancy near their ideal weight gain twenty-five to thirty pounds during pregnancy. Most African-American women should gain on the higher end of the recommended range, unless they are very overweight. Underweight women may need to gain as much as thirty-five pounds.

No matter how heavy you are, never gain fewer than twenty pounds during pregnancy. And don't try to keep your weight gain down in hopes that you will come out of pregnancy thin.

The weight you gain during the first half of your pregnancy goes into building up stores of fat and protein that the baby uses later in the pregnancy. Some is held over to sustain you after delivery and help produce breast milk.

Ideally, a woman should gain weight gradually and steadily throughout pregnancy, rather than in spurts. If you find yourself gaining too much weight, *do not cut back toward the end* of the pregnancy. Weight gain during the last three months is from the growth of the baby; reducing calories and nutrients at the end can seriously compromise the baby's health.

HOW MANY CALORIES?

Plan to consume about 300 to 400 extra calories a day, for a total intake of at least 2,300 to 2,500 calories per day.

But this is not the time to eat a lot of fatty or sweet foods, figuring that you're going to gain weight, anyway.

The best place to increase calories is in the protein category—adding three hundred calories from fish, skinless chicken, lean meat, skimmed dairy products or cheese, or a combination of beans and grains that add up to quality protein. Add more vegetables and fruits on top of this, and you should be all set. In addition, don't forget to drink plenty of water every day—at least six to eight glasses.

RETURNING TO YOUR NORMAL WEIGHT

For unknown reasons, black women have more trouble losing extra pounds after pregnancy than do white women. This weight retention after pregnancy seems to be part of the overall tendency of black women to gain more weight than others during their child-bearing years. Many researchers have reported on this phenomenon—most notably observed in the 1988 National Maternal and Infant Survey—but no one has been able to pinpoint the cause, except to say that the weight increase is probably due to environmental and cultural factors rather than to racial ones. It may be that African-American women continue eating the same number of calories after pregnancy that they were consuming during it.

It's important to get back to your normal weight. Excessive weight gain by African-American women during their middle adult years is a potentially serious health problem, because obesity often precedes diabetes. At the same time, you have to pay attention to getting adequate nutrition following pregnancy. Your body is still recovering from the demands of pregnancy while you're trying to adjust to the new demands of mothering. All new mothers need good nutrition to provide energy and positive health status. However, with a little care and attention, it's possible to get back to your previous weight without stress.

You will lose about fifteen pounds in the week following childbirth. From then on, if you're breast-feeding, you can expect to lose about a half a pound a week. This means if you simply return to your prepregnancy calorie intake—probably between 2,000 and 2,200 calories a day—you should be back to your normal weight in three to four months. Bottle-feeding mothers tend to lose weight more slowly. In either case, if you follow a healthy diet and a moderate exercise program, weight loss after pregnancy should be automatic and stress-free.

Most new mothers may begin exercising soon after birth, particularly if they had continued exercise during pregnancy. However, if your delivery required surgery, your doctor will advise when it's safe to resume your exercise program.

If you were overweight before pregnancy, or if you gained more than forty pounds during pregnancy, you'll be overweight after pregnancy. If you're bottle-feeding, you may want to eat a little less and exercise a little more, but don't try to lose more than about half a pound to one pound a week. No matter how heavy you think you are, do not engage in a crash weight-loss program.

TEEN PREGNANCIES

Many teenage girls are so poorly educated about sex and its consequences that they begin having babies as soon as they start menstruating, before their bodies are mature enough to support a healthy pregnancy. Teen mothers are less likely than older women to receive early prenatal care, and more likely to be poorly educated about pregnancy. They also tend to space children too closely. As a result, they often give birth to premature and very low-birth-weight infants.

This is why it's so important for expectant teen moms to receive early counseling and medical attention. I've had an opportunity to counsel teens in a prenatal clinic, and I've seen how stressed, confused, and unsure they are about their pregnancy and what the future holds for them.

Unfortunately, many teen mothers today are abandoned by the baby's father and possibly by their families, as well. If you are a teen mother or have a teenage daughter who's expecting, counseling by a social worker may help you cope with what's ahead. Counseling, along with the support of a gynecologist or obstetrician, nurse, and nutritionist can ensure the health of you and your baby. In this way, even a young and unplanned pregnancy can reap a positive outcome (see chapter 23).

In this chapter, we have looked at the important factors contributing to a healthy pregnancy: lowering risk factors, good nutrition, and early prenatal care. These should be routine for every pregnant woman, but sadly they are not. We know that African-American expectant mothers are often shortchanged when it comes to these basic needs. But being aware of the health problems you might face, and how you can go about preventing many of them yourself, means that you can do a lot to ensure a healthy pregnancy.

As you contemplate pregnancy and parenthood, you're embarking on the most joyous experience of your life, which can translate into having a happy, healthy infant. Giving your baby the opportunity to begin life on a positive note will have a lasting benefit.

Some mothers and fathers describe their childbirth experience as a miracle and a gift from God. It is indeed both. It is a miracle that a human being can be fully developed from a microscopic cell containing genetic material contributed by two different people. This cell will divide, thus creating a combination of millions of other cells that becomes a full human being who years later can make a great contribution to society. The childbirth process is pretty amazing and makes any woman and man feel humble. So take care of yourself and be ready for the precious gift that will be yours to have and to hold.

3

TAKING CARE OF YOURSELF
DURING PREGNANCY

As soon as you know you're pregnant—or even before—you need to find maternity care. You are looking for two things: a doctor and/or nurse-midwife to look after you while you are pregnant and a place in which to deliver your baby. High-quality obstetrical and delivery care can make the difference in outcome, especially when babies are born prematurely or are born too small despite a full-term pregnancy.

FINDING MATERNITY CARE

It's generally best to choose a doctor first. Then you can plan to deliver your baby at the hospital where he or she is affiliated. In some parts of the country, family doctors or general practitioners care for pregnant women and deliver babies. In other parts, family doctors refer their patients to obstetricians who specialize in pregnancy and childbirth. Many obstetricians also practice gynecology, a specialty that includes general health, and the diagnosis and treatment of diseases of the female reproductive system. Obstetricians may be board certified or board eligible, meaning that they have spent four to five years in residency training after obtaining their initial medical degrees and have passed, or are qualified to pass, a certifying examination.

Whoever you choose, experience, competency, and trust is what you're looking for. It's also important to choose a doctor whom you can get to easily for prenatal appointments.

BIRTHING OPTIONS

Hospitals. A number of hospitals in your area may provide services for delivery. In my own city, Baton Rouge, there are general and emergency care facilities and also a woman's hospital, all of which offer excellent delivery and postdelivery care. Be sure to find out which hospital your doctor is affiliated with. It's important to feel comfortable and confident about the reputation of the hospital, and it's also good to have more than one option, in case you have to alter your choice of delivery method at the last minute.

Most American women give birth to their babies in a hospital. Having medical technology instantly available helps ensure the safety of mother and child: When things go wrong during delivery, they often go wrong without warning. However, hospitals vary considerably in their approach to childbirth.

Many hospitals try to offer a personalized approach, in addition to the technological equipment that makes childbirth safer. Call hospitals in your area and ask to visit their maternity floors. People who work in high-quality maternity units are usually very proud of their services and will welcome a visit.

The hospital should also be able to give you a list of affiliated obstetricians, from which you can choose a doctor for your prenatal care, if you haven't already done so. Or the hospital itself may offer prenatal care in a special pregnancy clinic.

Hospital prenatal clinics. Prenatal clinics may be staffed by resident obstetricians, obstetrical nurses, and nurse-midwives. Your clinic visits include the same care that you would receive from a private obstetrician, offering prenatal checkups up until time of delivery. Clinics also offer childbirth-preparation classes. In many cases, a clinic means "one-stop shopping" and plenty of support.

Hospital maternity clinics also have available many different kinds of specialists, which make them a safe place for women with high-risk pregnancies. Another advantage is that although costs vary from place to place, clinics usually charge less than private doctors. And some clinics have a sliding pay scale that determines cost according to income.

Birthing centers. A birthing center is a small childbirth facility, often located near a hospital. Most centers offer full maternity care, including childbirth classes and delivery, in a friendly, personal atmosphere. Only low-risk mothers are accepted for care at a birthing center, which is often staffed by midwives. There are only 125 such facilities nationwide, so you may have trouble finding one near you. Look in the Yellow Pages of your telephone book under "Birthing Centers" or write to the American College of Nurse Midwives (see page 400).

Nurse-midwives. In the past two decades, midwifery has undergone a revolution that is bringing high-quality and highly personalized maternity care to growing numbers of women. Nurse-midwives are registered nurses who have completed advanced training in gynecology and obstetrics. Those who are certified nurse-midwives (C.N.M.) have passed a national examination and continue to attend education programs.

Nurse-midwives may deliver babies in hospitals, at birthing centers, and also at home. In some hospitals and birthing centers, the nurse-midwife sees the mother through labor and an obstetrician comes in toward the end to deliver the baby. In others, the nurse-midwife actually delivers the baby, with an obstetrician on call in case of complications.

Some obstetricians also employ nurse-midwives to perform a broad range of gynecological services for their patients, including Pap smears, breast and pelvic examinations, contraceptive and menopausal counseling, teenage pregnancy counseling, and assistance for new mothers.

Lay midwives. Lay midwives have acquired most of their skills from direct experience rather than academic training. The long, rich history of lay midwifery developed among many immigrant ethnic groups, but the tradition lasted much longer among African Americans. For hundreds of years, "grannies" practiced everywhere, particularly in the South, where they served countless pregnant women who were shut out from other medical care. They learned their skills from their grandmothers and mothers, or other midwives in the community. These women were sensitive to the cultural rituals surrounding pregnancy and birth, and they were said to have true callings.

With desegregation, many black women were allowed to deliver their babies in hospitals for the first time. The grannies were growing old, and young black women no longer had reason to learn from them. Lay practices faded into history.

Then, when the women's movement gained strength in the 1970s, many women began to demand more birthing options and more personal care. Suddenly, the idea of midwifery was reborn, albeit in a somewhat different style. The new generation of modern lay midwives, both black and white, continue to serve at-home births, but they tend to be younger and politically active in the birth-alternative movement.

Lay midwives today may practice legally in several states, although licensing requirements vary. If you choose to receive maternity care from a lay midwife, check her or his qualifications as carefully as you would any other health-care professional—and also check the qualifications of the midwife's physician backup. If the midwife doesn't have medical support, it would be unwise to choose her for maternity care, no matter how good and dedicated she is. Unexpected problems can arise during any delivery, and the need for prompt, effective treatment by a physician is always a possibility.

Home births. Delivery at home is safe for normal births; the problem is that you can't know ahead of time if a birth will be normal. If you choose home birth, make sure your midwife and obstetrician are experienced with home birthing. Your doctor should be affiliated with a reputable hospital, and you should have full instructions on what to do in case of an emergency. Make sure your professional prenatal care is as complete as any other mom's.

HOW YOUR BODY CHANGES DURING PREGNANCY

A woman's body undergoes amazing changes during pregnancy in order to nourish and give birth to a child. The uterus, normally a small organ weighing about two ounces, stretches into a capsule that eventually weighs two and a quarter pounds. (Don't worry. After childbirth, it returns to almost its original size.) Blood volume and other body fluids increase; the pelvic bones soften, and the rib cage widens. The nine months of pregnancy are divided into three equal periods, known as trimesters. During each trimester, the body goes through very distinct physical changes, each influenced primarily by pregnancy hormones.

FIRST TRIMESTER

In the first trimester (from zero to three months), hormones suddenly increase and you can expect to feel terrible. Fatigue and nausea are usual symptoms. Breasts feel tender, and sex is the last thing on your mind. Shifting hormones also mess with your emotions. A prospective father also goes through some changes about now, but his have more to do with the emotional aspects of becoming a father (although some men do have sympathetic aches and pains). Despite these unfamiliar feelings, early pregnancy is a wonderful time for sharing and offering support to each other, as well as anticipating together the changes that parenthood will bring.

SECOND TRIMESTER

Entering the second trimester (from four to six months) of pregnancy, most women begin to feel much better. These are usually the best months of pregnancy, and you will probably look and feel terrific. Many couples enjoy a special intimate relationship at this time. (Unless there are specific medical reasons, there is no need to avoid sex during pregnancy.)

You will probably be able to feel the baby moving by around week twenty. By the end of the second trimester, your blood volume will have increased by 30 to 40 percent and blood vessels throughout your body will be dilated. How do these changes affect you? For one thing, you're likely to develop varicose veins, especially in your legs. After the baby is born, these become almost invisible, though they reappear with every new pregnancy.

Almost every pregnant woman also develops hemorrhoids, a form of varicose veins, inside or around the anal area. Hemorrhoids are usually caused by the increased weight of the fetus and its downward pressure. Hemorrhoids may cause considerable discomfort, burning, and itching. Sometimes they rupture and bleed under pressure of a bowel movement. Hemorrhoids can be treated safely and promptly by your doctor, and they usually disappear within a few months following childbirth.

Pregnancy hormones also cause ligaments to soften and your joints to loosen. You can probably continue whatever exercise you normally do, as long as you avoid strains and stop if you begin to ache. Talk over your exercise regimen with your obstetrician or midwife. She may also recommend special pregnancy exercises to relieve backache and strengthen the pelvic muscles that will be involved in labor and delivery.

THIRD TRIMESTER

The last three months of pregnancy (from seven to nine months) bring yet another set of changes. You can expect your hair to feel coarser and your skin to feel dry and itchy. You may notice more hair growing on your arms and legs, even on your face and the lower part of your abdomen. This is simply a hormonal response to pregnancy. Pregnant women always feel warm, because the fetus radiates heat through the mother's skin.

The increasing weight of the baby puts pressure on all of the mother's internal organs, particularly the bladder and stomach. You will feel the need to urinate frequently, and you may have trouble eating a full meal in one sitting. Your blood pressure may fall and sometimes you may feel faint or nauseated. You may even find breathing difficult. General discomfort may make it hard to sleep at night, and you may rest better propped up with pillows. Resting or napping during the day is also helpful.

All of the extra fluid in your body causes swelling, especially around the feet and ankles. Moderate fluid retention is good for both you and the baby, because it adds to your blood volume and ensures adequate milk flow during early breast-feeding. But too much swelling can be uncomfortable and may affect your breathing and blood pressure. (See page 40 for a few things you can do to help relieve swelling.)

Changes in skin pigmentation are fairly common in the third trimester, including dark patches on the face and down the center of the stomach. You should never use bleaches or scrubs to try to erase the patches or streaks. These skin changes disappear after childbirth.

A few weeks before delivery, colostrum, a forerunner of breast milk, may begin to leak from your nipples. Wash your breasts gently with soap and water. If the leakage is heavy, fold breast pads or a soft tissue inside your bra to keep the colostrum from staining your clothing.

With all of the changes and discomfort in late pregnancy, it's natural for a pregnant woman's sexual desire to disappear. But most couples continue to grow closer in anticipation of greeting their new baby. They start making room, buying baby clothes and furniture. All of the things you do together now, especially expressing your anxieties, fears, hopes, and aspirations, add a new dimension to your feelings for each other.

CRAVINGS

No one knows why pregnant women crave certain foods. Some researchers say cravings are caused by hormonal influences on your sense of taste, while others associate them with vitamin and mineral deficiencies that may occur as the result of increased nutritional needs. Cravings are no problem as long as you crave

---

WHAT TO WEAR

- *Most pregnant women can wear regular clothing until the fourth or fifth month, as long as it's loose and comfortable. Avoid tight-fitting clothes or stockings that may restrict circulation. Support hose or leotards, on the other hand, can help reduce leg swelling, varicose veins, and leg cramps.*

- *Choose cotton underpants to lessen the chance of rash or itching caused by yeast infections.*

- *Breast size increases considerably in the first four months of pregnancy. Wearing a well-fitted maternity or nursing bra can provide extra support and relieve breast discomfort and upper backache. Nursing bras open in front to allow the nipples to rub freely against clothing, which helps a new mother prepare for nursing. This is also useful in the last month of pregnancy, when you want to "toughen up" nipples.*

- *Wear comfortable low-heeled shoes that help you balance your weight evenly, prevent backache and leg cramps, and maintain good posture.*

- *If you are very overweight, or if you have slack abdominal muscles from previous pregnancies, a maternity girdle can give extra abdominal support and also can help prevent backaches.*

---

fruits and vegetables or other health-promoting food. However, if you crave chocolate, as many pregnant women do, or other high-fat, high-calorie foods, you may gain a lot of weight. (Chocolate also contains caffeine.) The rule of thumb is, indulge your cravings unless you find yourself gorging on foods that are high in fat and low in nutritional value. Also, let your doctor know about your particular cravings so you can both keep track of your nutritional status.

OLD WIVES' TALES

Most women change their diets during pregnancy. Some changes are based on medical advice, and others on folk beliefs. Sometimes it's simply a matter of personal taste preferences, although taste is often a result of generations of cultural influences. Many of us hold on to a lot of myths our mothers and grandmothers taught us. Some women think eating certain foods, such as red meat, liver, and strawberries, causes birthmarks on a baby. Some traditions that relate to food choices can cause women to avoid nutritious foods. For example, in many African countries it is still a common practice for pregnant women to avoid eggs.

And some pregnant women say they crave nonfood substances such as dirt or clay or starch. The practice of eating such substances is called pica; it is not new, nor is it limited to any one geographic area, race, creed, culture, economic status, or even one sex. Clay eating is a tradition in West Africa, but pica is also practiced among many different groups in many other parts of the world, including the United States.

Pica is still fairly common among African-American women living in some parts of the rural South and in northern cities. In urban areas, laundry starch instead of clay is often the first choice, although some women eat milk of magnesia, coffee grounds, plaster, and paraffin. Pregnant women also have been known to crave ice, burnt matches, gravel, charcoal, ashes, mothballs, and practically anything else you can think of.

Pregnant women give various reasons for ingesting nonfood substances. Many tell me they eat clay or starch because their mothers did it, and for that reason it feels comforting to them. Some say these substances settle their stomachs or relieve nervous tension and hunger pains. And some say that clay prevents birth-marks, or that starch makes the skin of the baby lighter, or helps the baby to slip out during delivery.

The real biological effects of pica are, in fact, much less benign. Pica can cause serious health problems during pregnancy. These include lead poisoning passed on to the fetus; tender, irritable uterus, along with impacted fecal matter; small bowel obstruction in the mother, and parasitic infection caused by eating contami-nated soil or clay; and anemia in the fetus.

If you find yourself craving nonfood substances, don't be afraid to tell your doctor or midwife or dietitian about them—they're not all that unusual—and he or she may have some tips for you on how to overcome the cravings so that they don't interfere with the pregnancy.

If you tell your dietitian about the substances you crave, she can help you find substitutes that are high in nutritional value. Eating healthy foods that are of the same texture as the substances you crave can relieve the craving. For instance, if you crave a grainy substance like coffee grounds, try eating corn muffins or fat-free tortilla chips instead.

HOME REMEDIES TO RELIEVE THE DISCOMFORTS OF PREGNANCY

HELP FOR PREGNANCY SICKNESS AND HEARTBURN

About half of all pregnant women experience pregnancy sickness during the first trimester. (The term *morning sickness* is usually a misnomer: Nausea and vomiting can occur anytime, and it may last all day long.)

Heartburn is also common in early pregnancy. The same advice helps relieve both problems:

- Eat frequent small meals at two-hour intervals.
- Choose easy-to-digest carbohydrates like plain pasta, crack-ers, melba toast, baked potato, cooked cereal, rice, fruit, and vegetables.
- Avoid spicy foods.
- Avoid fried foods and any food that contains a lot of butter and fat.

- Eat a protein snack (such as peanut butter and crackers) before going to bed.
- *Before* you get out of bed in the morning, eat crackers, dry cereal, or dry toast.
- Get up slowly.
- Drink beverages between, rather than with, meals.

If you are vomiting more than twice a day, be sure to inform your doctor.

Later in pregnancy, when the baby's weight is pressing on your stomach, heartburn is likely to return. Follow the same tips you used in the first trimester, and add these:

- Don't lie down after eating.
- Do not bend from the waist or do vigorous exercise.
- Sleep with your head and upper torso propped up.
- Avoid taking antacids unless your doctor recommends them.

HELP FOR HEMORRHOIDS

Hemorrhoids are common during pregnancy, usually beginning during the second trimester. Here are some useful tips that will lessen their discomfort:

- Avoid becoming constipated.
- Drink plenty of fluids.
- Eat high-fiber foods (whole grains, vegetables, dried beans, peas, fruits, bran).
- Rest during the latter part of the day.
- Inform your doctor so he or she can prescribe safe treatment.

HELP FOR CONSTIPATION

Hormonal changes in pregnancy relax the gastrointestinal muscles. At the same time, increased pressure from the enlarging uterus may make bowel movements more difficult, especially during the last months of pregnancy.

- Drink at least eight glasses of water a day.
- Eat high-fiber foods (such as bran, whole grains, fruits, vegetables, dried beans, and peas).

- Exercise daily. (Walking is a good exercise during pregnancy.)
- Drink prune juice or eat prunes, figs, or other dried fruits that are natural laxatives. Add dried fruits to high-fiber cereals or choose cereals like raisin bran.
- Do not take laxatives unless prescribed by your doctor.

HELP FOR SWOLLEN ANKLES AND FEET (EDEMA)

- Do *not* take water pills (diuretics).
- Drink additional water—six to eight glasses a day or more. Water is a natural diuretic.
- Do not restrict salt in your diet, unless your doctor recommends it.
- Put your feet up, particularly when you're lying down or sitting for prolonged periods.
- Rest on your left side, which helps circulation.
- Wear comfortable shoes, even if you have to buy a size larger than usual.
- Remove tight-fitting rings or other items that might obstruct the flow of fluids in your hands and feet.

If swelling becomes severe, especially if you become short of breath, contact your doctor immediately.

WORKING MOTHERS

Healthy women can usually continue working through pregnancy. However, you can increase your comfort level by following these tips:

- Avoid sitting or standing in one position for long intervals. If you have a sedentary job, stand up and walk around at frequent intervals.
- Rest during your lunch and coffee breaks. Skip running around on errands, talking with friends, or making phone calls. Instead, put your feet up, close your eyes, and relax for five or ten minutes.
- Try to avoid physical strain, particularly lifting heavy objects.

- Avoid getting overly tired.
- It's important for everyone to be protected from on-the-job exposure to dangerous chemicals or physical hazards such as radiation or high levels of microwaves. It's even more important for a pregnant woman to be safe from these dangers because both she and her baby can be damaged. If you work in radiology at a hospital or clinic, make sure a full-leaded apron is available to shield you from exposure to radiation.

Ideally, pregnant women should cut back or even stop work if they become chronically fatigued or are under constant emotional stress. However, quitting work or taking a leave of absence isn't an option for everyone. If you find yourself in this situation, you may be able to make some adjustments at work that will give you additional rest and still let you keep your job.

If you are easily fatigued performing your regular duties, inform your immediate supervisor. He or she may be able to allow you to cut back on some of these duties or temporarily assign you responsibilities that are less taxing. A written doctor's order is usually given extra consideration and may save your permanent position.

If you work near your home, you may be able to go home on your lunch break and get in a brief nap.

If you are having problems that require longer or more frequent rest periods, it may be possible—depending on the nature of your job—to work at home, at least some of the time. Employers are likely to agree to this arrangement if much of your work is done at your desk or on the phone.

Finally, check your employee handbook or visit your personnel director to learn more about benefits or special work arrangements that you are legally entitled to, as well as those that are possible under certain conditions.

REDUCING STRESS DURING PREGNANCY

Reducing stress during your pregnancy is important, and small things can help enormously.

- Use daily relaxation techniques such as prayer, meditation, deep breathing, or yoga to relieve stress.

WHEN TO CALL THE DOCTOR

Doctors tell expectant mothers to contact them day or night if they experience any of the following symptoms:

- *Bright red blood from the vagina*
- *Water leaking from the vagina*
- *Blurred vision, double vision, or spots in front of your eyes*
- *Swelling of face or fingers*
- *Severe headache*
- *Soreness or aching in the muscles that lingers for long periods of time*
- *Convulsions*
- *Abdominal pain*
- *Persistent vomiting after the first trimester*
- *Chills or fever*
- *Burning during urination*
- *Unusual changes in the baby's movements*

- Pamper yourself—even if it's only a long warm bath or shower, a nap before dinner, a walk in the park, or an hour with a good book.
- Talk things over with your relatives and friends, and let them reassure and comfort you when you need it most.
- Rest yourself in the arms of your church and your community. They may also offer programs to help you learn more about new babies and coming parenthood.
- Listen to music you most love.
- Eat a healthy, nutritious diet.
- Look for ways to turn stress into positive action. Individual empowerment is a technique that speaks directly to race-based stress that black women suffer.
- Set aside quiet times with your partner to discuss your hopes, concerns, points of conflict, and plans for the future.
- For all of your questions and worries, seek advice and reassurance from trusted friends or health-care professionals.

- Attend a prenatal group or childbirth classes for support and information.

CHILDBIRTH CLASSES

In the second or third trimester of pregnancy, many couples attend childbirth classes together to learn what to expect in the delivery room. This is a wonderful opportunity for the baby's father to join in the birth process. Women without partners often ask their mothers or sisters or a close friend to go with them. Make sure that the person you choose is likely to be available at a moment's notice when you go into labor.

For information on availability of classes in your area, check with your local hospital, the YWCA, or your doctor. Classes are usually no more than ten couples. They meet for about two hours, once a week, for six weeks. A good class provides basic information about pregnancy, explains vaginal and cesarean deliveries, and discusses pain-relief options during delivery. It will also include discussions about various childbirth techniques. In addition, your teacher may also offer instructions on nursing your new baby, as well as other useful postdelivery advice. In childbirth classes, everyone has a chance to ask questions and to share their experience.

All classes emphasize relaxation and teach breathing techniques that release tension and facilitate labor. The emphasis is on being awake and aware during childbirth, but intensity and duration of labor pain vary from person to person. Never be ashamed to ask for, or to accept, pain relief during labor and delivery.

HOW YOUR BABY GROWS

A baby begins life as a single cell, a fusion of the mother's egg and the father's sperm. Within nine or ten days, the new cell has divided into a cluster of cells, called a blastocyst, which plants itself like a small clot in the lining of the uterus. The side attached to the uterus becomes the placenta, which will sustain the baby's growth over the next nine months. The opposite side contains the raw material from which the embryo will grow.

In these very early days, the embryo is especially vulnerable to damage from alcohol, cigarette smoke, and drugs. In the next four weeks of development, which is called the embryonic period, dramatic changes take place in the nervous system and blood supply of the fetus as sets of cells align themselves in ladderlike progressions; these lines of cells eventually become cartilage, bones, and muscles.

About twelve weeks after conception, the fetus is about three inches long, with discernible limbs and internal organs. Its sex can be determined by ultrasound.

For the remainder of the pregnancy, the fetus will grow rapidly. After five months, fine downy fuzz begins to appear on the head and eyebrows. It eventually covers the whole body. A creamy white substance called *vernix caseosa* appears on the back, scalp, and in joint creases; it, too, will eventually cover the body, protecting the thin skin and preventing it from becoming waterlogged by the amniotic fluid.

By the end of the eighth month, the baby is completely formed. It can open its eyes and move freely and vigorously. It is about sixteen inches long and, hopefully, weighs about three and a half pounds. However, the baby is still rather thin and its lungs and other vital organs are still immature. If the baby is born at this stage, there is a possibility the delicate skull could be injured during delivery.

In the last month, the baby fills the uterus and is probably lying with its head down toward the mother's pelvis, beginning to position itself for birth. It is about eighteen inches long now and weighs approximately five and a half pounds. If it is born at this weight, its kidneys will be fully developed, but its lungs will not be fully mature; such a baby would be classified as a low-birth-weight. Not until the final weeks of pregnancy does the baby reach its full development.

Sometime in the last two weeks, the baby's head moves farther down into the mother's pelvis, which usually relieves some of the pressure on her lungs and stomach.

The baby is almost ready to be born. In the last week of pregnancy, its body is round and plump. Most of the downy fuzz has been replaced by secondary hair follicles. The body is still covered with the protective coating except around the mouth and eyes. The baby's fingernails have grown beyond the ends of the fingers, and the toenails have just reached the toe tips.

CHILDBIRTH

Few babies arrive on the day they are expected. There is little cause for concern when labor begins three weeks before or two weeks after the estimated due date. The weight of the baby has something to do with the onset of labor. For example, a woman carrying twins will often go into premature labor because the combined weight of the babies triggers her body into starting labor.

Sometimes, but not always, the fetal membranes break just before the onset of labor. Often, the only sensation is a gush of water; the mother feels no pain, because the membranes have no nerves. Water breaking is a sign to call the doctor and get ready for labor.

Labor begins officially with the first contractions, which are usually felt as low back pain. The cervix begins to dilate and the plug of mucus sealing the opening is dislodged. A little show of sticky pink mucus may be the first noticeable sign of labor. Gentle contractions begin to move across the abdomen every fifteen or twenty minutes.

The *first stage* of labor lasts until the cervix is fully dilated. It usually takes a long time for the cervix even to reach the halfway point. After that, the contractions increase in frequency and strength until they seem to come in waves.

This is likely to be the most difficult part of labor. When the cervix is seven centimeters open, it is three-quarters dilated. If the fetal membranes did not break at the onset of labor, they will break now, and almost a quart of sterile amniotic fluid automatically cleans the birth canal as it escapes.

Now the contractions usually speed up as the baby's head exerts a firmer pressure against the cervix, encouraging it to open. This pressure further stimulates the release of the hormone prostaglandin, which spurs contractions. Bloodstained mucus is discharged from the vagina, and the contractions begin to double up, sometimes with no obvious pattern. The mother feels the need to bear down, although she will be cautioned not to, since the cervix is not quite open. This transition between stage one and stage two may last a few minutes, or it may last an hour. When fully dilated, the cervix measures eight to ten centimeters across.

The first stage of labor can last up to thirteen or fourteen hours, or even longer for a first baby. In subsequent pregnancies, it may last only seven hours or less.

Now, the *second stage* begins. This is the most energetic phase of labor, and bearing down now helps push the baby out. Contractions vary in intensity, lasting about sixty seconds each and coming every one or two minutes.

Many women like to move around into different positions during this phase. The most common delivery position is sitting propped up at a forty-five-degree angle. But kneeling, crouching, and sitting in a birthing chair are all positions used by women during the second stage of labor.

On its journey to be born, the baby will move in a downward curve, always presenting its narrowest circumference to the birth passage. The baby's head begins to show, then recedes again between contractions. The head looks like shiny black corrugated cardboard because of the wrinkling the scalp undergoes as the mother's pelvic muscles guide it through the birth canal.

With a few more hard pushes, the baby is squeezed farther down the birth canal; more and more of the head shows at the outer folds of the vagina. The moment the baby's head stays at the opening without receding is called the "crowning."

The skin between the mother's vagina and anus is tautly stretched at this point; if it starts to tear, the doctor will make a small incision—a procedure called an episiotomy—in the tissue to ease the delivery of the baby's head. Episiotomies can take a long time to heal after childbirth, and many women prefer not to have one unless absolutely necessary. *The question of an episiotomy should be discussed with your doctor during one of your regular prenatal visits—before you go into labor.*

As soon as the baby's head emerges, it naturally rotates to either the left or right, depending on which side the baby has been lying. Then the shoulders quickly emerge, rotating to ease their way out. Now that the largest parts have been born, the rest of the body slides out almost immediately.

If you are having your first baby, the second stage of labor usually lasts about thirty minutes to an hour, although it can be much longer. For subsequent pregnancies, the second stage of labor is usually shorter.

The *third stage* of labor involves the delivery of the afterbirth, or placenta. This is the easiest stage for the mother, comparatively speaking, although contractions can be quite sharp. The doctor clamps the umbilical cord and waits for the placenta to separate spontaneously from the uterus. He may give the person an injection of oxytocin, a drug that will strengthen the contractions that cause the empty uterus to shrink suddenly, forcing the placenta to shear off. The blood vessels that supplied the placenta will constrict and seal themselves off. These richly supplied vessels may leak some blood for several weeks after childbirth, until the raw area where the placenta has pulled away heals.

When the placenta is completely detached, it slides down and is expelled through the vagina. The doctor or midwife usually helps the process along by pushing down on the mother's abdomen in small circular motions and pulling gently on the umbilical cord. It's important for the placenta to be delivered intact. Any open or torn vessels on the placenta suggest that a piece has been retained and still requires removal.

This third, and final, stage of labor may take a few minutes to a half hour.

YOUR NEW BABY

Ideally, your baby will weigh between six and a half pounds and nine pounds. This healthy weight means that your baby is getting off to a vibrant start in life. I wish this wonderful outcome for every woman. I know that everyone doesn't have access to good prenatal care, nor does everyone have good nutrition that supplies plenty of vitamins and minerals. Nor does every woman have a loving partner to help her. But, as we've seen, there's a lot each of us can do individually to help our babies come into the world.

Your newborn will spend its time enmeshed in and absorbing all the aspects of your life as she experiences the basic rhythms of your household, the sights and sounds of your home and neighborhood.

The task now is to create a life of harmony that allows room for the personal growth and fulfillment of both parents while they meet the physical and emotional needs of the new baby. In addition to giving the baby the gift of life, both parents are also giving the baby the gift of their own lives. Your own happiness will form the foundation for your new baby's happiness.

Your baby becomes part of an elaborate chain of lives that

stretches back for generations. He learns from you, as you learned from your own parents. Play with your new baby, cuddle him, and devote your love and attention to him—and remember to love yourselves, too. The more parents can fulfill themselves and make their own lives happy, the happier the baby will be.

4

EARLY DANGERS

Despite lifesaving medical technology, and despite the eagerness with which we welcome new life, infancy continues to hold dangerous health hazards for black Americans. In 1995, the United States, which spends a higher percentage of its gross national product on health care than any other nation, ranked twentieth in infant mortality among developed countries. And African-American infants are still twice as likely as white babies to die before their first birthday.

The most important predictor of infant mortality is very low birth weight (less than 3.3 pounds) caused by prematurity. (Any baby born under thirty-seven weeks is "preterm," regardless of weight.) It's true that new, costly technologies are increasing the chances of survival for these very small, very premature infants, but survival does not guarantee quality of life. Superior technology cannot make up for all the deficits that continue to threaten very premature infants. Many of the survivors are left with permanent disabilities. *The real focus must remain on preventing prematurity.*

The infant mortality rate is defined as the number of babies (out of every one thousand) who die before they reach the age of one. Infant mortality is further divided into two main components: death that occurs in the first twenty-seven days of life; death that occurs between twenty-eight days and one year, called postneonatal death.

Very early death is usually caused by congenital abnormalities that are often present in very premature babies. (In chapters 2 and

3, we have discussed the many things you can do to help ensure a healthy full-term baby.)

Babies who make it past twenty-eight days are still vulnerable. And black infants, even those of normal weight, have a greater risk of postnatal death. Accidents are one cause. Other risks involve stress and infections (which are higher among poor mothers and babies, who often receive inadequate medical care). However, the leading cause of *post*neonatal death is sudden infant death syndrome (SIDS), which for unknown reasons is significantly higher among black infants.

SUDDEN INFANT DEATH SYNDROME (SIDS)

SIDS claims about seven thousand American infants each year. Most deaths occur quietly while the baby is asleep—often between the hours of midnight and 8:00 A.M. SIDS occurs more often during the winter than during the summer months. The baby is usually between two and four months old, rarely older than six months.

SIDS can happen to any baby. Asian babies appear to have the lowest risk, and black and Native American babies have a particularly high risk. Boys die more often than girls. SIDS tends to occur more than once in families.

No one knows why these deaths occur, nor if SIDS is one disease or many. It is no one's fault, and even if you take every possible precaution, it can still happen. SIDS seems to have no warning signs, and it is only determined as the cause of death after all other possibilities have been ruled out.

Although SIDS is relatively rare—the risk of the average baby dying of SIDS is about 1.7 in 1,000—its impact is devastating, leading researchers to focus intense work on this sad mystery.

Vaccinations, colds, and fevers seem to have no bearing on an infant's risk. Neither do occasional pauses in breathing, called newborn apnea, cause SIDS. SIDS is not caused by choking, and it is not contagious.

On the other hand, SIDS babies may not be as healthy as they appear at birth. Autopsies of infants who died of SIDS show slight pinpoint hemorrhages in their lungs, lung congestion, and mild inflammation of the upper airways. These vulnerabilities may be present at birth, undermining an infant's ability to thrive outside the womb. Other studies suggest that the breathing and heart rate of SIDS babies is poorly coordinated, indicating immature heart and lung function. Babies born with inadequately oxygenated blood, accelerated heartbeat (tachycardia), respiratory distress, or accelerated breathing (tachypnea) are known to be at higher risk. Other studies of SIDS babies have found that several had been sick with diarrhea and vomiting during the two weeks prior to death.

Nevertheless, after thirty years of research, the SIDS mystery still has no final answer. SIDS is not caused by neglect or abuse. Factors that appear to increase risk are these:

- Maternal smoking during pregnancy—for example, a population study conducted in Sweden showed that maternal smoking doubled the risk for SIDS
- Maternal drug use
- A family history of SIDS or a near miss (when an infant was rescued after breathing stopped)
- Low birth weight or premature birth
- Putting an infant to sleep in a prone position
- Soft, fluffy infant bedding

WHAT YOU CAN DO

Thanks to the intense attention being focused on this disease, parents do have a line of defense against SIDS.

Number one is altering your baby's sleeping position. Based on evidence from Norway, New Zealand, and Australia, where SIDS deaths have been reduced by half, the American Academy of Pediatrics now recommends healthy babies be put to sleep on their backs or on their sides. They call their new recommendation "Back to Sleep."

During the first six months of life, most infants cannot roll from one position to another, but if you worry that your baby will shift, prop him against the crib's side and bring his underneath arm forward at a right angle to stabilize him. By the time your baby is old enough to roll over by himself, the most dangerous SIDS period is past, and the baby can find the sleeping position that suits him best.

Second, never put your baby to sleep on soft bedding—no soft toys, no pillows or comforters, no water beds or sheepskin fluffies. Instead, use a firm infant mattress covered by a sheet or waterproof pad.

Third, try not to let your infant become overheated while sleeping. Since more babies die of SIDS in the winter, some researchers theorize that babies are unable to cool down because they're tightly wrapped or swaddled.

Fourth, and equally important, *make sure your baby's environment is smoke-free.*

EXCEPTIONS TO THE RULE

Certain babies do better sleeping facedown.

- Premature infants with respiratory disease
- Babies with symptoms of gastroesophageal reflux
- Babies with upper-airway malformations

Your doctor will advise you.

MONITORS

Some parents purchase an electronic monitor that sets off an alert if the infant's heart rate or breathing is interrupted. The value of these monitors is still uncertain. Since it's almost impossible to predict which infants are vulnerable, doctors do not yet recommend that every new parent purchase one.

Any family who has had the great misfortune of losing a baby knows how devastating the experience is. A SIDS death, which comes without warning and leaves so many unanswered questions, causes intense grief for parents and families. Police officers, emergency health professionals, counselors, and even members of the community become involved in the family's private life. At first, these strangers may seem intrusive. However, all are professionals experienced with SIDS deaths, and they can provide families with much of the support they desperately need. Families can also get help by joining a support group where others who have experienced a SIDS death can help them share their grief and express their feelings in a safe environment. In addition to peer support, a family physician, minister, nurse, or counselor can also provide consolation and assistance.

Remember, although SIDS is more common in African-American infants, it is still a rare phenomenon, and getting rarer every day. Parents have every reason to expect their new baby to survive and thrive—and most babies do.

5

AGES AND STAGES: FROM INFANCY THROUGH ADOLESCENCE

All babies are born with a well-developed set of reflexes. Place an object in the palm of a newborn's hand and she will clench her fist around it. Put pressure on the balls of her feet and she will curl her toes in response. Hold her upright over a flat surface and she will draw her legs up in walking movements. At any sudden noise or movement, the baby will throw out her arms and legs and probably cry. These reflexes largely disappear during the first three months as messages from the brain begin to control a baby's movements.

Although all children follow a similar series of landmarks in growth and development, every child is also unique. A healthy child may exceed average standards of growth and development in some areas and fall below standards in others. For example, the average child walks at twelve months, but a child who starts walking anytime between nine and sixteen months is still perfectly normal. In other words, "average" and "normal" are not necessarily the same.

Experienced parents know this. First-time parents, however, tend to be a little anxious about whether their baby is growing properly, and being aware of the normal range helps most parents feel more relaxed. In the rare event that your child's growth and development fall significantly outside the range, "well-baby" visits to the doctor will uncover problems early. (See chapter 6.)

Growth is the process of becoming physically larger and more mature; *development* is the process of becoming more physically and mentally complex. Growth and development are very much connected and move along in parallel fashion.

GROWTH

Immediately after birth, your baby's weight, length, and gestational age (duration of your pregnancy) are recorded. Your doctor compares this information with the normal values from growth charts compiled by the National Center for Health Statistics.

Here are the ranges for full-term newborns:

> *Weight: between 6 and 10 pounds*
> *Length: from 18.5 to 21.5 inches (46.2 to 53.7 centimeters)*
> *Head circumference: 13.2 to 14.8 inches (33 to 37 centimeters)*

Any measurements falling within these ranges are considered normal. As a child grows, weight is measured in relationship to height. For any given height, an ideal weight can be determined from a growth chart. An infant underweight for his height is failing to thrive. A child who weighs more than average for his height is overweight. Heredity and nutrition determine how quickly and how much your child grows.

Hunger is biologically determined, and babies have a strong survival instinct. The best advice is to feed babies on demand. This gives them an early sense of control over eating and sets up a healthy eating pattern for later life. (Inexperienced parents may have trouble knowing when their infant is "demanding" to be fed. See Part Two for guidelines.)

Babies grow very fast in their first year. Your baby's steady growth in height and weight is one of the best signs that he is healthy. Most babies gain about one-half a pound per week during the first few months.

On average, infants usually double their birth weight in the first four to five months, then triple their weight by the time they are one year of age. Height increases by a full 50 percent by the end of the first year. (A child's adult height depends largely on the height of his parents: Tall parents tend to have tall children, and short parents tend to have short children.)

GROWTH CHARTS

Your doctor will record the growth of your child on a growth chart, which becomes a standard part of your child's medical history. Your child's height, weight, and head circumference are plotted against standards developed by the National Center for Health Statistics; these show a range of normal measurements for infants and children. There are different charts for boys and girls. There are also special charts for prepubescence, when growth is quite rapid.

These charts have been devised from studies in which large numbers of healthy, normal children of the same race and same socioeconomic group were measured at various ages. The data have been ranked in percentiles. Most children stay in approximately the same percentile during infancy and childhood. Growth, however, does not always proceed in a smooth curve. Your child's growth rate may be occasionally high or low on the growth chart, due to his own growth lags and spurts.

The trouble with using growth charts for all American children is that the standards are based on large-scale surveys of the child population conducted in the late 1960s and early 1970s; the children were all white, and many, if not most, were from middle- and upper-income families.

The "standard" may not appropriately reflect growth expectations for some groups of children. For example, African-American infants at birth tend to be smaller than white infants, and most are going to weigh in on the low end of the growth chart, when in fact they may be average.

At least one study has questioned the growth charts and found them lacking. In a 1975 comparison study from the School of Public Health at the University of Michigan in 1975, height and weight measurements were collected on 1,233 black and white children from a child health clinic in Washtenaw County. Researchers found that in early infancy, African-American babies tended to be smaller than white babies. By their second birthdays, however, the black children tended to be heavier and taller than the white children. They concluded that different growth charts should be developed to reflect differences that may exist in different population groups.

Physicians continue to use standard growth charts because they are what is available; most pediatricians say that when assessing a child's health they focus mostly on the *rate of growth,* rather than where the child fits into the standard growth chart. Hopefully, your baby's doctor will do the same, and when looking at your child's overall growth take into consideration differences among population groups.

DEVELOPMENT

Your baby will go from a helpless little bundle to a walking, talking, unique person before you know it.

Motor development occurs in an orderly sequence, starting with lifting the head, then rolling over, sitting up, crawling, standing, and walking. Although the sequence is predictable—beginning with the head and following the maturation of the spinal cord downward—every baby matures at his or her own rate.

The sequence of speech development goes from cooing/gurgling, to babbling, to imitating speech sounds, to saying first words, then to using words together. Again, the normal rate varies considerably. The most reassuring and reliable characteristics of normal development are your baby's alertness and curiosity. Don't worry if your baby seems different from other babies of the same age; each baby develops in his or her own way.

Remember, there's no such thing as a spoiled baby. The more playing and cuddling you and your family give him, the better he will develop mentally and physically. If you have any questions about the way your child is growing and developing, ask his doctor or nurse practitioner.

NOTABLE LANDMARKS

Here are some events you can look forward to.

By six weeks, your baby will smile when you smile or play with her. She will look at mobiles and faces and notice sounds. She will also make a few sounds of her own (besides crying). Listen to her, and talk back to her. By the time she is about two months old, she'll be smiling and responding during your "conversations." She will wiggle so much that she can accidentally roll off a flat surface; always be sure never to turn your back on a baby who is lying on a table, bed, changing counter, or chair.

Babies cry *a lot*. It's their way of getting your attention so you can "fix it," whatever "it" happens to be. Wrapping the baby snugly in a soft blanket and cuddling her usually calms her down and helps her feel secure. She may want to suck on her thumb, fingers, or a pacifier. (Sucking is a natural reflex for babies, and most stop sucking by themselves before preschool.)

By about five months, she can hold up her head while lying on her stomach. This is a tremendous achievement, because neck muscles are weak at birth, and a baby's head is very large in relationship to its body. (At birth, a child's head size is already 60 percent of the adult size; by the age of three years, the head size will be nearly 90 percent of its adult size.)

She will laugh and giggle, reach for and hold objects, and—the biggest landmark of this period—learn to roll over. Your baby will be able to move around quickly and will try to put small objects in her mouth, so keep your eyes open.

At about six months, your baby may begin to stretch her arms out to be picked up. Baby teeth usually begin to come in about now, but don't worry if they don't arrive on schedule. Every baby is an individual, and yours has her own little time clock.

More safety precautions are necessary now because she is getting around a lot more. Cover all unused electric outlets with safety caps or tape, and keep all electric cords out of her reach. If your baby is around old paint that can chip or flake, be watchful that she doesn't chew or swallow it. Old paint may contain lead (see chapter 32).

By about eight months, your baby will respond to her own name, and if you place her in a sitting position, she can sit without support. She may creep by pulling her body with her arms and kicking her legs. Start baby-proofing your house (see chapter 33).

By about ten months, she understands the word *no,* and plays peekaboo. She can stand up if she holds on to something; she can also push her arms through when you are dressing her. By about one year, she waves bye-bye and has started copying your speech. She may be able to walk, if she holds on to something. When it comes to crawling and walking, there is a wide variation in time schedules. Some babies crawl before they walk, and they may be such good crawlers that they don't practice walking until a little later; others never crawl at all. If your baby isn't walking by sixteen months, let the doctor know.

When babies first discover walking, they are overjoyed and will wear you out by insisting that you give them a hand, literally, so they can practice. They especially love to practice walking up and down stairs.

Your baby doesn't really need shoes until she's walking outdoors, but shoes can steady her when she's pulling herself up and taking those first steps. When it comes to shoes, good fit is more important than cute style. Smooth leather on the bottom will give her more maneuverability than high-traction rubber bottoms, which sometimes pull early walkers up short and cause them to stumble.

By about eighteen months, she is probably walking, playing with a ball, stacking blocks, and feeding herself using a spoon and cup. She can say between twenty and thirty words.

Your baby's growth now begins to slow down and becomes more steady and gradual. By two years, you are looking at a whole new being. This is your toddler. She runs, starts to put words together, and talks incessantly. She likes to "help" with chores and feeds herself with a spoon or fork. Parents spend untold energy and time in pursuit of the adventurous toddler. Toddlers want to choose food, clothes, and toys for themselves, but their experience is limited. Parents can help by presenting attractive alternatives— dry cereal or hot oatmeal, the blue T-shirt or the red one, *Mother Goose* or *The Little Engine That Could*. Your toddler will choose what she likes best, and she'll enjoy the respect you give her as an individual.

TOILET TRAINING

Somewhere in the second year, babies become aware of their bodily functions. There are many different theories on toilet training, but the greatest success occurs when the baby becomes aware of when he is about to urinate or have a bowel movement. Generally, bowel training comes first. Cooperating with your baby, instead of insisting he uses the potty, makes toilet training easier and quicker. When your little one begins to use the potty, don't expect him to stay dry during naps or all night. Whatever you do, don't nag. Most children are fully toilet trained by the time they're ready for school.

YOUR CHILD'S BODY IMAGE

Children, like adults, come in a wide variety of sizes and shapes. Some kids are chunky, others thin, some muscular, some pear-shaped, some tall, some short—all shapes are healthy and all shapes are inherently good. Body *shape* is a matter of genetics; your child cannot do anything about his body shape. Weight is another issue entirely, and everyone has some measure of control over weight.

However, our culture, like every other society on earth, has its own ideas of what's beautiful and what isn't. None of this is rooted in reality, but children have no way of knowing that. A child's body image is intimately connected to his self-esteem. His view of himself changes in response to the feedback he gets from other people. No matter how a child grows, our job as adults and parents is to nurture self-esteem and promote a positive body image.

I can still remember how I felt as a young child when adults criticized me, and I also remember the positive words they used to describe my sister. Among African Americans, some of these words have to do with shape and size; others concern the color of our skin and texture of our hair. I was often described as skinny, nappy-haired, and dark. My sister had "good hair," and people said she was cubby cute or "fine." Her skin was also lighter than mine, which in the late 1950s and early 1960s was viewed as admirable. These comments hurt me and had long-lasting effects. Self-esteem based on the comments and opinions of other people develops early in children.

Even as we help our children accept that diversity in body shape is normal and good, we can also encourage nutritious eating and exercise, which promote healthy bodies in all children, regardless of their body shape. Bear in mind that growth in height and weight do not happen simultaneously. A child may look chubby, then grow into his weight. A tall, skinny child may fill out in a matter of months.

GETTING READY FOR SCHOOL

Children are born with an internal drive to master themselves and their environment. The central mission of your toddler is to become more independent. By around age two, he is likely to have a vocabulary of about 300 words, and will use two- to three-word sentences. By age three, his vocabulary has increased to 500 to 1,000 words; he uses short, four-word sentences with ease and asks questions constantly. He will talk for the fun of it, and there's no need to inhibit or correct him.

At around age four, a child becomes more logical. In preschool or kindergarten, he is learning to get along with new friends. Temper tantrums, in response to frustration, are normal at this age, although not every child has them. Parents can help by acknowledging the child's feelings, while putting limits on hitting others or hurting himself. The way you behave when you're upset has a tremendous influence on kids. Reinforcing a child's positive behavior and overlooking annoying acts—rather than punishing a child for outbursts—is usually the best way to go. Tantrums may persist for a year or so; then they usually disappear.

BEHAVIORAL PROBLEMS

Behavioral problems, if there are any, may start to show up during a child's early school years. You may have already noticed if your child seems hyperactive, but when he gets into a school environment, the teachers know it, too.

What we used to call hyperactivity is now often identified as attention deficit–hyperactivity disorder, or ADHD. ADHD is one of the most common behavioral disorders, one that puts children at a huge disadvantage in school because they can't concentrate long enough to learn. When they start falling behind other children, their problems are compounded daily.

When we were kids, neither we nor our parents had heard of hyperactivity. Most of us appeared to be well behaved and orderly. Exceptions were few and far between, and mostly boys (who were known to be "bad"). Today, many baby boomer parents find it hard to accept that ADHD is a real medical problem.

Almost every child could be described as hyperactive from time to time, but for children who suffer from ADHD, it's almost *all* the time. This disorder affects boys four to seven times more often than girls. In school, these kids have a hard time sitting still, they often talk loudly and continuously, they interrupt, and they have trouble listening and following directions. They don't pay attention to activities that interest other children, and they become agitated if they have to wait in line. They easily become frustrated, display sudden emotional outbursts, and persistently misbehave, despite repeatedly being told to stop.

If your child behaves this way on a regular basis, ask a pediatrician about the possibility of ADHD. ADHD is often confused with specific learning disabilities, hearing or vision impairment, mood and anxiety disorders, and other problems. New diagnostic guidelines can be used to separate these various disorders from one another.

Researchers have not yet found the precise cause of ADHD. Refined sugar and food additives do not seem to cause the disorder, as was previously thought. New studies suggest that ADHD has a biological basis—a child whose parent or sibling has the disorder is more likely to have ADHD, and a child exposed during fetal development to his mother's drinking or smoking also appears to have a higher risk.

Treatment may help some children. The drug methylphenidate, commonly known as Ritalin, can calm hyperactive children. The drug won't cure the problem or eliminate all the symptoms, but it helps some ADHD kids focus their attention and keep up in school, which prevents compounding the problem as a child grows up. This is a step forward, but side effects can cause problems. Talk it over thoroughly with your child's doctor before and during Ritalin treatment.

AS YOUR CHILD GROWS AND DEVELOPS

Between the ages of five and nine, a child's physical growth slows down. In fact, he may not seem to be growing at all. Nonetheless, children accomplish a huge number of developmental tasks during this period, particularly in terms of self-esteem and self-image. They will try to perform in ways that earn your respect, and they'll begin to understand that negotiation and compromise are signs of strength. They will also be attracted to other adult role models, and hopefully they will find positive ones.

Children in this stage will begin to test the limits of your rules in an effort to establish themselves as fully independent individuals. And they will do almost anything to be accepted by their peers, even at the expense of their own individuality.

Their mental skills are also developing, as they learn to maintain attention and complete boring tasks for the sake of long-term goals. Increased short-term and long-term memory allows them to compare and interpret complex situations. They continue to advance in reading, writing, and using numbers. Above all, they continue talking. By six or seven, a child may tell stories that go on and on and on. . . . Have patience. Listen. Try to hang on every word. Your child is practicing grammar and other language skills, accomplishments that can give him a huge boost in self-confidence and prepare him for future education and achievement. All of this mental development takes place before the next dramatic physical change in your child's life.

PUBERTY

It's difficult to say just when puberty starts. From birth through age eight or nine, boys and girls grow and develop rapidly, and they are very similar to each other, except for the outward evidence of their sexual organs. At a certain mysterious point, long before any physical changes are apparent, the body's hormonal system activates the reproductive system. The hormonal system is controlled by the brain, but what actually triggers the system is uncertain.

Some researchers believe that a child's body weight plays a part. We know, for example, that malnourished children often experience delayed puberty. We also know that modern American children, who are heavier than their forebears, go through puberty about four years earlier than children did one hundred years ago. Other possibilities include genetics and sunlight (girls living in countries where sunlight is vivid year-round tend to reach maturity at a younger age). All of these factors may be involved.

In any event, when children reach the threshold of puberty—about age nine for girls and age eleven for boys—the hypothalamus signals the pituitary gland to release—or hold back—certain hormones. The pituitary gland first releases hormones that bombard the ovaries in a girl and the testicles in a boy. These organs now begin to make their own hormones: The testicles begin to make testosterone, and the ovaries begin to make estrogen and progesterone. ,

The pituitary gland releases other hormones that stimulate other glands, which in turn produce growth hormones. Growth hormones encourage bones to grow longer, and they promote fat deposits in markedly different patterns for boys and girls. Growth spurts can be sudden and erratic as different hormones pour into the bloodstream in varying amounts. Early developers may grow at slow rates and late developers may suddenly shoot up. Genetic endowment is the strongest predictor of stature. In general, height and sexual development increase together, and when sexual maturity peaks, the body's height is fixed.

A girl may reach the threshold of puberty as early as age eight or nine, when her breasts begin to develop and her own unique biological time clock begins to tick. She begins to grow taller, and her waist slims, while her hips grow slightly fuller. By age eleven, most girls have grown several inches in height and soft hair begins to grow under the arms and around the pubic area. Many girls have a first period around this time.

Menstruation is actually a late sign of puberty, beginning after much of the dramatic growth of puberty is finished. By the age of fourteen, most girls are menstruating regularly. Once begun, puberty in girls takes from one and a half to four years from start to finish.

In boys, puberty usually begins later, between the ages of nine and a half and fourteen. The typical sequence of changes may be quite subtle and take place over a fairly long period of time. The hormone testosterone is responsible for the enlargement of the testicles, penis, and the growth of pubic hair. In most boys, enlargement of the testicles begins at about age eleven and continues until about age eighteen. Penis enlargement usually begins about a year later and continues until about age sixteen. The first signs of early pubic hair may be around age eleven, but they may not be really noticeable until about age thirteen and a half.

Testosterone is also responsible for the development of facial hair, voice changes, adult body odor, acne, and increasing muscle mass, all seen at about age fifteen. About half of all boys also experience some breast enlargement and may have a tender lump under one or both nipples. These breast changes are so common, and so embarrassing, that it helps to explain to boys that it's the result of normal hormonal changes and they will probably grow out of it within a year. If your son seems especially worried, or if the condition does not disappear, it's a good idea to suggest a visit to the doctor.

ADOLESCENCE

Puberty is a biological surge, defined by a specific set of physical changes that take a child into sexual maturity. A few medical conditions are associated with delayed or precocious puberty, but for most boys and girls puberty proceeds with predictable regularity. The experience of adolescence, however, varies widely among teenagers.

Adolescence is the psychological response to puberty. It is influenced by ethnic and cultural background, religious beliefs, moral values, family style, geography, politics, and economic status. Adolescence describes the whole time of growing up—emotionally, intellectually, and physically—from about nine to nineteen or twenty.

The physical changes of puberty have a major impact on emotions, behavior, and personality, which can result in unexpected mood swings out of proportion to any obvious provocation. The rising tide of sex hormones in early puberty also presses for fulfillment at a time when most youngsters are not yet ready to cope with sexual intercourse. Masturbation is common in both sexes and considered normal. Sexual experimentation with members of the same sex is also fairly common at this age. Both boys and girls are curious about sexual anatomy and they sometimes find it easier to explore their changing bodies and growing sex drives with friends of their own sex. It's one way to confirm that they are physically okay. This doesn't mean that a child is or will be homosexual. It is well documented that significant numbers of gay men and women first became aware of their homosexuality in early childhood. Experimentation often occurs early, before homophobia is taught and/or absorbed.

An understanding of the consequences of sexual activity is vital at this stage. But if we have trouble getting our kids to turn down the stereo or take out the garbage, how are we going to sit down and talk about sex? Educating teenagers about sex, without invading their privacy, requires sensitivity and respect on the part of parents at a time when most children are especially irritating. (For more information on discussing sex, see chapter 23.)

The teenager's mission is to become fully independent. They demand complete freedom and look for ways to develop their own resources and values outside the family system. The best way to do this is to create conflict between themselves and their nurturing, loving parents. This is the time when most kids break family rules and challenge everything their parents say and do. Conflict directly correlates with physical development: If puberty comes early, so does the conflict; if puberty is late, the period of tension is delayed.

Like all important life transitions, the degree of adolescent turmoil seems to depend on other crises that might coincide with puberty. Changing schools at a critical time, divorce of parents, or losing a parent through death can make adolescence more difficult than usual.

The adolescent in the African-American family faces an arduous set of developmental hurdles. He or she may feel very alienated from society. Adolescents living in poverty, white as well as black, are often very disillusioned with parents who have failed to make headway toward achieving the American dream. Some are drawn to antisocial, wealthier adult figures, such as drug dealers. Black adolescents often find themselves falling between the cracks of our society—without the guidance, nurturing, support, and parenting we experienced just a few decades ago. Yet the strengths of the black family, even those families living in poverty, can surpass these dangers. All African-American parents, in every situation, already know they have to give their children extra help to get them through the most complicated period of their lives.

The good news is that conflict—in the form of nagging, squabbling, and bickering—rarely damages the close emotional bonds a child has with his parents, nor does it lead most adolescents and parents to reject one another. In recent surveys, most teenagers admitted that their relationships with their parents did decline during these years, but they also said these relationships went from "very positive" to "less positive"—in other words, most teens didn't feel the parental relationship disintegrated into the negative.

With consistent, persistent attention and love (and a little luck), adolescence is a temporary passage that helps children grow up. As life-cycle theorists like to point out, if teenagers didn't argue with their parents about picking up their socks, they might never leave home at all. It is the adolescent's job to break away from the family circle. It is usually over by the age of fifteen or sixteen. This emotional breaking away eventually turns a child into a capable and achieving adult.

6

Visiting the Doctor

For generations, African-American families have raised healthy children with few or no visits to the doctor. In fact, this is how I remember my own childhood. My sister and I were rarely ill, and when we were, our mother used home remedies that had been passed down from her mother. She had remedies for colds, stomachaches, earaches, constipation, and diarrhea. Once a month, sick or not, we were given a tonic to get rid of parasites, just in case we had them. Most black mothers in our neighborhood used similar methods.

The current generation of African-American mothers seeks medical care for their children much more regularly than in the past. In many parts of the country, nurses and pediatricians are getting out the message that more frequent "well-baby" visits and examinations can keep kids healthy and thriving. One thing is certain: The sooner your child receives medical checkups, the better your chances of preventing or treating health problems.

WELL-BABY CHECKUPS

During the first two years, babies grow and develop quickly. Therefore, regular visits to your baby's doctor—well-baby checkups—will make sure she is growing normally. Well-baby checkups are scheduled by your baby's doctor or nurse practitioner in addition to the times you might take your baby to the doctor for illnesses.

The doctor will answer any questions you have, provide laboratory testing for diseases, and make certain immunizations are on schedule.

Age	Self-Check or Community Screening	Doctor Visits
Newborn		In hospital, includes first hearing exam*
Two weeks		Well-baby check
Two months		Well-baby check
Four months		Well-baby check
Six months		Well-baby check
		First eye exam
Nine months		Well-baby check
Twelve months		Well-baby check
Fifteen months		Well-baby check
Eighteen months		Well-baby check
Twenty-four months		Well-baby check
Children from two to thirteen		Physical once a year through age six; then every two years**
		Eye exam every two years unless child exhibits problems (squinting, sitting too close to TV)
		Hearing tested every two years
		Dentist every six months, beginning at age three
Teens from fourteen to eighteen	Check weight monthly.	Physical exam, vision, and hearing, every two years
	Follow balanced diet and exercise regimen.	Dentist every six months

*New tests can now detect hearing and eyesight problems in infants; therefore, these exams are now given much earlier in life, which allows for earlier treatment.
**During the first three or four years of puberty, most pediatricians like to see a child once a year, especially females (girls: age nine through twelve; boys: approximately eleven through fourteen).

Your baby's doctor can also provide advice and information about feeding and nutrition, as well as general health and well-baby care.

Ideally, according to the American Academy of Pediatrics, mothers should take their infants in for a well-baby check about five times in the first year and about four more times in the second. These visits coordinate with the recommended immunization schedule. (After the age of two, your child should continue to see the doctor about once a year until age six.)

Every pediatrician has a personal approach to well-baby checkups. The organization of the physical exam, the number and type of assessment techniques used, and the procedures performed also vary with the needs of the child. Your child's first visit may take place earlier or later than you anticipate, depending on her overall health at birth.

The Academy of Pediatrics and U.S. government guidelines recommend the following schedule of well-baby and well-child checkups.

DOCTOR VISITS DURING TEEN YEARS

Starting around age eleven, adolescents begin to encounter a host of potential health problems. Encouraging your adolescent to visit the doctor on a regular basis and allowing him or her to have private time with the doctor (confidentiality is guaranteed) can go a long way toward preventing physical, emotional, and behavioral problems. Teens can be screened for blood pressure, weight and stature, anemia, and various health risks (smoking, drinking, and sexually transmitted diseases, as well as sexual behavior).

The fact that many teenage health problems can be prevented has led to school-based and community-based health centers for teenagers, although these are not yet a widespread trend. Teens generally don't think about their health or about disease prevention. However, if your child is used to visiting the doctor, he or she is more likely to follow through in the teenage years. Sharing information within the family can also help. You can do this by leaving pamphlets and books around the house, taking the family to health fairs, and subscribing to such magazines as *Essence, Health Quest, Heart and Soul,* and *Ebony,* which regularly feature health articles.

WHEN TO CALL THE DOCTOR: INFANTS

Even though babies and young children will cry when they are not feeling well, they often cannot tell you what's wrong. As children grow up, most parents develop a sixth sense that tells them when to call the doctor. Until then, the best advice is to call whenever you notice a change in eating habits or bowel movements, or an increase in crying. In other words, if you're worried, call.

Before you do, jot down your observations and take your baby's temperature with a rectal thermometer. When you call, have a pad and pencil handy to write down the advice you get; also have the telephone number of a pharmacy, in case the doctor wants to phone in a prescription.

Call immediately if your infant displays any of the following symptoms:

> *Fever (higher than 100° F)*
>
> *Vomiting, more than spit-up*
>
> *Jaundice (skin has a yellowish cast)*
>
> *Diarrhea—very watery, loose, foul-smelling stools more than twice a day; even one large watery bowel movement if your baby is less than three months old*
>
> *Breathing problems—has to work hard to get air in and out*
>
> *Convulsions (shaking arms and legs)*
>
> *Blood in diaper*
>
> *Cries more or differently from the usual, or moans as if in pain, or is very fussy*

Also call if the baby:

> *Seems weak, has no energy to cry as loudly as usual*
>
> *Refuses to feed or nurses poorly, or wants only half of the usual bottle*
>
> *Doesn't wake up as alertly as usual*
>
> *Is not playful, even for a short time (for older babies)*
>
> *Just doesn't seem right, and you are worried*

EMERGENCIES

Choking. This is always a potential threat with infants and toddlers. Coughing is the most effective way to clear air passages. If the baby can't cough or breathe, and her face is turning blue, place her across your knee, facedown, with her body tilted, headfirst, at about a thirty-degree angle. Administer four sharp blows between the baby's shoulder blades. *Ask your doctor to show you this technique before you ever have to use it.*

Accidents can happen. If your baby gets hurt or becomes suddenly sick, stay calm and call for emergency help. Always have emergency numbers near your telephone for the doctor, fire, police, rescue, and poison control center. Make sure you know where the closest hospital or emergency center is and how to get there. (See chapters 33 and 34. As a backup, there is a place to write emergency numbers on page 386.)

WHEN TO CALL THE DOCTOR: OLDER KIDS

Call the doctor if your child shows any of the following symptoms:

> *Difficulty breathing, a stiff neck, severe fatigue, or purple spots on skin*
>
> *Any seizure*
>
> *Persistent fever that doesn't come down after proper medication or lasts for more than twenty-four hours*
>
> *Fever accompanied by other symptoms such as earache, rash, vomiting, or stomach pain*
>
> *Fever in a child who is not taking fluids or urinating normally*
>
> *Stomach pain that is incapacitating or persists for more than two hours*

IMMUNIZATIONS

At a time when other nations are making dramatic progress in immunizing children against preventable diseases, government statistics show that less than half of white American preschoolers and only 34 percent of black preschoolers are fully immunized. (Immunization statistics are reported state by state; they range from as low as 30 percent in Texas to as high as 84 percent in Vermont.)

Immunization is required for school enrollment in all fifty states, so by the time children are five years old, 97 percent are fully vaccinated. But this is often too late to protect against many childhood diseases. Parents in every tax bracket seem to put off inoculations until the last minute, even though this puts their children at risk in the meantime.

Doctors believe that low immunization rates are responsible for the increase in the incidence of potentially dangerous childhood diseases, including measles, mumps, polio, and whooping cough.

In 1992, more than two thousand cases of measles and more than two thousand cases of mumps were reported to the Centers for Disease Control and Prevention. As of January 1, 1994, 6,132 cases of whooping cough were reported—an 80 percent jump over the previous year, and more than at any time since the late 1960s.

Even babies who see their doctors regularly may not receive all of their vaccinations. Many parents take their kids to free clinics for vaccinations and are not sure what shots they received or when. Children may be seen by a different doctor at each visit, and unless the clinic is particularly careful about record keeping, it is possible for the doctors there to overlook immunizations.

Cost is one obvious factor interfering with immunization. The cost of inoculations has risen from roughly $10.96 for the full course to $235. Many parents try to have their kids vaccinated at public clinics, but funding cutbacks, inconvenient hours, and endless waits at overburdened clinics often mean no immunizations for children whose parents have inflexible work schedules.

Even when vaccinations are free and kids have access to private doctors, the mystery surrounding the lack of immunization remains unsolved. A study that tracked families employed at Johnson & Johnson, all of whom had health insurance, found that the majority of the children of their employees were also underimmunized.

One important cause of underimmunization is the failure of parents to appreciate the potential seriousness of childhood diseases—primarily because modern parents have never experienced these diseases themselves. (The efficacy of vaccines has been proved: There is no smallpox on the face of the earth; very little polio, whooping cough, or lockjaw.) A 1993 Gallup poll showed that nearly half of parents today are unaware that polio is an infectious disease; 36 percent did not know that measles could be fatal; and 44 percent did not know hemophilus influenza B is the leading cause of potentially fatal childhood meningitis. Nor do they know firsthand the terrors of whooping cough, the often fatal paralysis of tetanus, or the sometimes fatal throat infection caused by diphtheria.

The U.S. Public Health Service has set a goal of completely immunizing 90 percent of all infants by the year 2000. In 1994, despite opposition from vaccine manufacturers, Congress passed President Clinton's national immunization initiative, which says that no child can be refused immunization because the family is unable to pay. Additional federal money is being used to allow clinics to expand their hours and to help states to implement vaccine distribution programs.

HOW VACCINES WORK

Vaccines deliver a small amount of the infectious agent into the bloodstream to activate the body's natural defense mechanisms. Once awakened, these defense mechanisms create antibodies to fight off future exposure to the disease. These are the same antibodies the body would develop naturally if the child actually contracted the disease.

Vaccines are created from bacteria or viruses. They are either "live" or "killed." Live vaccines cause a very mild case of the disease they're meant to prevent; killed vaccines are inactivated by radiation, heat or chemical treatment, and do not cause infection.

Live vaccines are almost never given to children with weakened immune systems, for instance those who are HIV-positive or undergoing chemotherapy. Some vaccines are made from a part of the viral organism. The body builds up an immunity to this part, which in turn protects against the whole virus.

Reactions. Doctors observe few serious negative reactions to any immunization. For the most part, minor reactions are much less problematic than the disease itself. Local reactions, such as pain, swelling, and soreness, may occur around the injection site, but they usually disappear after a few days. Sometimes a hard nodule forms below the skin and may linger for several months. Systemic reactions affecting the entire body include vomiting, diarrhea, runny nose, ear infections, and coughing. Some of the most severe reactions are produced by the whooping cough vaccine, or DPT (diphtheria-pertussis-tetanus). DPT vaccine, which is said to be from 70 to 90 percent effective in preventing the spread of whooping cough, is given in three separate shots to infants between two and six months of age. Rarely, DPT vaccine produces seizures in infants.

A small, vocal minority in the United States claims that children do not need DPT or other vaccinations. They say that childhood diseases were already declining before the advent of immunizations, due primarily to improved living conditions and cleaner water supplies.

They also argue that at the very least it's sensible to wait until children are older before beginning vaccinations, based on the theory that as an infant grows, his natural immune system gets stronger. They suggest that vaccines might actually weaken the immune system and leave children more vulnerable to recurrent infections. This simply is not true. Delaying vaccinations until a child is older doesn't make sense, because most serious childhood diseases occur early in life. And there is no evidence that immunizations weaken the immune system.

Even when a disease is known to occur in a particular community, in this age of international travel diseases readily cross borders. By the time an outbreak is recognized it may be too late. In countries where DPT vaccination has been stopped for any length of time it has been followed by significant outbreaks of disease, and many deaths that could have been prevented.

The United States Health Department and the vast majority of American pediatricians agree that the benefits of vaccines, including DPT, far outweigh the rare instances of severe reaction. Immunizations are crucial for our communities. In 1989, a measles epidemic in Chicago struck over 2,300 people—71 percent were African Americans.

IMMUNIZATION SCHEDULE

Children can receive vaccinations from pediatricians, local clinics, or hospitals. Most kids (and adults, too) hate getting shots. You can make the experience less traumatic for your child if you hold him on your lap and don't fuss or cringe yourself. Be conversational and natural with the doctor, and act as if the shot is no big deal.

Vaccines are scheduled according to times children are most likely to catch specific diseases. For example, the chance of contracting hemophilus influenza B, which can cause spinal meningitis and other serious infections, peaks between six and twelve months of age. Vaccination is therefore recommended at two months, followed by two more injections given at two-month intervals.

Routine childhood illnesses, such as an ear infection or strep throat, are no longer considered reasons to put off vaccinations. The American Academy of Pediatrics says that only moderate to severe illness, or allergic sensitivity to a vaccine component, should delay a child's vaccination.

The following is the 1995 immunization schedule recommended by the Academy:

Key to Vaccines

DPT: diphtheria-pertussis-tetanus
Hib: hemophilus influenza B
HBV: hepatitis B
MMR: measles-mumps-rubella (German measles)
OPV: oral polio vaccine

Birth: HBV
Two months: DPT, Hib, HBV, OPV
Four months: DPT, Hib, OPV
Six months: DPT, Hib, HBV*, OPV*
Twelve–fifteen months: TB test, MMR, DPT, Hib*
Five years (or school entry): DPT, OPV
Twelve years: MMR**
Fifteen years: TD (adult tetanus-diphtheria); repeated every ten years throughout life
*Can be given anytime between six and eighteen months.
**In your area, this booster shot may be given at school entry, as recommended by the Centers for Disease Control and Prevention. If so, it's not necessary to repeat it at age twelve.

Which vaccines appear on the recommended schedule varies from time to time, based on the possible danger of a given disease versus the possible danger of reactions to the vaccine. The schedule also changes as new vaccines are developed. For example, a new version of the old injectable polio vaccine, based on killed virus, may soon be in use. The new injectable is expected to provide better protection and, at the same time, prevent the rare cases of paralytic polio that occur with use of the current live oral vaccine.

Another new vaccine that protects against chicken pox has recently been approved by the FDA. Chicken pox is a highly contagious disease that occurs in about 4 million people each year, mostly children younger than fifteen. While most cases of chicken pox are fairly mild, they are extremely disruptive because children must be kept out of school for two weeks or longer, and parents often have to miss work. The new vaccine is expected to appear on the next schedule.

New information also may result in a change in recommendations. For example, some physicans are just beginning to understand the importance of the timing of HBV, the vaccine that protects against the hepatitis B virus.

For a long time the hepatitis B virus, which can cause chronic liver disease and liver cancer, was thought to occur only in adults. But we now know that 90 percent of the cases occur in adolescents and young adults. (The virus may be acquired through sexual contact, sharing needles during intravenous drug use, or being born to a hepatitis B–infected mother—but 30 percent of adults and as many as 60 percent of adolescents have none of these identifiable "risk factors.") Three hundred thousand individuals become infected with the hepatitis B virus each year and 5,000 die. (This is more than five times the number of deaths that occurred from hemophilus influenza B infection before we started vaccinating infants with Hib.)

The American Academy of Pediatrics now recommends that all babies be immunized for hepatitis B, since it can easily be incorporated into the current infant schedule and it is a way of getting children immunized before they start engaging in high-risk activity. We know the vaccine lasts at least ten years, and probably a lot longer. This means that the vaccine will give at least some immunity through puberty, and will be easier to "boost" at a later age.

The American Academy of Pediatrics now recommends vaccinating eleven- and twelve-year-olds, as well as infants. The Advisory Committee on Immunization Practices of the CDC is also calling for routine adolescent immunizations against hepatitis B. This information is especially important for African Americans since we are at greater risk than other groups of this deadly infection. Dr. Karen Williams, a well-known pediatrician in Baton Rouge, and one of the medical reviewers of this book, recommends that all children receive HBV vaccination as early as possible. If your child, no matter what his or her age, has never received HBV, ask your doctor for the immunization now.

Be sure you maintain a detailed record (including dates) of immunizations. This is very useful if you move and/or change physicians or if you receive immunizations at a clinic.

If your child has any reaction from an inoculation, record it. If the reaction is so severe that your doctor says your child should not receive the full schedule of that particular vaccine, ask the physician to write out and *sign* a description of the vaccine and the reaction so your child can be admitted to school.

LEGAL LOOPHOLES

Personally, I support vaccinations because I believe the overall benefits outweigh the potential risks. However, if you have talked it over with your pediatrician and still do not want to immunize your child, the U.S. Public Health Service provides three possible exemptions: medical, religious, and philosophical.

Medical exemptions may be permanent or temporary and require the recommendation of your doctor, as well as approval by the health department. Temporary exemptions are reviewed each year. Medical exemptions may be granted for the following: a suppressed immune system either from disease or its treatment (tuberculosis, leukemia, lymphomas, or malignant tumors requiring chemotherapy); medication that lowers a child's resistance to infection (cortisone, prednisone, some cancer drugs); prior serious allergic reactions to vaccination or individual substances used in the vaccines. In addition, each vaccine has its own individual medical contraindications.

Religious exemptions are valid in every state except West Virginia and Mississippi, although the requirements vary. Check with local health authorities to find out your state's requirements.

You must write to the state health department or to your child's school principal to explain that immunization conflicts with your "sincere religious principles or beliefs." You need not itemize these principles, but be certain to include your child's name, the date, and a statement claiming you will assume full responsibility for his or her health. Take your letter to any notary and sign it in that person's presence. (Some states have a generalized religious-exemption form you can use.)

Philosophical exemptions cover the gray area between religion and issues of conscience. Philosophical exemptions are currently offered by twenty states, and the process is identical to filing for religious exemption.

Most requests for exemptions are upheld. If yours is rejected, get the reason in writing. Talk with the school principal, superintendent, or state health officials—sometimes you just have to reword the request to have it accepted. If you are hassled by officials, remember your right to an exemption is legally guaranteed. Present your case to the local school board for a vote. If it is still denied, and you feel strongly about not immunizing your child, consider hiring an attorney.

State and federal laws have been designed to protect the health and well-being of all children. However, your personal feelings about your child's medical care are also important. If you disagree with the treatment your child receives, it's always a good idea to share your concerns and objectives with your child's doctor. It's also crucial to listen to the doctor's explanation about the treatment or care he or she recommends. Together, you should be able to reach a choice that is in the best interest of your child. If you cannot, or if you simply do not like the way the doctor treats you and your child, make a change. You can easily change private physicians, and in some circumstances you can also change hospital clinics, depending on the choices available in your community. Your goal, and the goal of the pediatrician you choose, should be to make your child's well-baby visits a positive experience that will yield many years of good health in the future.

7

VISITING THE DENTIST

Tooth buds began to form while your baby was still in the womb. When he is about eight months old, some teeth begin to emerge from the gums. Molars appear between eighteen and twenty-four months, and canine teeth are usually in place by age two. When the set is complete, your baby will have twenty teeth.

Teething can be uncomfortable, and babies often show symptoms even before teeth break through. Gnawing on almost any hard *rubber* object can soothe pain. (Don't use plastic—it can shatter.) Never give your child a full bottle of milk or juice to teethe on—tooth decay and even gum infections can result. For the same reason, never put a baby to sleep with a bottle in his mouth.

When nothing else spells relief, baby doses of acetaminophen should do the trick. Avoid giving any other medication by mouth or rubbing anything on the baby's gums, unless recommended by your baby's doctor.

Teething itself doesn't make babies sick. Therefore, if your teething baby develops a fever, seems fretful, has diarrhea, or tugs at his ear (a sign of possible infection), call the doctor. Something more is going on.

As soon as little teeth emerge, it's time to take care of them. You can clean a baby's gums and teeth with a piece of wet gauze or a small soft toothbrush. Skip the toothpaste—babies just swallow it. Water will do the job. Even toddlers don't need more than a pea-sized dab of unfluoridated toothpaste until they are old enough to spit it out.

(Fluoride toothpaste plus fluoridated drinking water can add up to an overdose in very young children.)

Toothbrushes should be replaced frequently. Even a toothbrush that still looks new should be changed after six weeks or even less, because bacteria from the mouth accumulate on the bristles.

Baby teeth start falling out between ages five and six, and permanent teeth begin arriving, following roughly the same progression as baby teeth did. They keep coming until your child is grown up and has thirty-two adult teeth, usually sometime in his or her late teens or early twenties.

DENTAL CHECKUPS

It's important to take good care of baby teeth; baby teeth that become decayed may fall out early, and with nothing to push against, permanent teeth may subsequently come in crooked. But when does your child need to see a dentist?

Our medical reviewers, Dr. M. Mokiso Murrill and Dr. Karen Williams, both African-American pediatricians practicing in Baton Rouge, Louisiana, point out that many families simply are unable to afford frequent dental visits. They place more emphasis on preventive care, starting early in childhood. If your child has any noticeable dental problem before age four, take him to the dentist. Otherwise, concentrate on good dental hygiene.

After age four, most children should see a dentist annually for an examination and professional cleaning.

The concept behind regular dental visits is to treat small problems before they become large problems. Large problems in dentistry mean premature loss of teeth, enormous expense, and lifelong aggravation. It's a lot cheaper to prevent dental problems than it is to fix them after they have reached a crisis point.

Despite the pain-saving, money-saving benefits of visiting the dentist, about one in seven poor children *never* see a dentist. African-American children in all income groups are less likely to see a dentist regularly.

When I was a child, my mother, like most African-American parents at that time, knew very little about dental care or prevention. She always tried over-the-counter toothache medication first. If the pain persisted, she would take me to the dentist. This was also the way my friends dealt with tooth problems. All of us associated dental visits with pain, and a trip to the dentist was never welcomed by anyone. Besides, all dentists we visited were white and wearing white.

A recent revolution has been going on among dentists. Some specialize in treating children, and their offices are painted in bright colors and littered with toys and games. And guess what children's dentists are wearing these days? Cute, colorful "kid" T-shirts, sneakers, and jeans. No kidding.

If you're lucky enough to have a dental college in your area, you can get considerable financial benefit. Dental schools, such as the New York University Dentistry College, usually have clinics that offer services at reduced rates. Dentists in training are closely supervised by experienced dentists and professors. Patients can expect excellent care because one or more top professionals are consulting with the student dentist doing the work. Dental-school clinics also have the latest equipment and are up on all the newest techniques and technologies.

Going to the dentist is only one part of dental care. The larger, most important part is done at home. Parents can go a long way toward protecting their children's teeth and teaching their children how to do the job for themselves. The sooner you start, the better.

PREVENTING DENTAL PROBLEMS

The two best ways to maintain dental health are:

- Avoiding sticky, sugary foods
- Brushing and flossing after every meal

It's true that some lucky kids have fewer dental problems than others. But most cavities are caused by exposure to sugars and starches in food; these turn into enamel-eating acids. Bacteria can then multiply in the soft portion of the teeth and cause decay.

Solid sugar is worse for teeth than liquid sugars because it adheres to the tooth surface longer. This means that clingy, sugary foods, such as raisins or caramel-marshmallow-chocolate bars, do more damage than those that slip past teeth quickly, such as ice cream and soda pop.

Encourage your kids to follow these guidelines (especially when they're not able to brush right after they eat):

- Avoid sticky, sugary foods.
- If you do eat sweets, eat them with meals, rather than as snacks alone. Dried fruits, for example, cause fewer problems when they're combined with cereal, baked goods, or salads.
- Eat protein foods such as hard cheeses, nuts, eggs, and meat after eating starches or sweets; this also helps protect against cavities.
- At the end of meals, munch vegetables like celery, carrots, and lettuce; these serve as natural toothbrushes, clearing away sugars.
- Try chewing sugarless gum after eating starchy or sweet foods; this may help clean teeth and control acidity.

Remember, there's no substitute for brushing. Brushing after meals is one of the single-most-important lifetime habits you can teach your child. Little kids naturally love to watch everything you do and try to do it themselves. Encourage your child to imitate you brushing your own teeth. Give him a soft toothbrush with nylon bristles and show him how to scrub teeth *and* gums after meals.

Flossing can start after your child's second teeth come in. The purpose of flossing is to prevent gum disease. Left untreated, gum disease, which is caused by bacterial infections, can cause teeth to fall out and can even destroy the jawbone. Regular flossing removes food particles lodged between teeth, as well as the plaque along the sides of teeth. Again, the best way to encourage flossing is to *set a good example.*

FLUORIDE PRODUCTS

Adding fluoride to the water supply has vastly reduced the number of cavities children develop. Kids should still use a fluoride toothpaste approved by the American Dental Association. Beyond that, your child probably doesn't need any additional fluoride. If your community doesn't fluoridate the water supply, or if you use bottled water that does not contain fluoride, your dentist may recommend a fluoride supplement for your child. Supplements should begin as soon as possible after birth and be continued on a daily basis thereafter until about sixteen years of age. Some dentists paint on a protective sealant that protects teeth from cavities for five to seven years.

Some soft drinks and other foods also contain fluoride. Check with your dentist before routinely using these products. Too much fluoride for children leads to mottling of the tooth surface in developing teeth, a condition called fluorosis.

Remember, fluoride by itself cannot eliminate tooth decay and gum disease. A healthy diet, plus good home oral hygiene, will help keep kids smiling.

8

GETTING THE MOST FROM HEALTH CARE

In May of 1990, the Council on Ethical and Judicial Affairs of the American Medical Association acknowledged that even when African Americans can afford medical care, we are less likely than whites to receive the best treatment. When it comes to treating blacks and other minorities, many doctors still tend to settle for Band-Aid, or temporary, treatment that relieves immediate symptoms but does not address underlying health problems.

This adds up to a picture of a health-care system that does not begin to meet the needs of black children.

Even middle-income and upper-income blacks are wary of doctors, and with good reason.

Racism is still part of most medical care. Dr. Mitchell Rice and Dr. Mylon Winn, writing in *The Journal of the National Medical Association,* the publication of the premier medical society for black physicians, identified the following barriers between us and the medical system.

African Americans are reluctant to seek early help because care is usually provided by nonblacks who are often insensitive to our concerns. Only about 3 percent of physicians are African American. By contrast, 17.7 percent of nurses and 27.3 percent of nursing aides, orderlies, and attendants are black. As the pay scale and training requirements go up, the number of blacks in each profession goes down.

Even when we can afford to go to private doctors, we don't *feel* cared for. We are kept waiting longer for appointments than whites, especially if we are on Medicaid or Medicare. We sit waiting with our children, often treated as if we weren't really there. This sends a message, and it is not a message of quality health care. When we do get in to see someone, our concerns are often ignored or not taken seriously.

Finally, many private doctors simply refuse to provide services in poor communities or to Medicaid patients, leaving many of us with *no* practical access to health care at all.

Our problems with the medical profession didn't begin yesterday. Since the earliest years of enslavement, African Americans have been shut out of mainstream health care. Some developed their own healing arts, based on memories of Africa. The most gifted healers were usually women who had been given permission by the planters to learn "white medicine" and minister to ailing slaves. These black nurses secretly experimented with their own home remedies, and their recipes for cures were whispered from ear to ear and passed down from parent to child.

The hallmarks of health care in Africa—nutritional and herbal remedies, mental and spiritual healing, and family bonding and sharing—helped blacks survive in the New World. This separate system of health care continued to operate within the shadow of white medicine long after emancipation.

As late as 1930, only one hospital bed was available for every 1,941 black Americans (as opposed to one for every 139 white Americans). By now, everyone has heard about the infamous 1932 Tuskegee study, in which four hundred black men with syphilis were deliberately left untreated for *forty years* so researchers could observe the natural course of the disease. The deception was not uncovered until 1972, when a reporter for the *Washington Star* made it news.

The Tuskegee study was so unethical that some people believe it was an aberration perpetrated by singularly evil-minded individuals. In fact, it was probably not that unusual. In April of 1994, it was discovered that back in the 1960s and 1970s, researchers had forged signatures of eighty-eight patients on consent forms and then exposed them to intense doses of whole-body radiation. Many of the patients were poor and black. They were being treated for inoperable malignant tumors at Cincinnati General, a public hospital. Patients received whole-body radiation up to the equivalent of twenty thousand chest X rays; most became violently ill and died within a few months of treatment. Their surviving relatives said that the patients never knew they were part of an experiment, which had been financed in part by the Pentagon.

One hopes that public exposure of these unethical studies will put an end to medical experimentation at the expense of minorities. Even if it does, unequal treatment continues in the realm of research, prevention, early diagnosis, and treatment. It should surprise no one that many African Americans have an abiding distrust for the medical establishment and hesitate to seek medical attention until we absolutely have to.

Consequently, when an illness is finally diagnosed, it is harder to treat and may already be life-threatening. Medical anthropologist Eric J. Bailey, who investigated the way African Americans living in Detroit seek health care, found that even after illness appeared, they often delayed days or weeks before seeking medical help. Instead, they turned to relatives, friends, or ministers. They tried home remedies and hoped that the body would heal itself naturally or through prayer. Only when all else failed did they visit a clinic or see a doctor.

I think it's possible to draw on our powerful spirit of community and kinship to help our children today, and even use it to make the medical system work to our advantage. I believe that modern medicine can have a place side by side with our history and traditions of self-help.

A FAMILY-CENTERED APPROACH

Children are the prime beneficiaries of family-centered medical care. This approach can include your child's father, your mother, sister, or any of those who help you care for your child. Caring support from people who love them encourages children to follow medical regimens, improve their nutrition, and join in exercise activities.

Many health-care professionals are becoming more aware of cultural variations among Americans and will readily agree to let another family member or friend participate in a child's visit. If your doctor does not agree, let him know that is the way you and your child would be most comfortable. When you find a doctor or nurse who *listens* carefully to your child's complaint and circumstances—either directly from your child or from any of his kin—you know he's going to get good treatment. You can help this process along by being forthright and letting the health-care folks have a glimpse into your family's circumstances.

On the other hand, if a doctor or nurse practitioner seems insensitive to your child's needs, voice your concerns, or seek another doctor. If you feel it's important for your child to have an African-American doctor, call your local chapter of the National Medical Association and ask for a list of pediatricians and family doctors in your area.

WHAT YOU CAN DO: TAKING AN ACTIVE ROLE

The more involved you are with the medical team you choose to care for your child, the better your child's pediatric care will be.

Parents who speak up and ask questions get more attention for their children; they also remember more and follow recommended treatment better. This is important because it teaches your children—by your own example—how to speak up for themselves. By taking an active role, you and your child can improve communication with the physician.

A positive and honest relationship between you and your child's doctor is your child's passport to good health. *Every doctor-patient relationship benefits from a complete picture of what's going on with the whole family.*

Some parents worry that they will sound ignorant if they ask questions. They may not want to talk about sensitive issues like sex and drugs. Or they may be embarrassed to admit they were unable to follow the doctor's recommendations. Don't fall into this trap. The only way a doctor can help is to offer treatment based on your child's individual needs—not someone else's.

Fear can also stand in the way of open patient-doctor communication—fear of disease, treatment, costs, or side effects. And normal anxiety is heightened by crowded waiting rooms and hurried physicians.

Here are some important guidelines all parents can use to help children get the most out of their visits to the doctor:

- Write down your questions and concerns in a notebook ahead of time.
- Bring your notebook and take notes on what the doctor says so you'll remember. (Your note taking may make the doctor pay more attention, too.)
- Even when things seem rushed, try to remain calm.
- Make sure the doctor answers your questions and concerns.

Asking questions should never be a hostile exchange. If the idea of talking to a doctor makes you feel nervous or angry, bringing along a friend or relative can be reassuring and also gives you another pair of ears to listen to the doctor's information.

One more bit of advice: When you ask questions, listen to what the doctor or nurse says and then write it down in your notebook before going on to the next question.

You're the top expert on your child and your family situation. Be open and honest with the doctor. For example, if your work schedule makes it almost impossible to give your child medication several times a day, say so. Your doctor or nurse may have some creative solutions if you make this known. If you're concerned about the cost of tests and medications, say so. Your concerns are legitimate. Don't agree to something you know will be difficult or impractical for you just because you don't want to make waves.

If a doctor lays a lot of medical language on you, go ahead—interrupt him. Many doctors who should know better do this without thinking. Be nice. Just ask, "What does that mean?"

If your child has a chronic disease, ask the doctor to recommend a support group that deals with his illness, and *join it* (you *and* your child). Support groups help in many ways—they even help you deal better with doctors.

GETTING YOUR CHILD INVOLVED IN HER OWN HEALTH CARE

Children learn by example. Your child can either absorb your worries and anxieties about seeing the doctor or she can learn from you how to get the information she needs when she needs it. As your child begins talking clearly, encourage her to talk to the doctor and answer the doctor's questions herself. Encourage her to think of her doctor as a friend. Your child can:

- Prepare questions ahead of time
- Ask what she wants to know
- Get a notebook of her own (older kids)
- Tell the doctor about how she feels, and about any problems or reactions she has taking medicines
- Telephone the receptionist or nurse between visits to report how she is doing or to follow up with any new questions she may have (older kids, with your permission)
- Tell the doctor if she is unable to follow the instructions given
- Get acquainted with other members of the health team, such as the nurse or dietitian
- Learn to make appointments for her next visit before leaving the doctor's office

As your child grows older, encourage her to talk privately with the doctor and have her checkups without you in the room. This habit will be invaluable when she reaches puberty and has a ton of questions she is embarrassed to ask in front of you.

PAYING THE BILLS

Loss of health insurance—and the escalating costs of health care—is a major reason that levels of health care have fallen for all American children. Low-income minority children have suffered most. In 1991, more than 8 million children were uninsured (12.6 percent). Among black children, 15.1 percent had no coverage. The stats were even worse among Latino children—26.7 percent had no health insurance coverage. Millions of others went without health insurance for part of the year, and millions more had inadequate insurance that failed to cover important preventive care or preexisting conditions.

WHAT KIND OF INSURANCE

We used to take it for granted that the "full coverage" offered by carriers such as Metropolitan, Aetna, or Blue Cross/Blue Shield was the best and only acceptable way to go. This kind of blue-chip coverage lets you select your own physician, who can then order any diagnostic test or recommend any treatment or hospitalization at his or her discretion.

Today, it has become almost impossible for individuals to pay for this kind of insurance. Even many companies have dropped it from their benefits programs and are looking for more affordable options.

People who are self-employed or working at jobs where they must pay for insurance out of their own pockets are finding that they do much better choosing a managed-care program. These programs are easier on the pocketbook and still provide quality health care. Several states are now enrolling Medicaid patients in managed-care programs such as health-maintenance organizations (HMOs).

Some managed-care programs, such as HIP and Kaiser Permanente, have been around a long time. They often have their own facilities, with various departments and attending physicians on the premises. Other managed-care programs are composed of doctors in private practice who join the program and adhere to its rules and requirements.

Here's how most managed-care programs work: You select a primary-care physician from a group of participating doctors. The physician you choose is then in charge of all your health-care needs. If you need a specialist, the primary-care physician usually refers you to another member in the group.

Managed care emphasizes prevention. All family members are encouraged to see their primary-care physician regularly for screening tests and checkups to detect early signs of disease. The goal is to keep the whole family healthy, which reduces the need for more extreme and more expensive treatment later on, particularly from specialists or hospitals. If anyone in the family requires hospitalization, the managed-care provider must first approve both the procedure and the hospital.

Doctors and patients like the program because of its simplicity. However, because participating physicians receive set fees, they may limit the time they spend with each patient. They also tend to prescribe older, less expensive drugs, if drugs are included in the coverage. Otherwise, the quality of service is considered good.

If your child has no insurance coverage, you may be reluctant to take him to a doctor until he becomes very sick. Many families have too much income to qualify for Medicaid but not enough to pay for medical care. Eligibility requirements for Medicaid vary widely from state to state.

In most states, Medicaid recipients can go to any doctor or hospital that will accept them. But because of Medicaid's low reimbursement rates, many doctors and private hospitals accept only limited numbers of Medicaid patients, and some refuse to take any. As a result, Medicaid patients are often forced to seek treatment at overcrowded clinics where treatment is on a first-come, first-served basis. If this is the kind of service you and your family have to accept, it's important to use it to your advantage.

Don't wait until the symptoms of an illness become severe and debilitating.

If you must wait in the waiting room for hours, find a way to be productive while you wait. Use this time to catch up on reading, studying, or office work. Make sure you bring something to keep your child fully occupied, also.

Always take plenty of notes during the visit. Make sure you jot down the doctor's name. On the next visit, your child may be assigned a different physician, and it may be up to you to keep track of who's taking care of your child. Also write down the name of the nurse, in case you have questions after the visit.

FINDING PEDIATRIC HEALTH CARE

Whom you choose to care for your child is determined to a great extent by what you can afford or which insurance plan you belong to. Here are some of the services available to children.

PRIMARY PHYSICIANS FOR CHILDREN

A child's primary-care physician may be a pediatrician or a family doctor who cares for the entire family. Both doctors are trained to care for children, but pediatricians are specialists who treat only children and adolescents until the age of twenty-one. Your child may see a pediatrician or family doctor (general practitioner) in private practice or in a clinic setting.

Some pediatricians have a particular interest in adolescent health, and they may even have separate examining and treatment areas for teenagers. Even so, your adolescent may not want to see a "baby doctor," or he may think when he enters his teens it's time for him to choose a new doctor himself, "just because." This is your grown-up child speaking.

PEDIATRIC NURSES

These are usually registered nurses who have had additional training in caring for children. Pediatricians employ pediatric nurses to take complaints, call for prescription refills, draw blood for lab tests, perform EKGs, and carry out other procedures used to make office diagnoses.

The National Association of Pediatric Nurse Associates and Practitioners has many programs to reach minority children. You will find these professionals working in many public health clinics and schools.

SCHOOL HEALTH PROGRAMS

In many communities, nurses and other health-care professionals are assigned to schools. Their services may include taking temperatures, giving first aid, and referring children to doctors, all the way to large-scale immunization programs and screening for dental, hearing, and vision problems. School programs also provide health instruction and nutrition education to children, as well as to school administrators, teachers, and parents. These valuable programs promote preventive services for all children.

SCREENING PROGRAMS

Programs for early screening and diagnosis of many childhood diseases are often sponsored by city health departments and given free or at minimum cost. Screening programs help fill the gap for those who cannot manage regular doctor visits. Your local health department can usually provide information on screening programs available in your area.

FEDERALLY FUNDED NEIGHBORHOOD HEALTH-CARE CENTERS AND PROGRAMS

Community health centers are major sources of prenatal care and childbirth facilities. These clinics were first developed in the late 1960s—with federal and some private funding—to relieve overburdened hospitals. They play an especially important role in underserved areas, where there are high rates of infant mortality and not enough physicians to go around. Enlarging and upgrading this system with quality staff and equipment could go a long way toward creating equal access to health care for everyone.

Maternal- and child-care programs are also available in many neighborhoods and communities, although, like other federal programs, they tend to be badly underfunded. The aim of these programs is to provide quality nutrition for pregnant women, new mothers, infants, and children up to the age of five whose weight is low for their age or who are anemic or near anemic. They also offer instruction and counseling in prenatal care, infant care, nutrition, and family planning. To qualify, mothers and children have to be below a certain income level. But even when qualified, they may not receive the service because of cutbacks at the federal level.

We can all do our share to make access to health care for all a reality. Hopefully, the government will help by working to reduce costs and placing more emphasis on prevention. Health-care professionals can help by educating themselves about the cultural background of patients, as well as being sensitive to their personal needs. Everyone can be involved in creating a more equitable system.

COMMUNITY EMPOWERMENT

Community-empowerment programs of every size are trying to replace the old Band-Aid approach to medical care with one that emphasizes wellness and prevention. Local programs staffed by local people help African Americans renew their traditional holistic approach to health care. They also work to develop health-care facilities within the community. Dr. Marc Rivo of the Commission of Public Health in Washington, D.C., believes that government should spend more of its health-care money at this grassroots level. It's where the kids are.

There are dozens of community programs around the country struggling to provide services for African-American infants, children, and teenagers. They've got the right idea, and all can use an influx of federal and state cash. If you are interested in getting involved in a community program, you can receive help from a range of professional associations and government agencies (see pages 405–416).

Part Two

———

FEEDING KIDS

9

OFF TO A GOOD START

For generations, it was assumed that when we became new parents we would automatically know what and how to feed our children. In the past, African-American women learned about child rearing, feeding, health, and nutrition from their mothers, grandmothers, and aunts—all of whom never seemed to tire of saying, "What was good enough for you is good enough for your child."

Today we know a lot more about nutrition for infants and children. Even so, there are many ways to provide children from every cultural and economic background with good, nutritious food.

LOOKING BACK

Our African heritage is visible in our contemporary food choices. We know that Africans introduced black-eyed peas, okra, peanuts, and sesame to the colonies.

They invented one-dish vegetable stews that could be made to last an entire week. Some of these combined rice and vegetables with fatback, and occasionally fish or small game. Many other traditional African-American dishes can be traced back to the period of enslavement, where necessity was definitely the mother of great cooking invention.

No matter how meager their supplies, enslaved Africans used West African cooking methods. They dried corn kernels and boiled them whole (hominy) or coarsely ground them and then boiled them as grits. In Africa, they had used palm oil to fry or flavor food. Cooks working in the plantation owners' houses now used lard to fry chicken and fish. They roasted sweet potatoes, boiled green leafy vegetables with pork fat, and thickened stews with okra or filé powder ground from sassafras. In the process, they invented a new, vibrant kind of American food culture that continues to be popular throughout the South and many other regions of the country.

In the South today, the original style of black cooking reigns supreme among blacks *and* whites. Sharing these dishes continues to bind African-American families and friends in the many other regions of the country where they have settled. However, old traditions are often mixed with modern trends that don't always produce a positive result. A diet containing too much salt, too many fried foods, not enough fresh fruits and vegetables, and not enough cereals and grains has diminished our vitamin and mineral content intake.

In urban areas, many African Americans depend on quick-service restaurants and convenience stores for meals. In the home, many people seem unaware of valuable new nutrition information. Grocery shopping in poor neighborhoods is a nutritionist's nightmare. Fresh produce is scarce, and what is available is not only poor in quality but priced sky-high. It's rare to find low-cholesterol mayonnaise, whole-wheat bread, and skim milk in stores, and exceptionally rare to find low-salt or no-salt products. When more healthful alternatives are available, such as low-salt soups, they cost more than the regular brands.

Generally speaking, inner-city store owners say they don't carry healthier choices because these products "don't sell." They say that in order to change customers' eating habits, they need help from major food manufacturers, nutritionists, and advertisers. They have a point. But store owners could make more of an effort by ordering healthier products, creating appealing store displays, and asking for advice and help from suppliers and sales reps to stimulate sales. Their efforts would encourage manufacturers to start promoting healthier foods in their marketing and advertising campaigns.

Positive promotion is important. Most inner-city kids don't believe that nutrition information is for them. They seldom see themselves portrayed on television and billboards advertising healthful products. On the other hand, white bread; high-fat; high-calorie products; liquor; and cigarettes are aggressively marketed to adults and children.

HEALTH PROBLEMS RELATED TO NUTRITION

Important nutrition factors that affect African Americans are:

- Low levels of calcium, vitamin D, and iron in the diet
- High salt intake
- Lactose intolerance
- Excessive consumption of fatty and fried foods

Some studies show that blacks living near the poverty level receive less than half the calcium and iron whites do; their diets are also often low in vitamins A and C, magnesium, vitamin B complex, and protein. Even when income increases, we tend to choose meat and other protein foods over fresh fruits, vegetables, and grains.

Certain vitamin deficiencies affect us at every income level. Because of the melanin pigment in our skin, we absorb one-third less of the ultraviolet light that triggers the body's production of vitamin D. Vitamin D helps the body use calcium and magnesium, minerals that are already at low levels in our diet. Other Americans get extra vitamin D from milk, but many blacks are lactose-intolerant and tend to avoid fresh milk and milk products, leaving them at risk for vitamin D and calcium deficiency.

Another nutritional problem that affects us at every income level and every age is salt sensitivity. Most people release excess sodium through sweat and urine. But many African Americans do the reverse: Our kidneys retain salt. Salt retention may have begun to develop in Africa thousands of years ago; the torrid climate put extra demands on body fluids and retaining salt helped humans conserve fluids. During the slave trade, those Africans best able to conserve fluids were the ones who survived the arduous journey to America. Modern African Americans are descended from this survivor population.

When people with high salt sensitivity begin to eat more salt, as surely we do in the United States today, the helpful mechanism becomes a disadvantage. One form of hypertension (called low-renin hypertension) is aggravated by salt intake. This salt-sensitive hypertension is the kind most blacks, and some nonblacks, have. (High-renin hypertension, which is not affected by salt intake to the same degree, is much less common among blacks and more common among nonblacks.)

HOW FOOD PREFERENCES DEVELOP

Taste preferences, like choices in clothes and music, are heavily influenced by family and friends. Choices made repeatedly in childhood become habitual *brain signals*. We know that young children don't necessarily like the same foods as their parents, but their food preferences become strikingly similar as they grow up. Brothers and sisters also have similar food preferences.

Television advertising also influences food tastes. In a recent survey, 71 percent of TV commercials were for food products and 80 percent of those were for low-nutrient foods containing large amounts of fat, calories, and sodium. Not only are kids bombarded with nonstop images of candy bars, cookies, and highly sugared cereals but advertisements also carry messages that certain products are "cooler" than others.

Like adults, kids often become passionate about foods they like, particularly foods presented as treats. Some parents offer a sweet food or sugary snack when kids eat their vegetables, and they treat themselves to a similar reward at the end of meals. This is a real trap. Candy, desserts, and sugary stuff are foods just like any others. Parents should avoid loading them with special significance.

GUIDING KIDS TOWARD GOOD NUTRITION

Forget rewards, punishments, bribes, and other negotiations. Instead, serve up healthy food, in adequate portions, and trust your children to eat enough.

If you assume all the responsibility for what your children eat, they lose their inborn ability to control their own appetites. Mealtimes often become focused on *everything else*—mood, rebellion, anger, teasing, revenge—and cease to be simply about satisfying hunger and enjoying camaraderie.

Building good nutrition and positive eating habits means allowing kids to stay in touch with their own internal cues about food. When children are very young, the less said about their food choices and eating habits, the better.

The best way to build good nutritional habits in children is for parents to practice them, too. The most common mistake I see parents make is to advocate one diet for their kids and eat another themselves. I can remember my own mom and dad insisting that my sister and I eat plenty of vegetables, even as they kept them off their own plates. Children resent being the only ones who have to practice what you preach. So serve a variety of attractive, healthy foods, and eat well yourself. Set a good example by keeping foods high in fat, cholesterol, and sodium (and low in nutritional value) out of the house. Make sure you have plenty of alternative choices available.

If your family enjoys snack foods like potato chips, tortilla chips, cookies, and popcorn, substitute low-salt pretzels, fat-free (baked) tortilla chips, and air-popped popcorn. Add fresh fruit and raw vegetables to your snack list. Remember, if your kids see you eating a variety of nutritious foods, the good influence will rub off.

Don't worry if your eating habits or food choices are not always perfect for yourself or your children. After a hard day's work, it's tough to resist our kids' pleadings for quick hamburgers and soft drinks, candy bars, and cookies. Having two teenage boys around my own house makes me appreciate the pressure parents are under. In fact, I may be under even more pressure than you are to offer healthy foods that taste good: People expect a nutritionist and her family to eat healthy *all* of the time. Believe me, it's impossible to cover all the bases every minute of every day.

The best approach is to become more aware and better armed with information about diet and nutrition and pass it along to your kids as consistently as possible.

No matter what your circumstances, finances, work schedule, or environment, there are certain things everyone can do to make mealtime a more positive experience for everyone—yourself included.

- Have the meal ready when you call your kids to sit down at the table. Having to wait in their seats for food makes kids bored and anxious. Mealtime will be off to a rocky start.
- Don't nag kids about what or how much they eat.
- Avoid referring to individual foods as "good" or "bad." Every food has some useful nutritional quality. Words like *good* and *bad* only describe overall diets.

- Never use food as reward or punishment. Bite your tongue when you're ready to say, "No dessert until you eat your vegetables."

- Don't serve dessert with every meal. It's just another food—sometimes you have it; sometimes you don't.

- Don't overdo your efforts to improve behavior and nutrition. Family mealtime is sometimes an emotional situation that can influence which foods children will eat and enjoy. Take it easy. One or two meals deviating from a healthy diet will not make your child unhealthy. It's what a child eats over the course of several days and weeks that counts.

- Think about improving table manners. Kids learn most of their manners naturally through observation. So wash your hands before sitting down at the table, chew with your mouth closed, handle your knife and fork properly, try all the foods on your plate, pace yourself, and approach cleanup time cheerfully. Require your children to do the same, gently reinforcing the good and ignoring the bad. Be patient and consistent. At the end of the meal, let children help clean up, and praise them for it.

Make sure your kids understand that good table manners are not just for show. Explain how good manners make life easier and more pleasant for everyone, including themselves. Knowing how to handle themselves at the dinner table makes children feel comfortable when they go to someone else's home for dinner. Showing courtesy to other people sends the message, I respect you. I enjoy being with you. I sit up alertly, and I won't toss my salad in your lap. So you will enjoy eating with me and ask me back again.

- Make sure that mealtime is relaxed and stress-free. Try to set aside regular, unhurried time for family meals. Turn off the television or radio. Involve your kids in the conversation.

- Mealtimes should be neither too short nor too long. Allow slower children time to finish their meals. And slow down children who eat fast.

- Plan menus with balance, variety, and moderation. Moderation means letting kids occasionally choose foods they especially enjoy, even if they aren't always the lowest in fat, sodium, and sugar.

ARE WE HAVING FUN YET?

Should mealtimes be fun? Absolutely. Here's why.

We all learned to love fried chicken, potato salad, barbecued ribs, chocolate layer cake, and ice cream because we associated them with Sunday picnics, outdoor fun, goofing off, playing games, and having good times with family. Food is one of the most powerful memory associations we have.

If the healthy food you serve kids is associated with happy meal-times—at the table or in the backyard, with a prayer and a song in a relaxed atmosphere—that association is embedded forever.

The best way to get your child on a permanent track to good nutrition is to associate eating healthful foods with pleasure, family unity, and parental love. (By the way, most traditional "comfort" foods we learned to love as children can fit into a healthful eating plan just by altering the quantities you serve and the method of preparation.)

Does this mean sitting down to dinner every night at the same time with the whole family? It's a nice idea, but it doesn't always work out. I've known families who never sit down at all—everything is a snack. Some kids never have a regular meal at the table. Family members eat standing up or even sitting in different rooms, ignoring one another completely. But even families with the most hectic schedules can usually find two nights a week for everyone to sit down together. On other evenings, you can create some other special family moments: Perhaps there can be an evening when Mom and kids, or Dad and kids, eat together. There can even be a regular meal kids make by themselves.

LET'S EAT OUT

Quick-service restaurants and family full-service restaurants are extremely popular, particularly when parents work outside the home. Many quick-service and family restaurants offer a wide variety of choices and also provide nutrition information. Although some are chaotic at certain times of the day or evening, they usually have a pleasant atmosphere that lets you enjoy time with your children.

Let your child make his own food choices, just as he does at home. But gently guide him toward nutritious foods. This doesn't mean kids can't ever have french fries or a milk shake. It just means that the whole meal doesn't need to be fatty, salty, and sweet. If your child has a hamburger, suggest she balance it with a green salad (with low-fat dressing). If she chooses a milk shake or french fries, then suggest broiled fish or broiled chicken as the main dish.

PICKY, PICKY, PICKY: GETTING KIDS TO TRY NEW FOODS

It's normal for children to get into occasional ruts over their food choices. Giving children *too much* say in food selection promotes food jags. So, allow your child to make his own food choices, but *within groups that you suggest*.

One way to broaden a child's food choices is to prepare new foods in an attractive, colorful manner. Mix and blend textures and teach your child the nutritional value of each new food as she accepts (or rejects) it.

Allow children to taste new foods in small portions. If you insist that your child finishes a new food completely, she won't like it. Praise her for trying even a little bit of something new.

EAT YOUR VEGETABLES, OR ELSE!

If your child's not hungry for vegetables, how can he possibly be hungry for tortilla chips and chocolate cake? Don't hassle it—that's just the way most kids are.

Some children eat fruit (because it has a sweet taste), but getting them to eat vegetables can be like pulling teeth. Don't give up. There are lots of ways to help kids enjoy eating vegetables.

Try combining vegetables with fruit. For example, diced carrots with raisins, or baked, mashed sweet potatoes with a spoonful of pureed mango "sauce" might be all your child needs to tempt his palate. Place a smorgasbord of vegetables and fruits in the middle of the table. Eat them yourself. And before you know it, your child will try them, too.

Another way to get children to eat more vegetables is to change the method of preparation. For example, cooked and raw vegetables have completely different flavors. A child who hates cooked carrots may love raw carrots. Similarly, pureed cooked carrots taste different from sliced cooked carrots. Mashing or pureeing releases the sugars in vegetables. Pureed carrots taste like sweet potatoes. Pureed cauliflower tastes like mashed potatoes. Pureed broccoli, peas, or asparagus have light, fresh tastes that defy comparisons with their whole or sliced cooked counterparts. (When you puree vegetables, there's no need to add butter, margarine, or cream to the blender. If the mix seems a little dry, just add a tablespoonful or so of the cooking water to bring it to a creamy, smooth consistency.)

SPECIAL MEALS

Another good way to introduce new foods is to plan theme nights at mealtime. Mexican Hat-Dance Night obviously features Mexican food and Orient Express Night introduces foods eaten in the Far East and Asia. Homeland Night features foods commonly eaten in Africa. The celebration of Kwanzaa is a great time to go all out in setting the table and selecting foods that have special meaning for each day of the celebration. Birthdays and special achievements, backpacking trips, and holiday picnics also provide a chance to create a mealtime theme.

EATING BREAKFAST

There's no doubt about it: Breakfast really is our most important meal. For children, eating breakfast means the difference between mental sluggishness and mental alertness. Schoolchildren who eat breakfast learn and participate more in class. Children who eat breakfast also consistently showed a greater intake of *all* nutrients when compared to breakfast noneaters. According to the U.S. Department of Agriculture (Continuing Survey of Food Intakes by Individuals, 1989–1992), children who skip breakfast do not make up for the loss of nutrients later in the day. On the other hand, African-American children who eat breakfast tend to consume more calories from fat than those who do not eat breakfast—unless they choose ready-to-eat cereals. Cereal-eaters consume less fat and receive more nutrients.

Unfortunately, many American children go off to school without any kind of breakfast. Lack of time, nothing in the cupboard or fridge, or too few choices are the usual reasons. Some kids say they don't like breakfast or that they're not hungry in the morning. Skipping breakfast is often a habit that develops when parents don't eat breakfast themselves.

You can remedy this situation with a few important changes:

- Encourage your child to get school clothes ready the night before and to get up a half hour earlier in the morning.

- Routinely set the table at night with cups, bowls, and plates.

- Plan ahead. Make sure breakfast foods are in the house. Keep a shopping list and stock up on breakfast items each time you go to the grocery store.

- Choose simple, easy-to-prepare foods like ready-to-eat or hot cereal (microwavable), bagels, bread, rolls, yogurt, fruit, and fruit juices. The low-fat breakfast foods are high in the nutrients many African-American children are missing.

- Low-fat toaster pastry or breakfast bars are okay, and for rush jobs, liquid breakfast drinks will do the trick.

- No matter how late your child is, or how cranky he feels, something is better than nothing. Breakfast is one time when pushing (a little) can help.

KIDS JOIN IN

A big part of your family's nutrition plan should be showing children how to improve their own nutrition. In my ongoing work as a consultant to a national restaurant chain, I speak annually to thousands of African-American children in elementary and high schools around the country. I can tell by the questions they ask that they enjoy choosing healthy foods and are willing to learn more about health and nutrition. You can make nutrition interesting for kids by getting them involved in meal choices and preparation. Invite your kids to help you develop menus. Take them grocery shopping with you, and teach them how to read labels. Ask for their help in the kitchen.

Even young children can wash vegetables and fruits, sprinkle on seasonings, fill pans with water, set the table nicely (using small bouquets and creatively folded napkins), arrange food attractively, and take dishes to the table (see chapter 18).

For special theme nights, help your children do a bit of research and ask them to demonstrate a special cooking utensil or present a unique food during the meal. I like to invite a group of kids into the kitchen and show them a package of thin, dry rice noodles that look like old string. I throw the "old string" into a hot wok, and it instantly explodes into an enormous mass of big crunchy snow-white threads. This kind of teaching and learning is fun. If you're careful, you can even let an older child toss in the noodles himself. (Young children are usually too short and uncoordinated to perform this trick safely.)

In the following chapters in this part, we're going to look at your child's nutritional needs from birth through adolescence. We'll also explore some special nutritional challenges, including allergies and food sensitivities. This section concludes with some healthful recipes designed to appeal to children. Letting your kids learn to cook is one of the best possible ways to teach nutrition. The next chapter will familiarize you with basic nutrition facts that are useful as you shop, plan menus, and prepare meals.

10

Your Family Nutrition Bible

Forming healthy eating habits early is easier than trying to remake old habits that have taken shape over many years. If you give a young child nutrition information, as he grows up he will automatically apply what he's learned. This may sound like a fantasy, but believe me, it's an approach that really works. You may already know much of the basic information supplied in this chapter, but here is a refresher primer to use as reference as you teach your child.

WHAT FOOD CONSISTS OF

Carbohydrates, protein, and fats work in partnership with vitamins and minerals to help a child's body achieve physical, emotional, and mental well-being.

Carbohydrates, protein, and fats are the *macronutrients* that the body needs in large quantities for energy, growth, and repair.

Vitamins and minerals are *micronutrients*—nutrients needed in only small amounts to regulate the many chemical actions in the body. Minerals also play a vital role in forming new tissue, including bones, teeth, and blood.

Water is the third basic component of good health. Water makes the whole process of growth, development, and maintenance work by providing a fluid medium for chemical reactions and for circulating blood and removing waste.

Each nutrient group needs the others in order to carry out its functions.

CARBOHYDRATES

Carbohydrates supply energy to the body. Carbohydrates may be either *complex* (breads, starches, cereals, grains) or *simple* (fruits and vegetables, sugars).

Complex carbohydrates provide protein and are important sources of B vitamins. Complex carbohydrates form the base of the USDA's Food Guide Pyramid and should be the centerpiece of every meal your family eats. They also add bulk and make your child feel full and satisfied. All fruits and vegetables are also carbohydrates, but without the protein found in grains and starches. Fruits and vegetables are naturally low in calories and high in vitamins and minerals. Vegetables and fruits also add color and variety to meals.

With a few exceptions, carbohydrates are virtually fat-free, and unprocessed carbs are also high in fiber. This is the combination you're looking for. Low-fat foods provide double benefit if they are also high in fiber.

FIBER

Fiber is a food substance that does not break down totally during digestion and therefore is not absorbed by the body. High-fiber foods include cereals, grains, beans, fruits, and vegetables. In adults, fiber helps control weight and prevents constipation and diarrhea, helps digestion, reduces blood cholesterol, and also reduces food cravings. In Africa, where high-fiber foods are a way of life, people rarely suffer from ulcers, appendicitis, or colon cancer.

A child's digestive system is unable to handle large amounts of high-fiber foods. High-fiber foods are definitely not appropriate for babies and should be carefully controlled for very young children. Young children should never be given cereals or other foods that have pure bran added to them. Pure bran is too harsh for their intestines.

School-age children and adolescents can tolerate more fibrous foods. At this age, high-fiber foods such as bran cereals, grains, fruits, and vegetables help reduce the desire for sugary snacks between meals.

Choose whole-wheat, rye, and pumpernickel breads, low-fat crackers, hot and cold cereals (without extra sugar), rice, and potatoes. Oats have been good food for generations, and hot oat-meal is still one of the best breakfast foods you can offer kids. Choose either regular or quick-cooking varieties.

For years, starchy carbohydrates such as potatoes and rice were considered fattening, but this is not true. In fact, it's what we *add* to carbohydrates that increases fat and calories. The trick is to prepare high-fiber foods in a healthful manner:

- Skip the sugar on cereals, and add low-fat or skim milk instead of whole milk.

- Bake or steam potatoes instead of frying.

- Use low-fat or nonfat toppings like yogurt instead of sour cream or butter.

- Experiment also with different high-fiber grains, like corn-meal, barley, kasha or buckwheat, and millet.

- A host of important vitamins and minerals are present in all vegetables and fruits. The more intense the color, the greater the supply of nutrients.

PROTEINS

Proteins help body cells and tissues grow and regenerate. Protein is essential for all of us, particularly for growing bodies. The younger a child is, the more protein he needs. In the first two years of life, half the protein a child consumes is used for growth. At two to three years of age, this amount declines to 11 percent; by the time the adolescent growth spurt is over, protein is used for maintenance only, so the body needs less.

Protein is composed of substances called amino acids. Proteins from animal sources—meat, fish, eggs, and dairy products—are called *complete proteins,* because they contain all eight essential amino acids.

Grains and legumes also contain proteins, but none contains all eight essential amino acids. Therefore, plant proteins are called *incomplete.* In certain combinations (such as rice and beans), plant proteins complement one another and add up to complete proteins. (See chapter 16.)

While protein is good and beneficial, many high-protein foods also come with a downside: fat.

FATS

Infants and young children require fats for healthy growth and development. Fats help the body absorb and use important vitamins and minerals. From birth to age two, dietary fat and cholesterol should not be restricted. In older children, however, too much dietary fat causes weight gain and elevated cholesterol, both of which are associated with disease in later life. All fats are high in calories and all are used slowly by the body. Older kids who eat too much fat over a period of time *get fat.*

Children older than age two, especially those who have high blood-cholesterol levels or weight problems, can safely drink low-fat and skim milk; unsaturated vegetable fats are also an option at this stage, rather than saturated fats from animal sources.

Saturated fats, found in red meat and other animal products, contribute to raising blood cholesterol levels, even in children. Milk, cheese, butter, and other dairy products all contain saturated fats. A few vegetable oils (those called tropical oils) are also highly saturated. (Do not confuse "no cholesterol" foods with "no fat" foods. Snacks and bakery goods that claim they contain no cholesterol may actually contain saturated fat from tropical oils.) You'll see tropical oils listed on the label as coconut oil, palm oil, and palm-kernel oil. Keep an eye out for these kinds of fats in cookies, cakes, and snack foods.

Unsaturated fats are found only in vegetables; these generally do less damage to arteries than saturated fats. Two kinds are considered "heart-healthy": the *polyunsaturates* and the *monounsaturates.*

These fats are liquid at room temperature. However, if they are hardened, or *hydrogenated,* they become saturated. The harder a vegetable oil is, the more saturated it becomes. Therefore, stick margarine and vegetable shortenings—including canned Crisco, which we love to fry chicken and fish in—are saturated.

Any product label that lists "partially hydrogenated oil" contains *trans fatty acids,* or trans fats, which may be as harmful as saturated fat. Products likely to include trans fats are crackers, cookies, pastries, cakes, doughnuts, french fries, potato chips, puddings, and graham crackers.

When it comes to margarine, choose products that list liquid oil as the first ingredient. Generally, the softer the margarine, the less saturated it is. Liquid squeeze margarine is lowest in saturated fats. Tub margarine is next, and stick margarine is last.

Use monounsaturated (olive oil, canola oil) or polyunsaturated corn oil in cooking. But remember: Whether unsaturated or not, they are still fats and they still add a load of calories to foods. Use even these fats in small amounts. Total fat should be no more than 25 to 30 percent of total calories for each person in your family who is over the age of two. I use the lower number for myself and for kids, too.

PEANUT BUTTER NOTE FOR MOM

Peanut butter contains monounsaturated fat, so in theory it is an okay kind of fat. However, commercial peanut butter that you buy at the supermarket has been hydrogenated—that is, put through the process where it is made more saturated. Lower-fat versions are now available, but even these products are still relatively high in saturated fat when compared with natural peanut butter.

If your kids love peanut butter—and whose don't—your best bet is to grind the peanuts yourself, or have them ground at the

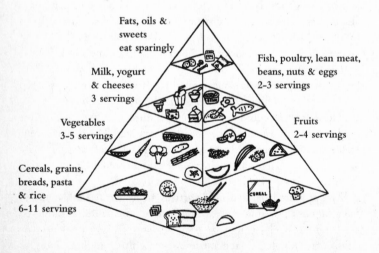

Fats, oils & sweets eat sparingly

Milk, yogurt & cheeses 3 servings

Fish, poultry, lean meat, beans, nuts & eggs 2-3 servings

Vegetables 3-5 servings

Fruits 2-4 servings

Cereals, grains, breads, pasta & rice 6-11 servings

KIDS' FOOD PYRAMID

This pyramid is adapted from the USDA's Dietary Guidelines for Americans. The recommended number of servings are the minimum.

health-food store. The oil rises to the top, so just pour it off before making those great sandwiches.

FAT SUBSTITUTES

Fat substitutes are products that mimic the flavor and texture of fat; they are made from both synthetic and natural substances, including proteins, starches, and soluble fiber. You may find fat substitutes incorporated into baked goods, some cheese and dairy products, ice cream, salad dressings, margarines, and cooking oils.

Children older than two years may eat products containing fat substitutes as part of an overall program to lower their consumption of dietary fat. However, there are a couple of things to watch out for: The flat taste of reduced-fat products encourages manufacturers to load them with extra sugar and salt. Some fat substitutes also contain eggs and milk, which should not be eaten by children with allergies to these foods. Read labels carefully. Be on the lookout for hidden negatives (such as high sugar and sodium) contained in "healthy alternative" foods.

NEW LABELS

Food labels received a major overhaul in 1993, and products now carry clearer, more useful labels. The new labels include basic information on calories and fat per serving, as well as the percentage of calories derived from fat in the product. Other mandatory information includes the amount of cholesterol, sodium, carbohydrates, and protein, as well as information on vitamins A and C, calcium, and iron.

Many labels state the "% Daily Value" offered by the product. Daily values are set by the government and reflect nutrition recommendations for a two-thousand-calorie-per-day diet. You can use the daily values to compare products and to see how the nutrients in one serving fit into your child's overall diet.

SUGAR

Sugar comes in many different forms and is found naturally in fruits and vegetables. Sugars that occur naturally in foods are not a problem for children. Children can also have refined sugar in moderation. But going overboard on sugary foods can certainly interfere with adequate nutrition.

Most researchers feel that the taste for sweetness is inborn in humans. But eating sweet foods is also a cultural habit. Most African Americans have developed one big sweet tooth, which started growing hundreds of years ago. The slave trade between Africa and the Caribbean began with the need for labor in sugarcane fields. Africans *breathed* sugar as they cut cane from dawn to dark, every day of the year. Molasses, a by-product of refined sugar, was a welcome addition to tedious, poor-quality rations. Later, molasses, along with cane syrup, was incorporated into traditional southern black cooking, and both are still considered staples in many of our homes.

Sugar should not be added to the formula or food of infants. Babies who drink sugared water or formula are prone to tooth decay and can become overweight from excessive calories.

For years, sugar was linked to hyperactivity in children. Although this theory has been largely disproved, the possible effects of sugar on behavioral problems in children continue to be studied. Overall, your child should eat sugared foods only in moderation, especially if tooth decay or weight is a problem.

Trying to avoid sugar isn't always easy. Manufacturers often use various forms of sugar in their products without having to list the word *sugar* on the nutrition label. Any ingredient ending in *ose*—for example, glucose or sucrose—is a form of sugar. Nutritionwise, all sugar is the same.

Sugar is one of those foods that conjures up pleasant associations; some of us reach for it when our emotions cry for comfort, even if we're not actually hungry. Sugar is a carbohydrate, and all carbohydrates increase the release of serotonin, a brain chemical that makes children and adults feel relaxed.

Fortunately, we can get the same "feel good" effect from eating complex carbohydrates, fruits, and vegetables. In other words, brown rice can be as satisfying as a candy bar (and the good effect lasts longer). A child who eats complex carbohydrates instead of sugar gets extra fiber and important vitamins and minerals to boot. Replacing sugary, fatty treats with complex carbs helps your child win all around. Good carbohydrate snacks include rice cakes, low-fat or fat-free crackers, pretzels, dry cereal, and trail mixes.

SUGAR SUBSTITUTES

Diet sodas and other foods containing sugar substitutes may not be harmful in moderate amounts, but they should never replace basic foods and beverages. Children and adults who are known to have phenylketonuria (PKU) or seizure disorders should strictly avoid diet products containing aspartame (NutraSweet).

SALT (SODIUM)

Salt is a combination of two minerals: sodium (40 percent) and chloride (60 percent). It's the sodium that we worry about. Sodium is an important mineral and is needed by everyone. It helps keep body fluids in balance, facilitates normal muscle contraction, and works with enzymes and chemicals to aid digestion. Sodium removes carbon dioxide from the bloodstream and dissolves other beneficial blood minerals, helping them go to work better.

Sodium is found naturally in most foods, and most children easily get enough to meet their daily needs. Excess sodium, however, provides no nutritional benefit. And too much sodium can actually be harmful, especially to very young children and children with higher than normal blood pressure.

Safety mechanisms are built into the body's systems to filter excess sodium through the kidneys and excrete it via urine. But some people, particularly African Americans, are "salt sensitive," meaning that their kidneys retain excess sodium. Some scientists believe salt sensitivity is responsible for the high incidence of high blood pressure in our population. In fact, some studies of infants, children, and adults have led researchers to conclude that reducing salt in childhood may prevent high blood pressure from ever developing.

Given the high incidence of hypertension in our population, I believe that reducing salt in your child's diet may be the single most important step you can take to ensure his future health. If a child is already hypertensive, the task force on blood pressure control in children recommends limiting his sodium intake to 5 to 6 gm a day.

Once children develop a taste for saltiness—which can begin as early as four months of age—the habit can be hard to break. When I was a child, I thought unsalted food was tasteless. My mother

---

SALT ALERT FOR KIDS

Here are some of the "kid foods" that have a high sodium content.

American cheese	Mayonnaise
Bacon	Mustard (prepared)
Barbecue sauce	Olives (green)
Beef jerky	Pickles
Canned soup	Pizza
Catsup	Salted chips, nuts, pretzels
Cheeseburgers	Salted popcorn
Cheese puffs	Sauerkraut
Chili sauce	Tomato sauce
Cocoa mixes	Vegetables, canned
Ham, luncheon meat	Worcestershire sauce
Hot dogs	

---

added salt to foods before, during, and often after cooking. She said that salt "brought out the flavor" in foods.

It's never too late to switch, but the earlier you start, the easier it will be to get your kids used to low-salt foods. Families with a history of hypertension should start as early as possible.

You can start to reduce sodium by reading labels on food products to develop an awareness of foods that have a high sodium content.

Then, remove the salt shaker from the table and replace it with salt-free seasoning mixtures such as Mrs. Dash original blend, McCormick (salt-free) all-purpose, or American Heart Association lemon herb seasoning.

Next, begin gradually to reduce the amount of salt you use in cooking.

Young children will never even realize they are on a low-salt diet. And older children eventually get used to it, because low-salt foods actually taste better than highly salted food. I realized this myself when I stopped using salt. After a lifetime of eating salty foods, it took a few weeks for my salt taste buds to subside, but eventually they did. I discovered that salt doesn't bring out flavor, like my mom said; it covers it up. Now I eat almost no salt at all, and I enjoy the difference.

VITAMINS AND MINERALS

A healthy diet that includes a variety of foods helps maintain an adequate intake of all vitamins and minerals. Vitamins and minerals do not give kids energy and pep. (Energy comes from calories consumed in carbohydrates, protein, and fat.) But they are essential to maintain normal body functions. New research shows that certain vitamins and minerals may also prevent and even reverse many deadly diseases, including cancer, heart disease, a weak immune system, and other chronic disorders.

Vitamins are organic substances found in food. Water-soluble vitamins—C and B complex—must be consumed daily, because they are rapidly absorbed and rapidly excreted through sweat and urine. Excess fat-soluble vitamins—A, E, D, and K—are stored in body fat, which means they can build up and become toxic if a child consumes too much.

Minerals are inorganic substances derived from metals and salt found in soil and water. Like vitamins, minerals are essential for your child's good health. But most minerals are needed in small amounts that are naturally present in the diets of young children.

However, lack of *any* nutrient can harm a child's normal growth and development. Children of low-income families are particularly at risk for nutrient deficiency because their food supply can be inadequate and poorly balanced.

Approximately fifty nutrients are required for good health. Your child can receive them all by eating a healthy diet containing a wide variety of foods. At the same time, there are circumstances in which children may not get all the nutrients they need, including poor or inadequate food sources, stress, and illness. It helps to be familiar with the major vitamins and minerals essential to a child's growth and development. Here is a selected overview of vitamins and minerals especially important in childhood.

A REVIEW OF SELECTED VITAMINS

Vitamin A (beta-carotene and carotenoid). Vitamin A promotes healthy eyes and clear vision. It also contributes to steady growth and a healthy immune system. Vitamin A is needed for proper bone growth, tooth development, and healthy skin and hair. It may help fight infections by protecting mucous membranes, which include the nasal passages, mouth, and intestinal tract.

Preformed vitamin A, called retinol, is found in animal foods like liver, eggs, cheese, and butter. All of these foods are high in cholesterol, saturated fats, or both. Consumed in excessive amounts, preformed vitamin A can be toxic, leading to blurred vision, loss of appetite, headaches, rashes, digestive problems, abnormal bone growth, brain and nerve injury, and liver damage.

However, when vitamin A is obtained from *beta-carotene,* which is prominent in fruits and vegetables, the body makes only enough to meet its needs. When consumed in very large amounts—for example, drinking large quantities of carrot juice—the yellow-orange pigment may give the skin a yellowish look. The condition is easily reversed by consuming less. Beta-carotene is not known to be toxic.

Beta-carotene is only one of a group of important compounds known as *carotenoid,* which are believed to work together to protect against certain forms of cancer and heart disease. The best way to get all the possible benefits of various carotenoids is to eat a variety of fruits and vegetables, especially those that are dark green, deep yellow, and orange and red: leafy green vegetables, carrots, sweet potatoes, winter squash, and cantaloupe.

Fats help the body absorb carotenoid, which is one reason why *small amounts* of fat should be included in every diet.

Vitamin D. Vitamin D enables the body to absorb and use calcium and phosphorus, therefore making it vital for building healthy bones and teeth. Vitamin D is also thought to affect the body's ability to secrete insulin, which means it may play an important role in preventing diabetes, a disease that afflicts blacks in huge proportions.

The ultraviolet rays of the sun that pass through the skin set off the production of vitamin D, making it the only vitamin that isn't derived solely from the diet. Dark-skinned children living in cold or very cloudy climates may not get enough of the "sunshine vitamin" to be healthy. A lack of vitamin D can cause irritability, muscle weakness, dental decay, and rickets (in youngsters) and bone softening (in adults).

Fortified milk and dairy products contain vitamin D. However, this doesn't solve the problem for African-American children who are lactose-intolerant. They must consume other D-rich foods.

Good food sources of vitamin D include eggs, butter, margarine, tuna and other cold-water fatty fish such as cod and herring, cod liver oil, and fortified milk. Beef liver and chicken liver also contain vitamin D.

(Vitamin D is fat-soluble, and therefore it is possible to get too much. If your child is getting too much of this vitamin, you may notice symptoms of excessive thirst, sore eyes, itching skin, and the urgent need to urinate.)

Vitamin C. Vitamin C was originally discovered as a preventer of scurvy, a disease whose symptoms include bleeding gums. New research suggests it helps prevent viral and bacterial infections, and it also appears to decrease the severity of common colds.

Vitamin C has many health benefits for children, and there are no proven toxic effects of high doses. Your child's body will excrete what it doesn't use. However, megadoses of C can deplete stores of vitamin B_{12} and folic acid. Occasional diarrhea, excess urination, skin rash, or kidney stones may develop if doses are extremely high (over 1,000 mg per day). Cutting back can usually relieve symptoms.

Excellent food sources of vitamin C include broccoli, brussels sprouts, cabbage, cauliflower, cantaloupe, citrus fruits and juices, tomatoes, mangos, papaya, peppers, spinach, strawberries, and many other vegetables and fruits.

B Vitamins. The B vitamins are a family of eight vitamins that complement one another; they fuel the nervous system, provide energy, and promote healthy skin and hair. For example, vitamin B_2 (riboflavin) is important for healthy eyes, cell respiration, good skin, nails, and hair. It maintains mucous membranes and preserves the nervous system. Folic acid, another member of the B-complex vitamin family, helps form red blood cells and is important in the prevention of anemia. Vitamin B_3 (niacin) supports a healthy nervous system, healthy skin, and the formation of sex hormones, thyroid hormones, and insulin.

The best food sources for the B vitamins are whole-grain breads, cereals, nuts, sunflower and pumpkin seeds, wheat germ, chickpeas, and other legumes. Other good sources are liver and other organ meats, brewer's yeast, milk, and eggs. Folic acid is also available in many uncooked fresh vegetables, particularly spinach and other leafy dark green vegetables.

A REVIEW OF SELECTED MINERALS

Calcium. Calcium is the most abundant mineral in the body and 99 percent of it is stored in bones and teeth. A small amount of calcium is also transported through soft tissues and body fluids to ensure proper nerve and muscle function and blood clotting. Calcium also helps the body use iron and absorb vitamin B_{12}. Calcium is the body's most important mineral and children need a *lot*.

Maintaining calcium stores can be tricky. The mineral is easily depleted, and too much sugar, fiber, or protein can decrease calcium absorption. (It is possible to overload, although this is *very rare*. A calcium overload is signaled by lethargy and confusion; with treatment, most children quickly and fully recover.)

Dairy products are excellent sources of calcium. So are canned sardines and salmon eaten with the bones. Tofu is a good food to include in your child's diet, because it has both calcium and magnesium. In fact, many foods high in calcium are also high in magnesium, including milk, cheese, dried beans and peas, kale and other dark green leafy vegetables, meat, nuts, seafood, and whole grains.

Magnesium. Calcium and magnesium work together to help build healthy bones and teeth. Magnesium also helps keep the nervous system, metabolism, and muscles functioning properly. For this reason, it's often called the "antistress" mineral. Magnesium helps your child's body use calcium, vitamin C, phosphorus, sodium, and potassium, so eating magnesium-rich foods along with calcium-rich foods can boost calcium absorption.

Food sources: Leafy green vegetables, apples, apricots, bananas, figs, grapefruit, and corn; cashews, almonds, and other nuts, seeds, grains, and dried beans and peas; tofu, milk, cheese, and meat.

Iron. Iron is one nutrient routinely lacking in the diets of young children and adolescents. Iron helps a child's body utilize its existing vitamin resources. It builds healthy blood and is therefore necessary to prevent anemia. Hemoglobin (red blood corpuscles), which contains most of a child's iron, is recycled and replaced approximately once every four months. Adolescent girls require even more iron than boys, because iron is lost each month in menstruation.

If you think your child is anemic and needs more iron, try offering more of these excellent food sources: liver, farina cereal, raw clams, dried fruits, red meat, egg yolks, nuts, asparagus, and oatmeal.

Iron-fortified foods, such as cereals, are also helpful ways to ensure adequate iron intake, particularly for strict vegetarians.

Potassium. Potassium is important to help keep the heart on a normal rhythm. It also teams up with sodium to become electrolytes, which are necessary for the kidneys to do their job. Electrolytes keep body fluids stable by regulating shifts and balances of water. An imbalance between potassium (55 percent) and sodium (45 percent) can throw off electrolytes and impair normal nerve and muscle function.

Food sources: bananas, potatoes, citrus fruits, watercress, sunflower seeds, dried fruits, bran, peanut butter, dried beans and peas, coffee, tea, and cocoa.

Zinc. We've known for some time that zinc has nutritional benefits for pregnant women and the developing fetus. Lately, we've been hearing more and more about its importance in growing children, too. Zinc helps ensure the proper development of sexual organs. Some nutritionists believe it increases mental alertness in children. And because it prevents sensory impairment, zinc is thought to improve the sense of taste and smell. Zinc also promotes the healing of wounds, cuts, and scrapes.

Zinc is a trace mineral, meaning that very small amounts are needed to do the job. All of the zinc your child needs can be gotten from food sources: lamb chops and other red meats, pork, wheat germ, pumpkin seeds, sunflower seeds, eggs, ground mustard, brewer's yeast and nonfat dry milk and cheese, seafood, and liver.

VITAMIN AND MINERAL SUPPLEMENTS

A well-balanced diet can provide all the nutrients a child needs to grow and develop in a healthy manner. But not every child gets a well-balanced diet. Many kids rush off to school without an adequate breakfast, and the nutritional value of lunches and dinners varies widely. Even children who are presented with a varied diet on a regular basis go through stages where they reject certain foods. For these reasons, parents often worry whether kids are getting enough nutrients from the foods they eat.

To be on the safe side, many parents give their children a kid's version of a daily vitamin/mineral tablet. Are children's supplements worthwhile? Popular kids' vitamins are often loaded with sugar and artificial colors and flavors. They may also have less nutritional value than regular vitamins.

However, supplemental vitamins and minerals can be very helpful under certain circumstances. But a child's body is too small and is growing too fast for one to make quick assumptions about which vitamins and minerals to supplement and in what amounts. Certain vitamin and mineral supplements (iron, magnesium, chromium, and selenium, for example) should never be given to children without careful medical supervision, and only then for specific health problems.

The decision on which vitamin/mineral supplements to give your child, if any, should be based on his lifestyle, his "realistic world" eating habits, and his health status. *I don't believe parents should give kids any kind of supplement without first consulting a pediatrician or registered dietitian, and then using the type and dosage he or she recommends.*

SYMPTOMS OF NUTRIENT DEFICIENCIES

Symptoms that suggest a child may be deficient in certain vitamins and minerals include:

> *Frequent fatigue*
> *Extremely dry and irritated skin and hair*
> *Constant irritability and crankiness*
> *Not growing and maturing according to growth charts*
> *Bleeding, cracked gums*
> *Chronic colds, infections*
> *Chronic hoarseness*
> *Frequent diarrhea*
> *Muscle weakness*

If your child displays any of these symptoms, start keeping a notebook and record what he eats for two or three weeks. Make an appointment with your child's pediatrician or a dietitian and bring the notebook along with you to the consultation. Only a professional can know which nutrients may be needed and which may interact negatively with foods or medication your child is taking.

Most nutritional deficiencies do not happen overnight. They often take years to develop to the point where you notice them. This also means that it takes time to turn them around. I always work with parents to evaluate a child's diet fully and to see if the problem can be solved by changing what he eats. If the symptoms don't subside after a fair trial of new foods, I might then suggest supplements, depending on the child's age.

However, giving your child a variety of nutritional supplements is the last approach one wants to take. Good wholesome food is the best way to go. Most foods are easy to digest and absorb, and they certainly taste better than pills or powders.

11

***

Your life following childbirth is full of excitement and contradictions. Here is the baby you've carried and nourished for months—tiny, precious, and utterly helpless. Most new parents feel simultaneously excited and terrified, gleeful and stressed. We're lucky to be able to profit from countless books, magazines, and videos on baby care, though much of what we learn about parenting still comes by way of on-the-job training. Whether we get our information from child-rearing experts or from personal experience, social and technological trends also influence our parenting styles and how we feed our babies.

NURSING TRENDS

Until the modern era, breast-feeding was the first choice for feeding a newborn. In this century, however, breast-feeding has cycled in and out of popularity. Women in the workplace weren't able to drop everything and rush home to nurse; wealthy women preferred not to be housebound. So bottle-feeding and infant formula became symbols of affluence and female independence. They provided convenient around-the-clock nourishment when mother could not.

Physicians, manufacturers, and advertisers jumped on the formula bandwagon, persuading mothers that robust-looking cow's milk formulas were as good as—even better than—human breast milk, which appears thinner and grayer in comparison. Gradually, when infant formula became available through federal and state-supported programs, poorer women also turned to bottle-feeding.

For a time, mothers who nursed were condescended to as if they were primitive.

In the late 1970s, breast-feeding got renewed attention as we learned more about its nutritional and health benefits. First affluent women and then, slowly, lower-income women started to breast-feed their babies. Today's widespread interest in breast-feeding is due to public education efforts sponsored by nutritionists, the U.S. Department of Health and Human Services, and such organizations as La Leche League International. Breast-feeding for full-term infants is recommended by both the American Dietetic Association and the American Academy of Pediatrics.

Despite these efforts, breast-feeding has not regained popularity with African-American women as quickly as with other groups. In 1992, only 27.2 percent of African-American babies born in hospitals were breast-fed, compared with 51.7 percent of Hispanic babies and 59.7 percent of white babies. The rates are especially low in the south-central and mid-Atlantic states.

Modern African-American women give several reasons for not breast-feeding. Some must return to work immediately and have no support in the workplace to bring their infants to the office. Others say that their husbands don't like them exposing their breasts in public. And some complain that it's just plain inconvenient. Nonetheless, breast-feeding is what nature intended for you and your baby.

BREAST-FEEDING

Human milk has at least a hundred ingredients that are not found in cow's milk and cannot be duplicated in a laboratory. In many different ways, human milk is ideally suited to the developmental needs of human babies. Breast milk is "individualized" to meet your baby's immediate and changing needs.

"First" breast milk is a thick yellowish fluid called colostrum, which provides all the water and nutrients the baby needs in the first few days. It also provides natural immunization against infection by conveying infection-fighting white cells that are so critical to good health.

More mature milk usually begins to come in around the second or third day after delivery, making the breasts feel hard and heavy.

This discomfort soon eases as the baby draws off the milk. After breast-feeding is established, the breasts will supply just as much milk as the baby needs, and it will be naturally composed of exactly the proper ingredients. Furthermore, breast milk is completely sanitary—and it's always the right temperature!

Breast-fed babies are less likely to be overfed than babies fed with formula. They are also less likely to develops allergies. Babies are almost never allergic to breast milk. (On the other hand, about one out of ten infants develops allergic reactions to cow's milk formula.)

Even though cow's milk contains relatively more calcium and phosphorus (it is designed to nurture a calf's large, rapidly expanding skeleton), the minerals in human milk are more easily absorbed by your baby. Breast milk helps digestion because it has properties that prevent the growth of harmful bacteria in the intestines; therefore, breast-fed babies are less likely to suffer from colic, gas, and excessive spitting up. Because breast milk has a natural laxative effect, your breast-fed baby is unlikely to become constipated or to have diarrhea. Breast-fed infants have bowel movements that are generally very soft, loose, and easy to pass. Breast milk also contains less sodium and protein than cow's milk, which means it's easier on an infant's kidneys.

Breast milk is always "in stock" and ready to use. If you must return to work soon after childbirth, you can extract and store your breast milk for feedings (in a bottle) at home or away from home. One more thing: Breast milk is free.

GETTING STARTED

The perfect time for you and your infant to begin sharing the breast-feeding experience is right after delivery. A newborn's natural sucking and swallowing reflexes are especially strong at birth. If placed close to the mother's breast, most newborns will nuzzle the breast and begin to suck the nipple immediately with surprising ease.

A new mother may not have much milk, but if she gently massages her breast and squeezes the nipple into the baby's mouth, the baby will probably continue to suck, which sets up a chain reaction that benefits both mother and child. Nursing creates an immediate, intense bond between mother and child. Suckling a newborn within minutes of delivery also helps the mother's uterus contract and get back in shape more rapidly. (By the way, before delivery, make sure the hospital nursing staff is aware that you intend to breast-feed, so that your baby will not be given formula in the hospital nursery.)

Breast-feeding does not *always* come right off the bat. Mothers who are extremely tired or have experienced a difficult delivery may need to delay breast-feeding for a few hours or even a few days. Some babies, too, need a little time before they're ready to begin breast-feeding.

IF YOU HAVE DIFFICULTY

It's not unusual to need a little help getting the breast-feeding process started. You may have already gotten some tips in childbirth classes, and some hospitals have get-togethers to provide new mothers with tips on breast-feeding. The nurse, midwife, or doctor can also help.

Sometimes, breast-feeding just doesn't take. If you cannot become comfortable breast-feeding, let it go. It isn't the end of the world. Some mothers simply don't want to breast-feed, and that's okay, too. Breast-feeding is best when it's right for you. Don't let anyone bully you into it. The most important part of feeding your baby is to feel comfortable with the choice you make—when you're comfortable, so is your baby.

HOW LONG TO CONTINUE BREAST-FEEDING

Different mothers stop breast-feeding at different times. Some new mothers stop breast-feeding after a few weeks or months. Some stop around six months of age, others around one year, and some wait even longer. Babies who stop during the first year can go from their mother's breast to drinking infant formula from a bottle, or sometimes even from a cup. You may wish to breast-feed right up to the time your baby is ready to be weaned.

TAKING CARE OF YOURSELF

When you are breast-feeding, it's important that you eat a diet rich in iron and other nutrients and that you take in at least eighteen hundred calories a day. You should drink a minimum of eight cups of fluids a day, including milk, juice, and water. Avoid caffeinated coffee, teas, and soda. Also avoid alcoholic beverages, because alcohol passes quickly into breast milk and can cause your baby to become jittery and irritable.

Concentrate on eating foods that are high in nutritional value and low in sugar. The idea is to eat moderate amounts of a wide range of foods. Anything in excess may cause problems for your baby. For example, fresh fruits are good, but eating *lots* of melons, peaches, or other fresh fruits may cause your baby to develop colic or diarrhea. Also, avoid gas-forming foods (cabbage, broccoli, dried beans) and foods strongly flavored with garlic and onions, which can cause your baby to develop colic.

WHEN NOT TO BREAST-FEED

Some new mothers are unable to breast-feed for health reasons. For example, a woman who has a new diagnosis of breast cancer should not nurse, because she may need to start chemical treatments that might alter the composition of breast milk or be passed on to the infant. Breast-feeding also stimulates hormones that can accelerate the growth of some cancers. (On the other hand, a woman who has completed radiation treatment for breast cancer in the past is usually able to breast-feed safely.)

Other reasons not to breast-feed include:

- If a mother has the HIV virus. The virus can be passed to infants through a mother's breast milk.
- If an infant has galactosemia, a congenital disorder that makes a baby intolerant to galactose, which is derived from the lactose in human milk. These babies must be fed lactose-free infant formulas.
- If an infant has phenylketonuria (PKU), a sensitivity to the amino acid phenylalanine, found in high concentrations in breast milk. A good alternative is the formula Lofenalac.
- If a new mother is taking any medication for chronic or temporary illnesses that can be passed through breast milk. This is a long list, which includes penicillin and other antibiotics. If you are taking any medication at all, check with your doctor and pharmacist before breast-feeding. If you take any over-

the-counter medications, read the labels carefully and still check with your doctor or pharmacist before breast-feeding.

- If a mother has heart disease, kidney disease, or severe anemia. A mother with any serious illness should consult her physician before deciding to breast-feed.

Also bear in mind that everything you eat and drink is passed to your nursing infant. If you are worried that the water supply in your community may not be safe, check with local public water authorities, discuss it with other mothers in your community, or drink bottled water.

BOTTLE-FEEDING

For various reasons some new mothers give up breast-feeding and some never plan to breast-feed at all. Bottle-feeding of infant formulas is the alternative. One major advantage of bottle-feeding is that it lets fathers share the intimacy of feeding the baby. Grandmas, other relatives, and friends can also feed the baby, which lets parents take time away if necessary. Bottle-feeding also makes it easier to monitor how much milk your baby is getting. It means you can take medications if necessary and be a little more flexible about your own diet. You needn't worry about baring your breast in front of other people, about soiling your clothing with breast milk, or about having to wear special bras to support your full breasts.

Bottle-feeding requires the same comfort and positioning as breast-feeding. Always hold the baby in your arms. Holding and touching makes your baby feel safe and secure. (Do not prop the bottle up artificially. Propping a bottle to feed a baby may cause tooth decay or predispose to ear infections if milk runs from the nipple across the baby's face and pools about the eustachian tube which leads to the middle ear.)

Tilt the bottle so that formula flows constantly into the nipple. This prevents the baby from sucking air, which can lead to gas. Always finish feeding the baby before putting her down for a nap. If she falls asleep while nursing, remove the bottle from her mouth. (You don't want her to choke.)

Formula-fed babies certainly thrive. And manufacturers are rapidly developing new products designed to make formulas more like mother's milk. The most widely used commercial formulas are Enfamil, Similac, and SMA. Most are made from cow's milk, but alternative formulas are available for infants who cannot tolerate cow's milk. Babies who cannot tolerate cow's milk, whether because of an allergy to the protein or an intolerance to the carbohydrate, may spit up large amounts of milk after feeding, have persistent diarrhea, or have colic. Babies with colic show pain, are restless, and cry after feeding. (Colic is not always caused by formula intolerance. In some instances, the cause is unknown and may be related to the immaturity of the digestive tract.)

Soy formulas and formulas made with hydrolyzed protein are the usual alternatives. Mothers who don't want to give their babies animal products can also use the soy formulas. Popular soy formulas are Isomil, Prosobee, Nursoy, and Soyalac.

Other formulas are available for babies who have special nutritional needs or who cannot tolerate either milk or soy formulas. Pregestimil, Nutramigen, and Alimentum may be recommended. Consult with your baby's doctor to make the best formula selection for your child's nutritional and growth needs. (For information on feeding premature and very small babies, see the next chapter.)

Infant formulas offer varying levels of fat, whey, vitamins, and minerals. Standards are based on recommendations from the American Academy of Pediatrics and regulated by the Infant Formula Act of 1980. You can buy most infant formulas in local grocery stores and drugstores. They come in powder, liquid concentrate, and ready-to-feed liquid. (Ready-to-feed formulas are the most expensive.)

Formula should be fed at room temperature. Leftovers can be refrigerated, then reheated to a lukewarm temperature for baby's next feeding. (Refrigerator shelf life for leftover formulas varies from twenty-four to forty-eight hours. Check the label carefully.)

To bring refrigerated formula back to room temperature, place the bottle in warm water. Don't heat bottles of formula in the microwave. Microwave heating may be uneven and the baby's mouth may be scalded. Always test heated formula on the sensitive skin of your inner arm or wrist. It should be close to room temperature, cooler rather than hotter.

For correct preparation, serving, refrigeration, and reheating of commercial infant formulas, always carefully follow the instructions on the can.

Your mother, grandmother, or thrifty-minded friends may suggest you give your baby regular fresh milk or evaporated milk as a less expensive alternative to infant formula. Don't buy it! Your aunt may claim to have raised eight healthy kids on household milk, but I do *not recommend* it for infants in the first year. Cow's milk lacks essential fats, vitamin C, zinc, and trace minerals your baby will get from formula. Infants who drink cow's milk may also become iron-deficient. Whole pasteurized cow's milk contains higher amounts of protein and electrolytes than formula, and for this reason it can put stress on an infant's kidneys. Skim milk is even worse for infants, because it has a yet higher ratio of protein to calories than whole milk.

WATER

Breast milk and formula usually provide a baby with enough fluid. However, you may wish to offer your baby one to two ounces of water *between* feedings to replace fluid lost from perspiration and breathing, especially in warm weather. However, water should never be offered in place of a formula or breast-milk feeding.

You may also want to give the baby some water before sleeping to wash milk from her mouth. Putting a baby down to sleep with a bottle of water may give her a sense of comfort, too, but make sure you remove it after she's fallen asleep.

Until your baby is at least four months old, tap water should be boiled before using in order to kill bacteria and ensure cleanliness. Bottled water is also acceptable and does not need to be boiled. But do not use sparkling or mineral water (such as Perrier). After the baby is four months old, household water can be used out of the tap, unless your water is not suited for drinking. In that case, continue to boil tap water or use bottled water for your child's needs. Never add sugar or other sweeteners to the baby's water.

FROM BIRTH TO SIX MONTHS

From birth to six months of age, human milk or infant formula is the only source of nutrition your baby needs. Breast-feeding moms should initially nurse every one to three hours, at least eight to ten times in every twenty-four-hour period. By age two weeks, most infants can go about four hours between feedings. By two months, many infants are sleeping through the night.

During each feeding, let your baby nurse for about ten to twenty minutes from each breast. Some babies feed faster and only need about five to ten minutes of nursing from each breast. Let your baby go at her own pace; don't try to rush her. She will tell you when she has had enough.

While you are nursing, you can hear and see the baby swallowing, which tells you she is getting the milk she needs. A diaper check is also reassuring—you should count six to eight wet diapers each day.*

If you are bottle-feeding, how much formula does your baby need? RDAs for the first year are a guide to the nutrient needs of healthy infants. The table below shows the approximate amount of commercial formula the average baby is expected to drink during the first year. Some babies will drink a little more or less, depending on individual rates of development. I recommend keeping a diary of the total amount of formula your child is getting so your baby's pediatrician can compare it with the baby's weight

Age	Amount (ounces)	Number of Feedings	Total Amount per Day (ounces)
Birth–3 weeks	2½–4	Every 2–3 h	16–24
3 weeks–2 months	4–6	Every 3–4 h	21–24
2–6 months	5–8	Every 3–4 h	24–32
6–9 months	6–9	Every 4 h	24–32
9–12 months	7–9	Every 4–6 h	28–32

Sometimes more than thirty-two ounces of formula will be needed to satisfy a baby's hunger. However, an infant who regularly drinks more than thirty-two ounces of formula in twenty-four hours also may be ready for solid foods (see page 134).

---

*A newborn's first bowel movements in the hospital are greenish black and sticky, which is simply an emptying of the residue collected in the infant's colon before birth. Within a day or two, stools become soft and yellow. A baby may have anywhere from several bowel movements a day to one movement every three or four days. As long as the stools are soft, your baby is not constipated.

Whether you bottle-feed or breast-feed, babies basically judge for themselves when they are hungry and how much they eat. After your baby has finished nursing from breast or bottle, pat him gently along his back to help release air that gets trapped as he suckles. It may erupt in a mighty burp or a series of little hiccups—you'll quickly learn your child's style.

Babies rarely need nutritional supplements or vitamins, except for the initial injection of vitamin K that all infants receive. The abundance of vitamins in breast milk or commercial baby formulas takes care of the rest of their needs.

Full-term babies usually have about a three-month supply of iron in their bodies. Breast milk usually contains enough additional iron until the baby is six months old. If you're bottle-feeding, your pediatrician will probably recommend a formula that has added iron. Pediatricians routinely start babies on iron-containing formulas from birth. If they didn't, some parents might get the impression that non-iron or low-iron formulas are okay during the first year of life, which they are not. Beginning with iron-containing formula ensures that no infant gets "left out" of being on the proper formula at the most important time.

Some pediatricians give new mothers drops of fluoride to add to baby formula if the local water supply is not fluoridated. Your doctor or public health department can tell you if fluoride is in the water supply.

AVOID OVERFEEDING

Overfeeding infants is one of the most common problems I encounter with my clients. Babies cry for many reasons and not every howl means "I'm hungry." Babies cry if they have a wet or messy diaper, if they want to suck or cuddle, if they have gas, if they're thirsty, and when they're ill. Before automatically offering bottle or breast, think about these other possibilities. Watch your baby for signs that she is full. She may turn her head away from the nipple or stop sucking. If your child refuses a scheduled feeding, don't force it. Just cuddle your baby instead and return her to the crib to sleep or play until she is ready to eat.

THE RIGHT TIME FOR SOLID FOODS

One common urge new mothers have is to introduce solid foods too soon. I've known mothers who try to feed cereal to their one- or two-month-old babies. To my horror, I've also seen mothers chew solid food and then offer it to their baby, as a bird does for her chicks. When I ask them why, they say, "My mother did it for me."

These are not appropriate tactics for an infant. Your infant's digestive system is still immature and can't digest the same foods that adults or older children eat.

Formula or breast milk supplies your baby with all the nutrition he needs for the first four months of life. Liquids are much easier for a young infant to process, digest, and absorb, and give his digestive system time to develop.

Holding off on solids also reduces the risk of allergic reactions, and it keeps your baby's digestive system from getting accustomed to excess nutrients and calories. Research indicates that childhood overeating can lead to obesity in adult life.

THE TRANSITIONAL PERIOD

Between four and eight months is a transitional period when you can begin offering your baby pureed and soft foods, in addition to the liquid nutrition to which he's already accustomed. If your infant does not accept solid foods at exactly four months, don't worry. Babies need to develop enough physically to accept the increase in texture, and each has his own individual rate of growth and development. This development is more complex than you may think, involving both physical and psychological advancement. Even when your infant is physically ready, new foods are a big step, and he will need reassuring support from you.

Between four to six months babies master early munching motions, which is your signal that she's ready for solid foods. You may also observe other physical cues: When your baby has doubled her birth weight, or is at least thirteen pounds, she is ready for more nutrition. When she can sit with support and can hold her head up, these physical skills also say, Go ahead. She may also indicate her readiness for new food by opening her mouth and leaning forward.

Start gradually by introducing iron-fortified infant cereal. I recommend rice cereals, which cause fewer allergic reactions than wheat or oat cereals.

At five to six months of age, your baby's chewing methods will improve. Now is also the time to begin introducing strained vegetables and strained fruits, in addition to cereal. Try strained peas, carrots, pears, or apricots. Avoid citrus fruits such as oranges, tangerines, and grapefruit, which commonly cause allergies in babies less than one year of age. Babies usually receive as much fiber as they need in pureed baby fruits and vegetables and in baby cereals.

It's important to keep a balance between vegetables and fruits. Parents who feed too much fruit and not enough vegetables sometimes find that as their children grow up they refuse vegetables in preference for sweeter foods. Good balance now encourages balance later.

At this point, your baby may be able to accept milk from a cup that you hold. Start with small amounts in a cup, but continue giving breast milk or formula (in the bottle). (Some babies are not ready to drink from a cup for several more months—so don't worry if your child rejects the cup.)

Between six and eight months, add strained plain baby meats. Zwieback or hard toast is another good choice for this stage, since it encourages your child to chew.

As a general rule of thumb, use single-strained foods instead of combinations. For example, choose strained chicken over a combination of strained chicken and noodles. Pick strained bananas over apple-bananas. In this way, if your child has an allergic reaction, you can more easily identify the cause.

FROM EIGHT MONTHS TO ONE YEAR

By the eighth or ninth month, your infant is probably ready for thicker foods. This is called the "modified adult" period, in which your baby's digestive system is able to tolerate foods with greater texture. By now, your baby can hold a bottle, as well as grasp small pieces of food and baby utensils. You guessed it: She is becoming much more independent and prefers to feed herself. This is a great time to introduce finger foods such as cheese sticks, dry cereal, tender diced or sliced vegetables, and tender finely chopped meat or liver.

A BASIC MODEL
FOR THE FIRST YEAR

The American Dietetic Association recommends the following schedule for introducing solid foods to your baby. Remember that throughout the first year, all new foods are *in addition* to breast milk or formula.

Age and Development	*What to Feed*
From birth to four months: Baby can suck, swallow, and stick out tongue.	Feed breast milk or formula prescribed by doctor, as well as water.
From four to six months: Baby stops pushing food out of mouth with tongue. Can support head and sit up with help.	Add one tablespoon of iron-fortified baby rice cereal two or three times a day.
From five to six months: Baby can eat from a spoon. Lips can close.	Add one to two tablespoons of plain strained baby vegetables or fruit two or three times a day (peas, carrots, squash, and green beans; bananas, applesauce, peaches, pears, and apricots). Introduce one new vegetable or fruit every three to four days and watch for food allergies (rash, spitting up, or diarrhea).
From six to eight months: Chewing motion is present.	Add one-half to one tablespoon plain strained baby meats once or twice daily (beef, veal, lamb, turkey, chicken, egg yolk, or liver). Try one new food every three to four days and watch for food allergies. Increase cereal to four tablespoons or more per day. Increase strained vegetables and fruits to two tablespoons or more per serving.

| From eight to nine months: Teeth are present. Chewing improves. Can grasp food with hands. | Begin trying junior foods (half jar) or mashed and chopped table foods (four tablespoons or more per day), such as egg yolk, meat, poultry, potato, or well-cooked pieces of vegetable. Finely chopped canned fruit may replace strained fruit. Increase amounts of food according to baby's hunger. |
| From ten to twelve months: Baby has more ability to chew and swallow foods; better grasping skills. | Add cut-up pieces of cooked vegetable, fruit, or lean meat (four tablespoons or more per day). Casseroles (four tablespoons or more per day) and cheese slices may be used. Continue iron-fortified cereals (four tablespoons or more per day). Increase these solids according to baby's hunger. |

Adapted from *Nutrition and Meal Planning in Child-Care Programs: A Practical Guide.* Used by permission, copyright © 1992 by The American Dietetic Association.

Chewing is an essential part of proper digestion. So, as your baby's teeth develop, you can progress from finely chopped to diced, then to small pieces of food cut in strips.

While your baby is eating, make sure you sit with him, even if he's doing pretty well handling his own food. Babies and children choke easily on foods. If your baby seems to be having difficulty chewing or swallowing, continue with softer, pureed foods until he can handle solids more easily. There's no rush.

Canned fruits packed in their own juice are acceptable. Cottage cheese and potatoes are good now, too. Continue offering new colors, textures, and tastes, but steer clear of spices and condiments. If you prepare food yourself, don't add salt or sugar.

Eggs can also be introduced about this time. You can offer mashed hard-boiled egg yolk, or scrambled or soft-cooked egg yolk. Egg whites are much more likely to cause allergic reactions and should not be given until the end of the first year.

Many adults are concerned about eggs and cholesterol, but a one- to two-year-old child does not need to have eggs restricted.

After age two, children can still have three or four eggs weekly without worrying about cholesterol, even in families at risk for heart disease.

Clinical studies have found that between one-third and two-thirds of infants who have allergic reactions to various foods will lose these sensitivities in early childhood, so don't worry if your child has an early food allergy. There's a good chance that it will disappear.

HOW MANY CALORIES?

The number of calories your baby needs each day is based on his growth and energy use. Growth spurts typically occur in the first year of life, then again between ages nine and thirteen for girls and ten and fifteen for boys. Following are the number of calories recommended by the National Academy of Sciences for babies in their first year:

Age	Calories per Pound	Calories per Day
Birth–6 months	49	650
6–12 months	45	850

FRUIT JUICES

One to four ounces of fruit juice can be added after five months of age but should not be given in place of breast milk or formula. Apple juice is the most popular juice for babies. (Do not give babies orange juice or any other citrus fruit juice because of the possibility of an allergic reaction.) Limit juices to four ounces per day for babies under one year of age.

VEGETARIAN BABIES

If you choose not to introduce pureed chicken or meat, you will want to make sure that all of your baby's nutritional needs are being met. The main thing is to make sure your child is getting enough iron and vitamin D. Iron-fortified cereals are widely available and are a good way to add iron when meats are avoided. Consult with your baby's doctor or dietitian to review an infant vegetarian diet. (For further information, see chapter 16.)

PASSING THE FIRST-YEAR MARK

This is a very important and impressionable stage. Your baby will be drinking less formula or breast milk by this time and eating more pureed and chopped foods.

During this stage, you will be setting the tone for mealtimes throughout the rest of your child's life. Allow your child as much control as possible, and provide supportive backup to her efforts. Go with the flow.

Accept your child's individual progress from one type of food to the next—from pureed foods to mashed and then to chopped—and do not push new food on her. Instead, encourage her to go at her own pace. Be sure your baby is never alone while she is eating. If your child gags or chokes on food, help her clear her mouth and take smaller amounts. By using "assist and allow" control, the learning process will be a breeze. One sure sign that your child is adjusting well to table food is when she is sitting up, unassisted, and feeding herself with her own hands.

If you haven't already done so, your child's first birthday is the time to introduce utensils. Start with foods that are easy for a baby to handle with a spoon—mashed potatoes, applesauce, and cooked cereal are good choices. Be prepared for spills! And don't worry if your baby wants to play with food more than eat it. Children instinctively eat enough to satisfy their hunger. Always start with small portions. If your child is still hungry, she'll let you know!

By fifteen months, your baby should be eating a variety of foods and eating at least three ounces of solid foods at each meal. By now, foods can be in slightly larger pieces and hand-held.

WEANING TO REGULAR MILK

Around your baby's first birthday, you can wean him away from breast milk or infant formula. Weaning is usually a gradual process. When the baby is around six months old, start offering less formula or breast milk as he begins eating more solid foods. Once your baby is drinking fewer than thirty-two ounces of formula a day, or has been taking two or three fewer breast-feedings, you can introduce "weanling" milk.

There are three choices: commercial weanling formula, pasteurized whole milk, and evaporated milk. I don't think commercial formula is really necessary, and in the long run it may be more expensive, because your baby isn't using the same milk as the rest of the family.

Evaporated whole milk should be diluted with water in a one-to-one ratio. Whole pasteurized milk can be served as is. Whether you choose evaporated or regular milk, make sure it is fortified with vitamins A and D. Wait until after two years of age for switching to milk with 2 percent or 1 percent fat.

HOMEMADE BABY FOOD

Today's jarred baby foods are safe and nutritious and low in sugar and salt. But if you are thinking about making your baby's food at home, go for it! Your main investment will be a blender or food processor, which makes it easier and faster to puree or chop food. Make certain that foods have been washed well before cooking, then cook them thoroughly and puree to a consistency that your baby will tolerate easily. Do not add any seasonings or spices to homemade foods. Babies readily accept foods that adults would consider bland. That means no added sugar or salt, and definitely no preservatives.

12

NOURISHING PREMATURE AND LOW-
BIRTH-WEIGHT BABIES

One of the most perplexing health problems facing the African-American community is infant mortality, which occurs most often in babies who are born too soon or are severely underweight. Our nation's rate of low-birth-weight infants is embarrassing, considering our per capita income and the amount of money we spend on health care. Moreover, the number of African-American infants born at low birth weight is twice that of the number of white infants. More research is needed to discover all the causes of low birth weight, and more effort needs to be spent to correct the causes we already know about, including inadequate prenatal care and poor maternal nutrition.

This chapter provides an overview of how to improve the overall health and nutrition of a baby who is born very small. If a low-birth-weight infant can survive the first year, he is well on the way to recovery and has the potential to grow and develop normally. Medical care and supervision obviously help improve an infant's immediate health status, but only parents can provide the moment-by-moment love and nourishment essential to a child's survival.

Low birth weight is one of the most crucial factors in the abnormal growth and development of an infant. Any newborn weighing less than five and a half pounds is called a low-birth-weight baby. A low-birth-weight baby may be born prematurely or may be born after full gestation.

The small stomachs of low-birth-weight infants and the reduced rate at which foods are broken down and moved through the gastrointestinal tract make it hard for them to take in the food they need to catch up. They tend to get tired just from eating and being handled. Premature babies, especially those of *very* low birth weight, also suffer from difficulties related to immature organ systems—particularly lungs, heart, kidneys, and digestive systems. As a result, they often have trouble sucking, swallowing, and breathing.

The diet for a premature and/or low-birth-weight baby must provide:

- Sufficient calories and carbohydrates to meet energy needs
- Enough protein for growth in an easy-to-digest formula
- Adequate dietary fat to meet increased growth needs and to help the body absorb fat-soluble vitamins and calcium
- Enough vitamins and minerals to make up for any nutrient deficiencies—particularly calcium, phosphorus, iron, and vitamin E
- Enough fluids to prevent dehydration, but not so much that the heart and kidneys are overburdened
- Sodium and potassium to replace electrolytes lost through perspiration, urination, or diarrhea

If nutrition management is not started immediately, the infant's health problems often continue throughout childhood and adolescence. Some chronic illnesses may cause your child to grow too slowly or become under- or overweight. Feeding skills may be slow to develop, or a child may be unable to tolerate various foods because the development of the digestive system—the mouth, esophagus, stomach, and colon—has been delayed. When nutritious foods cannot be tolerated or properly digested, the child's growth and development will be affected.

ASSESSING YOUR BABY'S NEEDS

Nutritional assessment and regular health screenings should begin immediately after your baby is born. At birth, the baby's weight, length, and gestational age (length of time of your pregnancy) is recorded and compared with "normal" values from national growth charts (see chapter 5).

African-American infants naturally tend to be smaller than white infants, so if your baby weighs only five and a half to six and a half pounds (the low end of the normal range), he is usually considered healthy. If you have other children, your pediatrician may compare the newborn's weight with that of his siblings at birth. The doctor will also look at the baby's family history.

Early on, while your newborn is still in the hospital, your doctor and health-care team—nutritionist, pharmacist, and nursing staff—will make sure your baby's nutritional needs are being met. Once the baby is developing well and is stable enough to go home, your baby's doctor or nutritionist will recommend a commercial, easily available infant formula that will continue to meet your baby's nutritional needs. The doctor will also ask you to bring the baby in for frequent checkups to make sure he is progressing satisfactorily.

SPECIAL INFANT FORMULAS

Formulas for premature infants differ in several important ways from standard baby formulas. Both regular and premature formulas come with and without iron, and both are designed to be gentle on your infant's kidneys. However, premature formulas give the baby extra support for growth and bone mineralization. Premature formulas contain the following:

- Extra calories
- A blend of long-chain fats and medium-chain fats (regular formulas contain only long-chain fats)—medium-chain fats are easier for a preterm infant to digest
- Both lactose (milk sugar) and glucose as a source of carbohydrates—regular formulas use only lactose
- Vitamins and minerals that are specially adjusted to premature needs

Most premature infants are able to tolerate any of the three common commercial premature formulas: Similac Special Care, Enfamil Premature Formula, and Preemie SMA.

If your baby's doctor recommends a particular formula, that's the one you should use. Don't switch formulas without discussing it first with your pediatrician.

For certain rare conditions in which an infant cannot absorb the nutrients in regular premature formulas, your baby's doctor might give you a prescription for a special formula. Again, your doctor knows best.

Depending on how your child progresses, it may be possible for you to breast-feed. Breast-feeding has its advantages: It's easier on the kidneys than regular infant formula and it contains proper protein for growth. However, human milk does not meet a very small baby's need for additional calcium and phosphorus, so if you do breast-feed, your pediatrician may recommend a nutritional supplement.

Your pediatrician will also tell you how much and how often to feed your small baby. Generally, all babies should be fed on demand, because this allows the baby to get calories when he needs them. A hungry baby should never be ignored for the sake of a feeding schedule. Some tiny newborns require more than eight feedings a day in order to take in the full amount of breast milk or formula they need. An extra one or two feedings at night may have to continue for several months.

The catch-up phase for a small baby is usually completed within one to two years, and your baby will gradually be able to tolerate a regular diet. Exceptions depend on the severity of any health problems, especially those that affect digestion and absorption of nutrients. For example, infants who have difficulty swallowing and chewing and who also take special medications for health problems will have multiple special nutritional needs.

SPECIAL PROBLEMS

Here is a summary of problems that require special nutritional attention in the first two years:

- Low weight for height and lack of appropriate weight gain
- Excessive weight gain in relation to length and height
- Iron-deficiency anemia
- Refusal to eat foods, even when able
- Eating nonfood items (pica)
- Lack of appetite
- Excessive appetite

- Gagging or vomiting with feeding attempts
- Food allergies and intolerances
- Too little fluid intake
- Constipation
- Inability to chew or swallow
- Inability of the child to grasp foods and feed himself
- Limited attention span or disruptive behavior at mealtimes

These and other problems may be caused by the presence of an underlying disease, or by developmental deficiencies caused by premature birth or low birth weight. Other causes include not eating enough food (poor oral intake), lesions in the mouth, infections, medications (such as steroids), diarrhea, fever, or physical handicaps and neurological impairments.

If your child has any of these problems, your health-care team can offer you a tremendous amount of guidance in making certain that your child receives adequate nourishment for growth and development.

INCREASING FOOD INTAKE

If not eating enough is the problem, observe your child's food preferences, then increase the amounts of preferred foods that are high in nutritional value and high in calories. Frequent small meals, in textures baby can digest easily, are usually more effective than larger, fewer meals.

If your baby's nutritional needs cannot be met by food intake alone, your pediatrician may recommend a multivitamin or liquid nutritional supplement. *Do not give your baby vitamins or nutritional supplements without first consulting your doctor.*

The first priority is to help your child eat normally. However, if your child's feeding problem is so severe that adequate nutrition cannot be achieved by mouth, your doctor may recommend temporarily feeding the baby with a nasogastric feeding tube. This tube conducts liquid nutrition through the nose into the esophagus and stomach. Alternatively, a liquid feeding tube can be surgically implanted into the stomach through the abdominal wall. Feeding tubes are used only if absolutely necessary.

MOUTH LESIONS

If your child has sores or lesions in her mouth, check the textures of foods you're offering; switch to nonirritating soft foods and beverages served at room temperature. Avoid serving your child acidic juices such as orange, grapefruit, or pineapple.

CHRONIC INFECTIONS

If your child suffers from repeated infections, colds, or flu increase the amount of calories and protein in his daily diet; this will prevent weight loss. Also increase water and fruit juices (particularly if fever is present).

MEDICATIONS

If your child is taking one or more medications for illnesses, your pediatrician will know how they might affect your child's nutritional status. Some medications can cause fluid and sodium retention, loss of electrolytes, and loss of vitamin C and calcium. In some cases, nutritional supplements will help replenish vitamin and mineral losses, but supplements must be given in amounts that are not toxic to a small baby.

PICA IN CHILDREN

Eating nonfood substances is considered a behavioral problem by most physicians, although the exact cause is unknown. Pica may be associated with stress from family instability, neglect, or inadequate supervision. Some medical experts speculate that children who crave nonfood substances may lack minerals such as iron or zinc in their diets.

When I began seeing patients in an inner-city hospital, paint chips were the most common nonfood substance children ate. (Lead-based paints are no longer used, but they may still exist on the interior walls of old buildings. Eating dust or chips from lead-based paint can cause lead poisoning.) Even harmless nonfood substances can compromise nutritional status if they take the place of healthy foods. They can also cause digestive problems and bowel obstruction.

If pica is a problem for your child, the best advice is to watch him closely and give him extra attention throughout the day. If you observe your child chewing and swallowing nonfood substances, distract him by presenting him with food you know he especially likes. And always let your doctor know.

DIARRHEA (POOR ABSORPTION OF NUTRIENTS)

Diarrhea or other physical problems that interfere with the body's ability to absorb nutrients can be life-threatening to an infant or very young child. Diarrhea in a small baby should be reported to the baby's doctor right away, since dehydration can occur quickly. The doctor may suggest that you restrict or eliminate lactose-containing formula or foods and replace them with lactose-free foods that are easier for some babies to digest.

DEVELOPMENTAL PROBLEMS

If your growing child has a physical and/or neurological impairment, you may need the help of a speech therapist, physical or occupational therapist, or dietitian. Special spoons, bowls, and drinking cups are available to help toddlers and older children who have trouble feeding themselves. Your pediatrician can usually recommend one of these specialists, or you can check the Yellow Pages or call your local health department.

GETTING HELP

Parents may find that health care and support resources are not readily available. It can be very difficult to give a premature or low-birth-weight child the special care and attention she needs. Support services and frequent doctor visits can be expensive. Health care insurance may not cover consultations with a nutritionist or registered dietitian, or with physical and occupational therapists. If you have health insurance, always get your doctor's order for services/consultations before making appointments for such services.

Working parents will need to find special day care for a child who has special feeding needs. Social workers, occupational therapists, or dietitians may be able to recommend a qualified individual or child-care center.

Your child may qualify for special state and federal health care benefit programs designed to provide medical support for those with physical and/or mental disabilities. Public health programs also provide a variety of services through Title V of the Social Security Act, which established the Program for Children with Special Health Care Needs. This program is listed in the Blue Pages under federal agencies: "Health and Human Services Department of the Social Security Administration."

Some city and state public health agencies also provide for home visits by a public health nurse, social worker, and nutritionist. These agencies are listed in the Blue Pages under "Health Department." The city listing also gives the names of child health clinics and school health services, as well as lead-poisoning prevention centers. State health departments oversee maternal and child health programs and the WIC (Woman, Infants, and Children) Program.

Finally, some hospitals and clinics (and some health-care professionals in private practice) have created "feeding teams" to assist parents in learning how to feed children with physical and psychological problems. Be sure to ask your baby's pediatrician if such a team exists in your community.

If your child has special needs, whether because of prematurity, handicaps, development delays, or chronic illness, you will need to have realistic expectations about how he will grow and develop. While your child may eventually achieve normal or near-normal growth and development, you should learn what to expect early on. While feeding problems may be resolved by the time your baby becomes a toddler, this is not always the case. Eating problems can continue until adolescence.

The sooner you receive guidance from your health-care team, the better you can meet short- and long-term needs. The team can help you assess your child's developmental levels as they occur and adjust feeding techniques to meet different challenges as they arise.

As your child grows and matures, he should be an active part of the health-care team, too. Ultimately, only he can decide which foods are acceptable for him. Your role should always be supporting and guiding. When feeding problems seem insurmountable, try not to lose patience or force your child to eat. Remain positive. And if you need help, seek it.

13

FEEDING TODDLERS AND
PRESCHOOLERS

Active, energetic, and *curious* are words to describe preschoolers, and all are apt to apply to your child from now until she's out of the house and headed for school. After the first year, your child is walking and easily distracted, so you will have more of a challenge. You will find that being a patient, reasonable, and yet a firm teacher will go a long way toward achieving success in feeding your child. You're looking for a middle ground to help your child establish good attitudes about eating.

NUTRITION FACTS

Young African-American children enrolled in the Bogalusa Heart Study were reported to consume a higher total fat and cholesterol intake than white children. (The white children were reported to eat more complex carbohydrates.) So the amount of fat your child gets, even at this age, is important, since we know hardening of the arteries associated with fatty deposits begins in childhood.

Getting adequate amounts of calcium, vitamin D, iron, and vitamins A and C are crucial. A diet with plenty of fruits and vegetables will provide the vitamins A and C; low-fat milk (after age two) will take care of vitamin D.

All young children are at risk for iron-deficiency anemia, particularly low-income children or those eating a total vegetarian diet. Between the ages of one and three, your child will need 15 mg of iron each day. Good amounts of iron are found in meat, poultry, and fish. The best sources of iron are liver and red meats. However, liver may provide too much vitamin A for your child at this young age, and it should only be given occasionally until he's older.

HOW MANY CALORIES?

How many calories do your toddler and preschooler need? The average child in these age groups needs about:

Age	Calories per Pound	Calories per Day
1–3	46	1,300
4–6	41	1,800

Very active children may require slightly more calories. Carbohydrates should comprise from 50 to 60 percent of total calories; protein from 10 to 15 percent; and fat from 25 to 35 percent.

SERVING SIZES

Serving sizes for young children are obviously not the same as for an adolescent or an adult. A good rule of thumb is to use one-fourth to one-third the adult portion, or one tablespoon per each year of age. The following are the serving sizes recommended by the U.S. Department of Agriculture. Bear in mind these are approximate guidelines, and children vary in the amount of food they can eat. Start with a small serving and allow your toddler to tell you if she wants seconds.

Food	Age: 1–2 years	Age: 3–5 years
Milk, whole or low-fat (including chocolate milk)	½ cup	¾ cup
Cereals, enriched		
Cold cereals	¼ cup	⅓ cup
Cooked cereals	¼ cup	⅓ cup
Breads	½ slice	½ slice

Crackers	2–4	2–4
Rice, noodles, pasta	¼ cup	¼ cup
Fruit and fruit juice (Grapes and figs are not recommended for young children, since they may cause choking.)	¼ cup	½ cup
Vegetables (Bean sprouts and sauerkraut are not recommended for toddlers ages 1–3 for safety reasons.)	¼ cup	½ cup
Meats Beef, pork, lamb, organ meats	1 ounce	1½ ounces
Poultry Chicken, turkey, duck, turkey or chicken franks, low-fat luncheon meat	1 ounce	1½ ounces
Fish or shellfish Fresh, frozen, canned	1 ounce	1½ ounces
Eggs, white or brown	1	1
Cheese Hard or soft, cheese food spread, American, ricotta, cottage cheese	1 ounce	1½ ounces
Yogurt (snack serving)	¼ cup	¼ cup
Dried cooked peas and beans Garbanzo, kidney, black, mung, lima, navy, baked beans, lentils, black-eyed peas	¼ cup	⅜ cup
Nuts Smooth peanut butter (Other nuts and seeds are not recommended for children under age 5 because they may choke on these foods.)	2 tablespoons	3 tablespoons

How Many Servings Each Day?

Food Group	Minimum Servings	Key Nutrients
Breads, cereals, rice, pasta	6	Carbohydrates, thiamine, iron, niacin
Vegetables	3	Vitamin A, vitamin C
Fruits	2	Vitamin A, vitamin C
Milk, yogurt, cheese	3	Calcium, riboflavin, protein
Meat, poultry, fish, dried beans, eggs, smooth peanut butter (Other nuts and seeds are not recommended for children under age 5 because of choking hazard.)	2	Protein, niacin, iron, thiamine

TODDLERS: FROM ONE TO THREE YEARS

Between the ages of one and three, children begin to grasp and manipulate food better. They use eating utensils and can drink from a cup in a fairly steady manner. (Left- or right-handedness is established after the first year of age.) At first, a child may not do a great job at the table, and he will probably still have difficulty lifting and tilting a cup and lowering it to the table after drinking. But he'll enjoy practicing! Toddlers like to explore foods and they enjoy feeding themselves. They're interested in how foods feel, and therefore use their fingers more often than utensils. Expect mealtimes to be messy. As your child's strength and coordination improves, drips and dribbles gradually decrease.

About now, your child will develop food preferences. She may suddenly reject foods she used to like, and she may even lose interest in eating altogether. Don't worry; these tastes aren't fixed for life. Your child will not starve herself.

By now, you should have replaced formula with regular milk. Children over age two thrive on either whole or low-fat milk. (I don't recommend skim milk until after age three.) Two or three cups of milk meet most children's daily needs. If your child cannot tolerate the lactose in cow's milk, try goat's milk (which is easier to digest), or soy or nut milks. Each option supplies ample protein and calcium.

If your child simply objects to the taste of milk, try blending milk with fruit or adding it to soups, puddings, cooked cereal, and mashed potatoes.

What else should your child be eating? The watchword is still *variety;* concentrate on the largest section—bottom—of the food pyramid (complex carbohydrates: breads, cereals, starches, grains).

During these years, your child's favorite foods will be ones that are easy for him to handle. Many parents tell me that their toddlers enjoy meat, cereals, dairy products, baked goods, yogurt, fruits, and snacks such as cookies, crackers, and fruit juice.

MEALTIMES ARE HAPPY TIMES

Feeding your toddler should be done with a watchful eye, patience, and care. Communicating with him on his own level is just about as important as good nutrition. Allow your child to have his own plate, bowl, and cup. This encourages the sense that meals are happy times to look forward to. And even with very young children, take the time to choose attractive and colorful foods, as well as colorful, eye-catching place mats and table settings.

PRECAUTIONS

Because toddlers are willing and able to put *anything* in their mouths for the sake of exploration, you must keep a watchful eye on your child to prevent him from choking on foods or nonfood objects. Death from asphyxiation or choking is most common in children less than two years of age.

Foods most often responsible for choking include hot dogs, candy, nuts, and grapes. But children can choke on many types of foods, particularly if they are hard or slippery or if they're just the right size to plug or obstruct the opening of the throat. Choking occurs because the child cannot cough or bring the item back up into his mouth. Foods that are sticky and thick, like peanut butter, candy-coated foods (like caramel popcorn), and hard pieces of cheese can cause problems, too. To help prevent your child from choking, make certain that someone is always there to supervise mealtimes. Young children should not eat alone.

You should also insist that your child sit down while she is eating. This will help her to concentrate on chewing and swallowing without getting distracted. Choose well-cooked soft foods that are easy to swallow.

If your family frequently eats in the car, use extra caution when a very young child is aboard, because it may be difficult to help him or get to the side of the road quickly if he starts to choke.

Also be careful if you apply rub-on teething medications (which should only be used on your doctor's recommendation). These can sometimes cause a child's throat to become numb, which can hinder normal chewing and swallowing.

PRESCHOOLERS: FROM THREE TO SIX YEARS

If you and your child have gotten through the toddler stage with flying colors, the preschool years (between ages three and six) will seem like a breeze. After all of her striving to become independent, suddenly you have in your midst a child who is eager to learn. The preschooler is out to please you, as well as other grown-ups around her. Although your child isn't likely to sit back quietly and watch, she will start to think more logically and will try to act a bit more responsibly.

Now is a good time for you to set limits, while still offering plenty of encouragement and praise. She will spend lots of time moving around, shouting, running, and playing. That means she'll also be burning plenty of calories and will need a good supply of protein, calcium, vitamins A and C, and iron to help her body keep up with the extra demands all this motion requires.

Fruits and vegetables in her diet are especially important. If your child rejects vegetables, experiment with different ways of preparing them. Perhaps it's the taste of boiled veggies she doesn't like— try offering them raw, lightly steamed, or stir-fried instead. Kids in this age group prefer crispy rather than stringy vegetables. Sometimes a creamy sauce (made with buttermilk or low-fat yogurt) successfully disguises the taste or aroma of a dreaded vegetable. Ask

your child why she dislikes a particular food and then offer to prepare it some way she might like.

Preschoolers usually continue drinking milk, and two or three
glasses a day is still average, generally at breakfast, lunch, and as a
late-evening snack.

WHAT TO OFFER PRESCHOOLERS

Preschoolers love finger foods like chicken drumsticks and wings,
hot dogs, hamburgers, and fish sticks. Don't overdo it with spices
and messy sauces that can irritate young eyes and sensitive palates.
Don't be surprised if your child requests the same food over and
over, day after day. Food jags or preferences are common and they
disappear without intervention. Protein foods (including certain
meats) may fall out of favor now. Don't discourage your child from
eating the foods she likes; and don't overwhelm her by introducing
too many new tastes at once.

Most preschoolers enjoy grain-based foods like cereals, crackers,
and breads. Encourage your child to try grains with different flavors
and textures, including rice, amaranth, rye, pumpernickel, and oat.
Get him to taste cereals that aren't presweetened. Try topping them
with fresh fruit instead. Nut butters are a great complement for
grainy breads, and they have lots of protein and vitamins. Keep
peanut, almond, or sesame-seed butters in the pantry.

A good rule of thumb with kids this age is to keep it simple. Single foods are better than combinations like stews, casseroles, and
multiingredient soups. Preschoolers prefer foods they can identify,
each with its own distinct taste, texture, and color.

At the preschool age, your child is learning a lot about foods and
eating behavior. This is also the time when your child is being
exposed to social eating situations in and outside of the home. She
will mimic others' behavior, so this is a perfect opportunity to
introduce and reinforce table manners.

At this time, your child will discover many new foods never
tried before. Give her a chance to accept new foods gradually. But
don't be surprised if she becomes a finicky eater at this age. Be
thrilled if she takes as little as a bite or two. If she rejects a food the
first time, or even several times after it's offered, that doesn't mean
she will continue to reject it forever.

When I worked as a pediatric dietitian at a Washington, D.C., hospital, the foods served there were quite different from the food the kids were used to eating at home. This, combined with the fact that an ill child often is not interested in eating at all, made mealtimes difficult. Sometimes the overworked nursing staff would get impatient trying to get one child to eat.

I decided to try feeding the children as a group instead of singly. When one or two children would try new foods, particularly vegetables, the others would join in. You can duplicate this same behavior at home. If a young child's parents and siblings enjoy eating a variety of foods, sooner or later the child will try them, too.

Start out with small portions and allow your child to ask for seconds when the time is right. Also, be careful not to categorize foods as "good" or "bad," and never use certain foods as a reward or punishment for behavior.

Vegetarians. Vegetarian diets are high in fiber, which can be a bit hard on the digestive system of young children. Also, these higher-fiber diets are more filling and may cause your child to eat less food. The key in this age range is to encourage your vegetarian preschooler to drink plenty of water and juice. Dried fruits are good snacks for this age; they are nutritionally rich and loaded with iron. Since toddlers may be eating fewer calories, you'll want to make sure that everything they do eat is packed with vitamins and minerals. (See chapter 16.)

Snacking. Should you allow your preschooler to eat between meals? Certainly. Children's energy needs are high, and they are still growing by leaps and bounds. Two or three snacks during the day and one after dinner should do the trick.

Encourage snack foods with good nutritional value, and keep a vegetable or fruit bowl on the table or in the refrigerator. Keep these healthy snacks on hand:

> *Fruit (bananas, apple slices, strawberries, melon)*
> *Cereal with low-fat milk*
> *Bagels*
> *Graham crackers*
> *Low-fat yogurt*
> *Raw vegetable sticks (kids older than four)*

String cheese
Turkey slices
Vegetable soup

Although you may not be able to eliminate completely chips, candies, cakes, and high-sugar treats from your child's diet (particularly if he receives them in preschool or day care), you can bring him back to high-nutrition foods at home.

How much should you worry about sugar in your child's diet? You should be concerned, although not panicky, if your child occasionally eats foods that include sugar. Sugar is hard to avoid. Each American man, woman, and child eats or drinks an average of 130 pounds of sugar per year. This amounts to about one-quarter of a cup of sugar per person per day, and it means that about 24 percent of the calories in the average diet come from sugar.

Sugar has been blamed for several health-related problems. Some parents report that foods containing sugar make their children irritable and hyperactive. While research has not shown this to be the case for the majority of kids, it's certainly worth working with your child's dietitian and the people who supervise the school breakfast or lunch program to see if a difference does occur in behavior if sugar is eliminated for a period of time.

All experts agree on sugar's harmful effects on dental health. Sugar promotes tooth decay by supporting the growth of acid-growing bacteria in the mouth (see chapter 7).

The best way to keep a handle on the amount of sugar your child consumes is to use sugar sparingly wherever you can. For instance, you should avoid cereals that are coated with extra sugar, as well as those that get more than half of their total calories from sugar. But if your child has eaten a cereal with sugar for breakfast, simply make certain that lunch and dinner foods are low in sugar. Don't save sugary desserts as treats for good behavior or special occasions. If you do, your child will soon start thinking of sweetened foods as a reward.

If you wish to omit sugar completely from your child's diet, look out for ingredients on labels ending in *ose*. Sucrose and all those other words ending in *ose* are forms of sugar. The list also includes honey, corn syrup, corn-syrup solids, maple syrup, molasses, and cane syrup.

Some food manufacturers use artificial sweeteners in many foods, but I don't advise you to give these products to kids routinely. Instead, offer cereals, cookies, and other foods that are sweetened with dried fruits or fruit juices. There are plenty of cereals that use little or no sugar.

EASY TIPS FOR YOUNG KIDS

MILK AND DAIRY PRODUCTS

- Some children do not like ice-cold milk. Pour milk a short time before serving.
- If your child doesn't like milk, he can still get excellent calcium provisions by drinking low-fat chocolate milk, milk with cereal, or eating milk-based soups, low-fat yogurt, low-fat cheeses, custard, or cheese sauces over vegetables.

BREADS AND CEREALS

- Let children prepare their own sandwiches and cereals. They're more interested in food they make themselves.
- Select unsugared or only slightly sugared cereals.
- Add fresh fruit to cereals. Bananas and peaches are the best.
- Serve whole-grain cereals, breads, buns, and rolls to children over age two. (Children under two cannot tolerate these coarse grains.) Do not choose all-bran cereals or bran-added foods.
- Instead of sugary desserts, try low-fat blueberry muffins or raisin bread as dessert.

FRUITS AND VEGETABLES

- Use brightly colored fruits and vegetables.
- Serve crunchy vegetables to older children. (Do not give raw or hard pieces of vegetables or small pieces of fruit, such as grapes, to children younger than four years old. They can choke.)
- Serve older children raw vegetables with a low-fat plain yogurt dip.

- Serve vegetables separately. Most kids find combined vegetable dishes like succotash and carrots and peas revolting.

TIPS TO REDUCE FAT
(KIDS WILL NEVER NOTICE)

Serve the following:

> *Low-fat chicken or turkey hot dogs*
> *Lean luncheon meats, or chicken and turkey luncheon meats*
> *Tuna salad with low-fat mayonnaise*
> *Plain, lean hamburger with lettuce and tomato*
> *Baked potato with low-fat plain yogurt or low-fat or fat-free sour cream*
> *Bean burrito*
> *Low-fat pudding or frozen yogurt*
> *Unsalted pretzels*
> *Angel food cake*
> *Plain pizza*
> *Baked chicken*
> *Low-fat mayonnaise*
> *Low-fat cottage cheese*

EDUCATING KIDS ABOUT NUTRITION

Now is a good time to begin teaching your child about nutrition and the importance of eating a variety of foods. Start early—every child needs to understand why a diet like this is important for good health. Even if you work outside the home, it's well worth your while to find time to educate your child about nutrition. If your child is in day care, you may have to assert yourself a little more to be involved in what she eats away from home.

Out-of-home child care has a significant impact on a child's nutrition. Menus at child-care centers are usually planned by the center director or the cook, and some employ home economists or dietitians. The important thing is that menus are planned by someone who has basic nutrition training and knows its impact on the growth and health of young children. Currently, nutrition experts are trying to help establish national standards and criteria for planning child-care diets.

Talk to those involved in food service at your child's day-care center so that you know what your child will be served for meals and snacks throughout the day. Find out if the foods offered are part of a well-balanced diet and if they meet the growth and development needs of your child. Feel free to talk to the director of the center about your child's specific food preferences and any sensitivities he may have.

Some day-care centers provide lunch and two snacks (one mid-morning and one midafternoon). Toddlers and preschoolers usually enjoy sharing meals and snacks with their playmates, and day-care mealtimes often bring lots of fun and play. You should try to extend that pleasure to mealtimes at home.

14

KIDS GO TO SCHOOL: AGES SIX
THROUGH TWELVE

Children grow steadily between the ages of six and twelve, long ago dubbed "the formative years" by a clever advertiser. They're also more active because they have a lot more to do. As they grow, their need for calories increases. By the time your child is twelve years old, she will be consuming as many calories as most adults.

Going to school and meeting new friends who may have entirely different eating habits will be interesting for your child. Food preferences are now hugely influenced by other children, teachers, sports heroes, and television. Between-meal snacking will be hard for you to control now. And the most convenient and kid-friendly snacks are often low in nutrition and high in fat, salt, and sugar.

How can you keep kids on the right nutritional path when they're eating one or two meals away from home every day? I can't stress this enough: Preaching doesn't work.

Kids know more about nutrition than we think. According to a 1991 nationwide survey of fourth through eighth graders conducted by the International Food Information Council and the National Center for Nutrition and Dietetics, 94 percent of children agreed that the food they eat can affect their future health. Ninety percent were familiar with the basic food groups, and 80 percent could identify at least three groups. Their percentages were higher than adults polled in a similar survey! In a 1990 Gallup poll, only 77 percent of adults knew the food groups, and only 55 percent could name three.

Of great concern in both surveys was the notion that certain foods were labeled intrinsically "good" or "bad." Parents influence children to believe some foods must be shunned because they're "bad"—and most kids (65 percent) said they were sick of hearing about it.

Food isn't good or evil. Certain methods of preparation are more or less nutritious, but all foods can be enjoyed in moderation and all foods can be included as part of a healthy diet. Since preaching doesn't work, lighten up. Let kids enjoy the foods they like and let them see how you prepare meals and manage your own portions.

Unfortunately, a new 1995 survey of 3,112 children in grades two through six, showed that a general acquaintance with food groups did not always translate into eating adequate amounts of the foods most recommended. Twenty-five percent of the children surveyed had eaten no fruit and 25 percent had eaten no vegetables the previous day. Forty-eight percent said they thought apple juice, which contains no fat, has more fat than whole milk, which has a lot. Moreover, 36 percent said watermelon has more fat than American cheese. The survey was conducted by the American Health Foundation, a private New York–based research organization, and Scholastic, Inc., a publisher. The survey's sponsors say the message is clear: Bad health habits as well as good ones start early.

If you allowed your young child the freedom to explore new foods, he will continue to do so now. With a little luck and reinforcement, your child's good food choices and table manners will carry over to school. A school-aged child is ready for much more independence, yet good nutrition guidance still comes from home. If each of you gives and takes a little, the new information and behavior coming into the house from the school environment shouldn't cause problems. Planning family meals together is a particular joy for this age group. Remember, everything you do together and talk about together is valuable and leaves an indelible impression.

One vital element of building healthy bodies is exercise, and this is the perfect time to instill good exercise habits in your child. Even though your child needs a lot of calories, physical activity is important to balance any excesses. Nevertheless, many kids return from school and plop down in front of the television or Nintendo screen, turn up the stereo full blast, or talk on the telephone (or do all four at the same time). Encourage your child to get outdoors and play outdoor games and sports with friends and family. Check out the youth clubs in your area. Some offer sports programs or at least supervision on public playgrounds. In some areas, it may not be easy to find after-school athletic programs, but it usually isn't impossible. Ask at your child's school or look in the Yellow Pages under "Youth Organizations and Centers."

NUTRITION FACTS

How Many Calories?

Age	Calories per Pound	Calories per Day
7–10	32	2,000
Boys: 11–12	25	2,500
Girls: 11–12	21	2,200

Very active children who regularly participate in exercise or sports may require more calories.

SERVING SIZES

Serving sizes increase in this age group. Here are the basic categories and serving sizes recommended by the U.S. Department of Agriculture. Bear in mind that these are approximate amounts. Serving sizes given here are for lunch or dinner. Amounts for snacks and breakfast may be smaller. Skim milk and other low-fat or non-fat dairy products are recommended for this age group.

Food	Amount
Milk	
Whole, low-fat, skim	1 cup
Buttermilk	1 cup
Chocolate milk	1 cup
Cereals	
Cold cereals	¾ cup
Hot cereals	½ cup
Breads	1 slice

Crackers	4–8
Rice, noodles, pasta	½ cup
Fruit and fruit juice	¾ cup
Vegetables	¾ cup
Meats Beef, pork, lamb, organ meats	2 ounces

Poultry
   Chicken, turkey, duck, turkey or
   chicken franks, low-fat luncheon meat
	2 ounces

Fish or shellfish Fresh, frozen, canned	2 ounces
Eggs, white or brown	1

Cheese
   Hard or soft, cheese spread, American,
   ricotta, cottage cheese
	2 ounces

Yogurt (snack serving)	½ cup

Dried cooked peas and beans
   Garbanzo, kidney, black, mung, lima,
   navy, baked beans, lentils, black-eyed peas
	½ cup

Nuts and seeds
   Peanut butter
   Various nuts and seeds
	
	4 tablespoons
	1 ounce

Number of Servings Each Day

Food Group	Minimum Servings	Key Nutrients
Breads, cereals, rice, pasta	6–11	Carbohydrates, thiamine, iron, niacin
Vegetables	3–5	Vitamin A, vitamin C
Fruits	3 or more	Vitamin A, vitamin C
Milk, yogurt, cheese	3–4	Calcium, riboflavin, protein
Meat, poultry, fish, dried beans, eggs, nuts	2	Protein, niacin, iron, thiamine

WHY IS BREAKFAST SO IMPORTANT?

Breakfast is an important meal for everyone, particularly for school-children, who must maintain alertness in a learning environment.

Breakfast should contribute at least one-fourth of the RDA for each day. Your school-age child has a lot to do before lunch, and breakfast provides the energy he will need for all of his morning activities. According to the U.S. Department of Agriculture (Continuing Survey of Food Intakes by Individuals, 1989–1992), children who eat breakfast consistently receive a greater amount of all nutrients than children who skip breakfast. In other words, kids who do not eat breakfast do not make up important vitamins and minerals later in the day.

When they're young, African-American kids actually do pretty well at the breakfast table. The survey reports that below the age of eleven, 92 percent of African-American children are eating breakfast, although slightly more than half are eating high-fat breakfasts. Those who stuck to ready-to-eat cereals consumed less fat, and more vitamin A, more of all the B vitamins, and more calcium. The additional calcium is presumed to come from the milk accompanying the cereal. The survey concluded that eating cereal in the morning increases a child's nutrients and reduces overall fat consumption.

Offer your child quick and easy choices, such as ready-to-eat cereal, hot cereal, bagels, toast, frozen waffles, low-fat breakfast bars, and fresh fruits and juices. Most school-aged children can prepare their own breakfast as long as the groceries are in the house.

SCHOOL BREAKFAST AND LUNCH PROGRAMS

Parents who don't have the means or the time to provide breakfast for a child may get help at school. In 1966, the School Breakfast Program was initiated by the U.S. Department of Agriculture. The program has been supported locally by many consumer groups and has slowly expanded since it began. Some states passed legislation requiring breakfast programs in school districts where a high percentage of children come from low-income families. In 1991, more than half of the schools participating in low-cost or free lunch programs were also offering breakfast. Once established, breakfast and lunch programs are open to all students, regardless of family income.

Over the years, school lunch programs have been criticized because their menus have not always met the nutritional needs of children, and they've also been high in fat, sodium, cholesterol, and sugar. School lunch menus are intended to meet the guidelines set by the National School Lunch Program, yet budget cuts and poor planning sometimes contribute to shortcomings. The American School Food Service Association is working hard to implement the Dietary Guidelines for Americans (reflected in the new food pyramid) and act on all of the nutrition-related objectives of Healthy People 2000, the national health goals set by the federal government for the next five years.

School lunch planners (dietitians and food-service managers) say it's tough to focus on nutritious foods because kids won't eat them. Kids themselves say they like food to look good and taste good, and they also want a variety of foods to choose from. Some schools have hired outside restaurants or vendors to make meals more appealing, and others have expanded food choices by getting kids involved in planning menus.

Bringing lunch boxes or brown-bag lunches from home is largely a thing of the past. However, kids and parents can participate in menu planning by offering suggestions to cafeteria managers. (Be alert for anticipated budget cuts at federal and state levels, which may reduce or eliminate school breakfast and lunch programs.)

In any event, you can make sure your child knows how to select healthy foods from school and restaurant menus.

GOOD MENU CHOICES

Choose Most Often	Choose Occasionally
Baked potato	French fries
Low-fat yogurt/milk shakes	Ice cream and milk shakes made with whole milk
Baked or grilled chicken/fish	Fried chicken/fried fish
Bagels, English muffins, whole-grain, low-fat muffins	Doughnuts, Danish pastries, croissants

Graham crackers, animal crackers, vanilla wafers, fig bars	Chocolate-chip cookies, cupcakes, cream-filled cookies
Pretzels, air-popped popcorn, rice cakes	Potato chips, corn chips, crackers with peanut butter or cheese

AFTER-SCHOOL SNACKS

As we've said in earlier chapters, snacking makes up an important part of every child's nutrition. Children have high energy needs and need to eat frequently. If the foods chosen are healthy, snacks are an excellent way for our kids to get all the nutrients they need.

All kids are hungry after school. Instead of keeping a supply of high-sugar, high-fat bakery products on hand (or chips, candy, and soda pop), stock the house with fruits, whole-grain low-fat crackers, nut butters, dried fruits, rice cakes, and fruit-sweetened cookies. You never know—your child might even enjoy munching on crisp carrot sticks, celery, or cucumber wedges.

DINNER

Dinner is an important time for the family to get together. If you take time in planning menus, dress up the table occasionally, and get the kids involved in both, dinner will be a time to look forward to.

According to the Harris poll for Dixie Kids Everyday Paperware, the majority of kids interviewed said that breakfast was boring, lunch was "lusterless," and dinner was dull. What a trio of meals to look forward to!

This needn't be the case at your house. With a little effort, even the smallest or simplest meals can be enjoyed. Offer a variety of foods for dinner, and increase the amount of food according to your child's fast-growing needs.

HIGH-FAT TV

Between preschool and junior high, most American children spend between twenty-four to twenty-seven hours per week watching television. This means that the average child is watching about three hours of food commercials each week, or approximately 19,000 to

22,000 commercials per year. The most frequently advertised product is sugared cereals, and there are few positive messages regarding nutrition on television.

The first positive nutrition message aimed at children has been produced by McDonald's Corporation and the Society for Nutrition Education. These public-service messages appear in between regular Saturday-morning shows and are aired nationwide on CBS affiliates. The nutrition-related "What's on Your Plate" message features clay-animated characters. They are upbeat, fun, and colorful, with simple messages that young children can comprehend. More positive efforts like this are gravely needed.

ROLE MODELS

Parents must be healthy-eating role models for children. How you choose or reject foods in your own diet will influence how your child chooses or rejects those same foods.

My mother and father did not like asparagus, beets, cauliflower, or squash, so we never had a chance to enjoy these foods when I was a young child. It wasn't until I went away to college that I finally tried them. I expected them to taste awful, but, much to my surprise, they were good. I admit that I still don't eat asparagus very often; I think this is largely due to the negative feelings that were fostered early on in my childhood.

I try not to be preachy about nutrition with my stepsons, although I always keep a variety of nutritious foods available in the house. If you are a stepparent, you know that eating habits differ from one household to another. If more nutritious foods are featured at your house, you won't get anywhere by criticizing the food available at your child's other household. In the long run, children exposed to a variety of foods will generally try them out and form their own opinions.

DIETING

After your child has been in school for several years, you're in for another surprise. Suddenly, you'll hear her start talking about dieting. Studies have shown that girls as young as nine, ten, and eleven years old are dieting to lose weight. At the same time, these girls are

KEEPING SCHOOL-AGE KIDS ON THE GOOD NUTRITION TRACK

- *To boost realistic nutrition awareness, talk with your child and keep a record of what he's eating on a daily basis.*

- *Skip the negative comments ("Your trouble is you eat too much junk!") and emphasize the positive ("Let's try for five citrus fruits this week!").*

- *Keep the pantry stocked with fruits, raw vegetables, nuts, and whole-grain snacks. When it comes to low-nutrition snacks, "out of sight, out of mind" often works.*

- *Don't scold. Encourage good eating habits, but be willing to compromise sometimes. Moderation is the key to success.*

- *Change recipes. If your child feels certain foods are unappealing, treat him (and yourself) to a new version. Vary cooking styles, spices, and combinations.*

- *Allow your child to help you shop for food and learn to read package labels on food.*

- *Teach your child to cook, or let him assist you. Give him chores like chopping and peeling vegetables. Acquaint him with your favorite recipes and give him one special food to prepare for the family meal. I admit this is easier to do with girls, but boys who have a male role model who cooks will join right in. If you don't have such a male at your house, find other opportunities for your son to observe a man who enjoys working around the kitchen.*

- *Watch the soft drinks. Encourage water or juice instead. Blended juices are good-tasting and nutritious, and they offer a festive change from carbonated beverages.*

exercising less. When a couch potato hits puberty, the result is often a full-blown case of the "I'm too fat" blues. Don't panic unless you observe behavior that suggests an eating disorder. (See chapter 20.)

Your boy or girl may be carrying a little extra body fat as puberty approaches. Reassure a child that this is normal growth and development and that excess fat is likely to go away as energy needs and activity increase. Don't start children on low-calorie diets at this age, unless they are so obese that it interferes with their normal activity or worsens an existing health problem. If you feel a diet is necessary, seek the advice of a registered dietitian or nutritionist first.

Continue to encourage your child to play sports and engage in other activities that offer daily physical exercise. Check menus and look for more ways to reduce the amount of fat, sodium, and sugar in recipes and cooking methods. These combined efforts will curb any tendency to gain excess weight.

15

NUTRITION FOR TEENAGERS: AGES TWELVE THROUGH NINETEEN

Adolescence is one of the most challenging periods of human development. After a period of slow growth in late childhood, the adolescent begins changing very rapidly. His body is growing so fast, you probably wonder if your teenager will ever stop eating—or growing. It's always amazing to me to see how much food my teenaged sons are eating. I mean *huge* amounts. When we eat out with the two of them, the table is covered from end to end with plates. They eat everything on every plate; then one or two hours later, they're ready to eat again. They are both already over six feet tall, and not overweight. This is completely typical. Most adolescents gain 20 percent of their adult height and 50 percent of their adult weight during this time. Body composition also changes. Both fat and muscle (lean body mass) increase along with sexual development.

For all of these reasons, adolescence is also a time when a child's nutritional needs shift. More calories and more nutrients are needed to nourish the adolescent growth spurt. Unfortunately, social pressures and changing eating habits make teenagers less likely than ever to get adequate amounts of nutrients in the food they choose.

WHAT IS YOUR TEENAGER EATING?
AND WHY?

Many parents see their teenager eating a *lot*—and thus they assume he is getting all the nutrition he needs. That's often not true. The biggest problem facing teens is overconsumption of calories and fat. The trouble lies in the kinds of foods teenagers choose. Teens are eating most of their food away from home, and their choices frequently are dominated by their friends. Peer pressure is a very strong factor at this age. Teens want to fit in; anyone who's different in the teen world is subject to ridicule.

All of this is made worse for teens who live below the poverty level. Young teenagers who don't get enough nutritious food may suffer from iron-deficiency anemia, which is especially prevalent among adolescent females. Adolescents are also prone to folic acid (folate) deficiency. Researchers in the National Health and Nutrition Examination Survey (NHANES II) found this deficiency most common among girls between the ages of ten and nineteen. Teenagers may also be getting inadequate amounts of calcium, B vitamins, vitamins A and D, and zinc.

Another factor affecting your adolescent's food choices is stress. Adolescence has never been an easy time. Teens have always felt pressure about their body image, scholastic and athletic achievements, relationships with friends and family, finances, career decisions, sexual changes, and coming to terms with their new adult self-image. But today's teens suffer from more stress than any other generation in history. When we were teenagers, we didn't worry that our fellow students were armed and dangerous. Drugs may have been around, but, unlike today, they were not as prevalent as schoolbooks.

Be aware of the stress in your teenager's life, and be careful not to add to it through unreasonable expectations and criticism. Try to be supportive, open-minded, and engaged instead of focusing on shortcomings. We can all afford to give our expectations a reality check and to offer positive reinforcement rather than additional pressure. (See chapter 19.)

Weight control also takes on new implications in this age group. Weight gain is a potentially serious health problem for African-American girls. For reasons no one can pinpoint, black women are likely to gain significant amounts of weight between the ages of twenty and forty-five, which increases the risk of developing diabetes, hypertension, heart disease, and other health problems. It's therefore important for *teenage* girls to learn how to control their weight (and keep it within normal range) before they start gaining extra pounds. Teaching adolescent girls positive-body-image weight control can enhance their health and forestall weight-related health disorders in later life.

Parents have to be aware of the tremendous pressure both boys and girls are under concerning their body image. As their bodies quickly change, teens often become uncomfortable with themselves. Teenagers are obsessed with their appearance. Every teenager wrestles with these particular fears, but some become overwhelmed. Your child may feel pressure to have a "perfect" body and he may go to extreme lengths to achieve it. Studies show that more than one-half of all adolescents are on self-imposed diets, although fewer than one-third are actually overweight.

Say your teenager decides one morning she's going on a diet. She skips breakfast, maybe even skips lunch, and by midafternoon she's so hungry, she binges on every high-fat, sugary, salty food she can get her hands on. This is what the average teen calls dieting. They think, Skip meals and save calories. They forget that one single high-fat and high-sugar meal can supply a whole day's worth of calories.

Such unsound dieting may interfere with growth and lead to dangerous eating disorders. Until recently, eating disorders (like anorexia and bulimia) were seen almost exclusively among upper-middle-class white female teens, but that picture is changing, and African-American teens are by no means immune to this problem.

If your teen thinks she's overweight, don't leave it to her to work out a sensible weight-reduction plan. A registered dietician (R.D.) or nutritionist can help create a food plan that includes many of her favorite foods, as well as appropriate amounts of calories and nutrients for growth and development.

If you suspect your adolescent is already suffering from anorexia, bulimia, or bulimarexia (the combination of both), inform her doctor and seek appropriate treatment. This should be a team effort involving a psychotherapist, registered dietitian, and physician. (See chapter 20.)

WHAT'S THE GOOD NEWS?

I'll tell you up front: It's not easy to convince adolescents to eat a healthy diet, especially when peer pressure is so high. Nutritionists like me have an even harder time with their own teenagers. It's typical for our teens to rebel and eat the complete opposite of what they know they should. Lecturing about nutrition doesn't work in my household, and from what other parents tell me, it probably won't work in yours, either. But this doesn't mean that you will always lose, especially if you have laid the groundwork in earlier years and set a good example yourself.

I maintain my own selection of foods and have them in the house for everyone. After several years of doing this, I have started finding my sons and my husband eating "my" rice cakes, trail mixes, fat-free salad dressings, and fat-free cookies. When the boys are with us, I notice we're always running out of "Barb's health foods."

GETTING THE MESSAGE

Continuing to eat a variety of foods with good nutritional value is crucial, and education about nutrition and health *can* positively influence the food choices a teenager makes. Teenage boys often get excited about nutrition because they want to start building a muscular body to excel in sports. Many girls will get interested in nutrition because they don't want to gain weight. So there is a window of opportunity in an adolescent's life where nutrition education can slip through.

Unfortunately, most of the media messages aimed at teens concentrate on soft drinks, burgers and fries, and a host of sugary, salty, and fatty fried foods—all being lavishly consumed by slender girls in bikinis and boys whose bodies ripple with muscles. The few healthful foods anyone is likely to see advertised on television are cereal, milk, and yogurt—and even these seem to be aimed at small children or health-conscious adults. I haven't seen any ads featuring black teens eating cereal and skim milk with fruit. In fact, black teens are often seen in commercials eating large sandwiches, chips and other snacks, and drinking soft drinks. Teens are exposed to some nutrition information through school courses in health or home economics, but there's little nutrition information aimed at African-American youth in the media.

Try to sit down to breakfast or dinner with your teenagers. Maintaining mealtimes takes some doing. Rather than leaving it loose—"Be here if you can make it"—make it a family rule for everyone (including you) to eat breakfast and dinner at home. A firm rule is useful. It gives teens something to complain about to their friends ("Aw, my mom says I have to be home for dinner").

Your teenaged daughter may be more apt to skip meals than your son, but insist that everyone show up. Even if dinner is take-out, sit down at the dinner table and eat as a family. The dinner table is a great setting for reviewing the day's events. Include your teenager in the process of menu planning, shopping, and meal preparation, encouraging his input even when it's unorthodox.

If conflicting schedules make it impossible to get everyone to the dinner table at the same time every evening, set a schedule of several nights each week that are always family night. Encourage your teen to bring a friend to dinner, or have a friend sleep over and share breakfast.

While it doesn't do any good to lecture kids, it does help to set a good example. A parent's self-example is important for children of every age, but it's absolutely vital for teenagers. Parents trying to change a teen's eating habits may need more time and patience, but even the worst food habits will eventually turn around.

HEALTHY TIPS FOR TEENS

These are the points to get across to your teenagers:

- *Eat a variety of different foods each day.*
- *Eat more whole-grain breads and cereals, as well as fruits and vegetables.*
- *Keep moving. Exercise to stay in shape.*
- *Remember the power of moderation.*
- *Choose nutritious snacks.*
- *Start each day with a good breakfast.*
- *Don't diet without professional supervision.*

NUTRITION FACTS

Every teen should consume between 39 and 56 gm of protein a day, which means three or more servings of foods like milk, cheese, eggs, fish, meat, and other high-protein foods.

Calcium is crucial. About 45 percent of total bone growth occurs during the adolescent period. Calcium requirements are higher during adolescence than at any other time of life except pregnancy. Calcium deficiencies in this age group are often caused by the dietary substitution of carbonated beverages for milk. However, calcium needs can easily be met by other low-fat and skim dairy products. Nuts, seeds, green vegetables, canned salmon, and sardines with bones will also contribute to satisfying overall calcium needs.

BOYS AND GIRLS

The nutritional needs of adolescent boys are higher than those of girls. Boys hit their growth spurt later than girls, but when they do, they grow even faster and are also building more muscle. They need greater amounts of B vitamins (thiamine, riboflavin, and niacin), and vitamins A and E. These can be gotten from additional servings of carbohydrates (particularly whole-grain breads and cereals) and larger portions of meat, poultry, and fish.

Girls, on the other hand, need more iron. Adolescent girls lose a small amount of blood during each menstrual period, which means they lose a certain amount of iron. Encourage your teenage girl to eat foods high in iron and vitamin C (which enables the body to absorb iron better). She should choose from lean meat, fish, and poultry, green leafy vegetables, dried beans, and iron-fortified breakfast cereals. Good sources of vitamin C include oranges, strawberries, red and green peppers, cantaloupe, tomatoes, broccoli, cabbage, and cauliflower.

How Many Calories?

Age	Calories per Pound	Calories per Day
Boys: 12–14	25	2,500
Girls: 12–14	22	2,200
Boys: 15–18	22	3,000
Girls: 15–18	18	2,200

SNACKS FOR TEENS

Theoretically, in this period of rapid growth, numerous small meals are healthier than a few large ones. Moderate snacking doesn't seem to spoil a teenager's appetite. In fact, it's much easier to meet a teenager's increased need for calories and other nutrients with frequent snacks. Nevertheless, you probably hope your kid will choose air-popped popcorn over greasy chips, or an apple over apple pie.

To some extent at least, hungry teenagers eat whatever's available. Keep raw vegetables, rice cakes, crackers, and fresh fruits and juices around the house. The *less* you say about eating them, the better. If your teens are already used to eating these kinds of foods, they'll certainly continue to eat them now. Even if healthy snacks are new to them, they'll eat them anyway, because *teenagers are always hungry.*

QUICK-SERVICE RESTAURANTS

Teenagers are big consumers of foods from quick-service restaurants, convenience stores, and vending machines. Fortunately, quick service today has come a long way. Menus have expanded, and customers are now able to choose from steamed and broiled foods, more vegetables and fruit juices, low-fat dairy products, and whole-grain breads. Some vending machines sport a variety of items including yogurt, dried fruits, fresh fruit, milk, and low-fat muffins, and special efforts have been made to have these machines placed in schools.

None of this guarantees that your child is grazing at the salad bar instead of munching on a burger and fries, but at least it's possible. Don't be alarmed if your teen chooses quick-service restaurants. If your teenager's *overall* diet meets the important nutritional guidelines, quick-service restaurants are popular places for teens to meet friends, the food is tasty and served in a flash, and the price is right. As long as kids are not eating the same foods every day in the same restaurants, you can be reassured that variety (and maybe even an occasional trip to the salad bar) can be achieved.

YOUR VEGETARIAN TEEN

It's not unusual for children to change their food preferences as they grow up. In one sense, they are simply declaring their status as separate individuals who can operate autonomously. They are also apt to be highly conscious of the environment and other animal life. When it comes to these issues, teenagers are often better informed than adults.

For these and many other reasons, it's not unusual for teens to pursue a vegetarian diet, which may be a temporary or permanent dietary change. If your child chooses to become a vegetarian and the rest of the family isn't, make sure that you educate yourself—and your child—about vegetarian eating and cooking so that his diet is sound.

A vegetarian teen may have some information about various vegetarian diets or he may be flying blind. He may or may not feel confident about making choices. But you can and should be supportive if he wants to try. If you do most of the family cooking, you can help by adding more vegetable and grain dishes. (The meat eaters in your family will benefit from these additions, too.) Your teenager can and should help you by looking for new recipes, taking responsibility for choosing what he wants to eat, helping with the grocery shopping, and helping out in the kitchen. (If your teenager doesn't go grocery shopping with you, he should at least make sure that the foods he chooses wind up on the grocery list. This is true of all children in the family, regardless of their food preferences.) (See chapters 9 and 16.)

When it comes to nutrition, the adolescent years can be trying times for parents. The effort you devoted to teaching your young child about nutrition may really pay off now—or good eating habits may temporarily disappear. Teenagers, like adults, want to do things their own way. Place the emphasis on variety, a wide range of foods, and encourage any physical activity your teenager is interested in. Make healthy eating and fitness a family affair without making a big fuss. (See chapter 21.)

16

Your Vegetarian Child

A 1992 survey revealed that over 12 million Americans consider themselves vegetarians. Although increasingly popular today, vegetarianism is not new. For centuries, people all over the world have subsisted on a near-vegetarian diet. In Africa, our own ancestors understood the benefits of foods that enhanced digestion and improved health; their diets were high in fiber and whole grains, as well as in native-grown fruits and vegetables. Meats and other animal foods were eaten much less frequently, probably because of limited availability. After several decades of encouraging red meat, cheese, and other high-fat foods, modern health experts of every kind are recommending the old nutritional wisdom of our forefathers and mothers.

Many African Americans find it familiar and appealing to turn back toward diets that contain little or no animal foods.

If you have chosen this way of eating, chances are you will want to raise your children the same way. New parents often wonder whether a young child can grow and develop normally on a vegetarian diet. Friends and family members may be telling you that feeding children a vegetarian diet deprives them of nutrients essential for growth.

The fact is, eating mostly fruits, vegetables, legumes, and grains can be healthy for children, as long as milk, other dairy products, and eggs are included. If they are not, it is more difficult (although not impossible) to plan meals that provide adequate nutrition, especially for a toddler.

Without dairy products, children cannot get enough calcium for bones and teeth or enough iron to support the development of red blood cells. Moreover, preschoolers who eat fruits, vegetables, and grains exclusively may not get enough calories to meet their basic energy needs.

To plan a sound vegetarian diet for a child, you need to know which foods contain which nutrients and how to balance foods in combinations that offer the best nutritional package. In the following pages, I will give you suggestions for feeding vegetarian children from infancy to adolescence. We'll also discuss how to educate your child to make healthy choices on his own.

WHY BE A VEGETARIAN?

The reasons someone chooses to become a vegetarian usually dictate which form of vegetarianism she will practice and how restrictive the diet is. Many people become vegetarians because they wish to live and eat more healthfully. They may be trying to lower the amount of fat in their diets to lose weight, lower cholesterol, or to protect themselves against certain forms of cancer, arthritis, and heart disease.

Some vegetarians are concerned about the humane treatment of animals and the preservation of the environment. They may abandon eating meat, and they may also avoid clothing and various other products that use animals for testing.

Muslims and Seventh-Day Adventists choose vegetarianism because of religious and spiritual convictions. They cite biblical guidance as a reason for abstaining from eating meat and other animal foods, although some allow dairy products in moderation.

Bearing in mind the various reasons for choosing vegetarianism, let me summarize the different categories:

Zen macrobiotics follows a grain and vegetable diet that in its original form progressively leads to eating primarily brown rice. Today, however, the American practice of macrobiotics has widened its scope to include significant amounts of specific vegetables.

Vegans rely on grains, fruits, vegetables, nuts, and seeds exclusively. Because they do not include any meat or animal products in their diets, vegans call themselves true, or pure, vegetarians.

Fruitarians eat only fresh and dried fruits, nuts, honey, and sometimes olive oil. They do not eat grains, vegetables, milk, or meat products.

Lactovegetarians allow milk, cheese, yogurt, and other milk products, but exclude all other sources of animal proteins.

Ovovegetarians allow eggs but exclude dairy or milk products and all other sources of animal protein.

Lacto-ovovegetarians allow eggs, milk, and other dairy products but do not eat other sources of animal protein.

There are several other subsets of vegetarians. Those who allow fish are called *pescovegetarians*, and those who allow poultry are called *pollovegetarians*. Those who abstain from eating red meat may allow fish, seafood, and poultry, however.

For many years, traditional dietitians, nutritionists, and physicians did not consider vegetarian diets nutritionally sound. But thanks to impressive modern research, we've learned that this past position was inaccurate with regard to most vegetarian diets.

In July of 1980, the American Dietetic Association changed its official position on the vegetarian approach to eating. The association now recognizes that "well-planned vegetarian diets are consistent with good nutrition status." The key words are *well-planned,* particularly when it comes to children and adolescents, whose nutritional needs are greater than those of adults.

Vegetarian diets that do not allow *any* animal products or fish (in other words, no milk, other dairy products, or eggs) require more careful planning in order to meet the nutritional needs of children. Nutritional supplements are often needed to provide important vitamins and minerals and adequate amounts of protein.

Fruitarian and Zen macrobiotic diets pose even more problems. Neither of these diets can meet the needs of children, and I do not recommend them, even when nutritional supplements are added. Nonetheless, Zen macrobiotics is part of a philosophy, and macrobiotic practitioners adhere to their own nutritional guidelines for children. It is not unusual for them to disagree with Western nutritionists. Individuals who follow the principles of macrobiotics are usually fully aware of the nutritional drawbacks associated with the diet, but they see other rewards that we do not.

If you choose a fruitarian or Zen macrobiotic diet for yourself, be very cautious about choosing it for your children. If you're serious about raising your child this way, consult with an experienced practitioner of the diet, and also a registered dietitian/nutritionist. Be open enough to listen to different points of view and educate yourself thoroughly before proceeding.

Let's look at the nutrients that require special attention in any vegetarian diet, particularly diets that exclude milk and milk products and eggs.

QUALITY PROTEIN

Vegetarian diets that include milk and milk products, eggs, and some fish or poultry easily provide enough protein for children, as much as any diet featuring red meat. The more restricted the diet, however, the more you have to rely on plant proteins.

Plant proteins do not have the same nutritional value as animal proteins. Animal proteins are complete, meaning that they contain all eight of the essential amino acids. Plant proteins are missing various amino acids. However, as experienced vegetarians know, if the right plant sources are eaten together or in the same day, the mixture can provide all the essential amino acids, just as meat, eggs, or milk do.

For example, beans are low in the amino acid methionine, but they are adequate in another, lysine. The reverse is true of wheat, rice, and corn. If you combine beans with any one of these three grains, the result is a fully balanced complete protein.

Here are the categories of vegetable proteins, followed by a summary of their balanced combinations.

CATEGORIES OF VEGETABLE PROTEINS

Grains
> *Barley, buckwheat, bulgur, corn, millet, oats, rice, rye, and wheat*

Legumes
> *Beans (black, broad, kidney, lima, mung, navy, peas, soy), black-eyed peas (cowpeas), chickpeas (garbanzo beans), lentils, peanuts*

Seeds
> *Pumpkin, sesame, squash, sunflower*

Nuts
> *Almonds, Brazil nuts, cashews, coconut, filberts, macadamia nuts, pecans, pine nuts, pistachio nuts, walnuts*

BALANCED PROTEIN COMBINATIONS

- Combine legumes with grains.
- Combine legumes with nuts and/or seeds.
- Combine eggs or dairy products with any vegetable protein.
- Combine nuts with wheat, oats, corn, or rice.

CALCIUM

Everybody knows that children get most of their calcium from dairy products. It's true that other foods besides dairy products also contain calcium. Other foods relatively high in calcium include:

> *Fortified soy formula*
> *Fortified soy milk*
> *Legumes*
> *Tofu*
> *Sesame seeds*
> *Dark green leafy vegetables*
> *Broccoli*
> *Almonds*

It's very difficult for a growing child to consume these foods in amounts large enough to get adequate calcium. Therefore, if the vegetarian diet you have chosen excludes dairy products, consult a nutritionist who will assess the amount of calcium your child is getting. Calcium supplements may be necessary to compensate for missing dairy products.

IRON

Meat products are the best known sources of iron, but iron can also be found in plant foods. Grains, fortified cereals, breads, some nuts, and dried fruits are good sources of iron. Legumes, green leafy vegetables, and other vegetables also contain iron.

The problem is that only about 3 to 8 percent of the iron in vegetables and grains is absorbed by the body (versus 20 percent of the iron in meat, poultry, and fish).

Obviously, the human body gets no benefit from what it doesn't absorb. How can you help increase iron absorption? The best way is to combine iron-rich vegetables and grains with foods high in vitamin C. Vitamin C helps your child's body use and absorb iron more efficiently. Iron-fortified cereal combined with fruit is a perfect example. (A glass of fruit juice along with a bowl of cereal will get the same result.) Adding grapefruit sections to green salads achieves a similar effect.

Iron absorption is also improved by reducing or eliminating the amount of sugar your child is eating. Finally, always choose iron-fortified packaged foods, such as bread and cereal, over regular ones.

OTHER VITAMINS AND MINERALS IMPORTANT IN VEGETARIAN DIETS

RIBOFLAVIN

This B vitamin can be lacking in vegetarian diets that do not contain milk. Legumes, whole grains, breads, cereals, vegetables, and fortified foods can help provide riboflavin. Some soy milks are fortified with both riboflavin and vitamin D.

VITAMIN B_{12}

Of all the nutrients that might be missing in a vegetarian diet, vitamin B_{12} is the one you hear about most. There are no known vegetables that provide vitamin B_{12}.

Vitamin B_{12} is produced by microorganisms in the gut, then absorbed by animals and secreted in their milk or eggs, or stored in their body tissues. It's important that vegan diets use products fortified with this vitamin. Soybean milk and soya meats fortified with vitamin B_{12} usually can be found in health-food stores and in the specialty foods section of supermarkets.

ZINC

Zinc is another nutrient that is found mostly in meat and meat products. However, nuts, beans, wheat germ, and cheese eaten on a regular basis can provide adequate amounts of zinc. Watch out for the excess *phytates* in zinc-containing foods like whole grains and nuts, though. The phytates can actually interfere with zinc absorption. Unleavened breads contain more phytates than regular breads made with yeast.

VEGETARIAN SERVING SIZES FOR VARIOUS AGE GROUPS

Foods	Ages		
	1–2 years	*3–5 years*	*6–12 years*
Milk	½ cup	¾ cup	1 cup
Cheese	1 ounce	1½ ounces	2 ounces
Egg	1	1	1
Fish	1 ounce	1½ ounces	2 ounces
Nuts	None	None	1 ounce
Peanut butter	2 tablespoons	3 tablespoons	4 tablespoons
Soybeans	¼ cup	⅜ cup	½ cup
Whole-grain breads	½ slice	½ slice	1 slice
Whole-grain cereals	¼ cup	⅓ cup	¾ cup
Legumes	¼ cup	⅜ cup	½ cup
Fruits and vegetables	¼ cup	½ cup	¾ cup

Adapted from *A Planning Guide for Food Service in Child Care Centers*. The U.S. Department of Agriculture, Food and Nutrition Service, 1989. Publication FNS-64.

HOW MANY SERVINGS?

You can use a modified version of the food pyramid to help plan vegetarian menus for growing children.

Foods	Servings per Day
Milk and milk products	3–4
Fish or eggs	2
Combined vegetable proteins	2
Whole-grain breads or cereals	4
Vegetables and fruits	4

As your vegetarian child approaches adolescence or is more physically active, he will be eating adult serving sizes. Vegetarian teenagers should have three regular meals a day, as well as three additional, slightly smaller meals. Vegetarian diets provide more bulk and cause children to feel full, even if they haven't eaten much. Adolescents must eat protein sources such as legumes, seeds, and nuts through the day so that the total quantity is large enough to meet a teen's nutritional and caloric needs.

QUICK TIPS FOR PLANNING VEGETARIAN DIETS

- *Reduce "empty-calorie" foods that do not provide needed nutrients. Use whole-grain breads and cereals as much as possible.*
- *Serve dairy products, eggs, legumes, nuts, and soy-based meat look-alikes. Use proper plant-protein combinations to make certain that your child is getting complete proteins.*
- *Use nonfat and low-fat milk products for older children.*
- *Increase the amount of grains and vitamin-enriched breads and cereals. Serve in small portions several times a day.*
- *Use a variety of fresh fruits and vegetables, raw or cooked, according to your child's taste preference.*
- *Use unsweetened fruit and vegetable juices between or with meals. Vitamin C will help increase iron absorption.*
- *Use fortified soy-milk drinks.*
- *Use nutritionally fortified foods wherever possible, especially those with extra calcium, vitamin D, vitamin B_{12}, and riboflavin.*
- *Add small amounts of brewer's yeast (high in B vitamins and the mineral chromium) to shakes and other foods.*

Vegetarian diets have a tendency to become monotonous because the choices are fewer. It helps to plan meals on a weekly basis. Write down menus and consider how you can vary colors, textures, and flavors.

In feeding your child a vegetarian diet, the most important consideration is to provide nutrients in adequate amounts for normal growth and development. Even if you are very experienced with a vegetarian diet for yourself, it's a good idea to sit down with a registered dietitian or nutritionist to review foods and amounts important for young children and adolescents. A child's nutritional needs are different from your own, and seeking advice early—even before, or just after, the birth of your child—will put you on the road to success.

17

Allergies and Food Sensitivities

Food allergies have become one of the most common undiagnosed health problems today. Some researchers speculate that more than half of the people in the United States suffer from symptoms brought on by food allergies. My own sensitivities to foods have become a real challenge, and at times they are downright troublesome. As a young child, I used to get skin rashes after eating certain foods. My mother said I would grow out of them, and she was right. By the time I was grown, my allergies had disappeared. But a few years ago, they reappeared. This experience is not uncommon.

Unfortunately, many African-American parents feel the same as my mother did, expecting their children to just grow out of allergies. For this reason, children may not receive diagnosis and treatment from medical specialists who can help them. While some allergic reactions may cause only minor discomfort, others can be life-threatening. When a child shows a possible allergic reaction to certain foods, the best approach is to get a handle on it as soon as possible.

An allergy is a hypersensitivity to a specific substance that doesn't bother most other people. The allergy-causing substance is called an *allergen* (it may also be called an *antigen*). Allergens may be swallowed, inhaled, or touched. Therefore, allergic reactions can be caused by food and the artificial flavors and colors added to food; by pollen, dust, and cat and dog dander; by feathers and other substances that come in contact with skin, such as dyes, fabrics, and plants. In addition, allergic reactions can be triggered by emotional stress, changes in weather, and infections.

We hear a lot about food allergies, because food is something everyone has to have. Food allergies may be obvious or hidden. Obvious food allergies cause a child to break out in a rash, swell, wheeze, sneeze, or develop headaches soon after eating a specific food. Strawberries, shellfish, nuts, eggs, chocolate, and citrus foods are common culprits.

Hidden food allergies occur in a more gradual manner. Symptoms may appear so slowly—taking anywhere from twelve to forty-eight hours—that it's almost impossible to associate the reactions with the particular food or ingredient that caused them. Sometimes a hidden allergy develops only if a child eats the same food several times in a row or on several consecutive days. Foods that commonly cause hidden symptoms include those mentioned above, plus milk, corn, wheat, sugar, and various others. The cause may also be your child's favorite food, even if it's not a commonly known allergen. My own allergies are still triggered by my favorite childhood foods that I would eat quite often.

A suppressed immune system is behind most food allergies. Allergies may first appear after a child has been ill with chicken pox or some other ailment that suppresses the immune system. Once an allergic reaction occurs, it can settle in for life, appear sporadically, or disappear entirely.

COMMON SYMPTOMS ASSOCIATED WITH FOOD ALLERGIES

Common reactions in children include bed-wetting, persistent colds, hyperactivity, recurring nosebleeds, cough, irritability, leg and muscle aches, puffiness and swelling, as well as constipation, diarrhea, and fatigue. Symptoms vary widely among children and are often confused with other childhood ailments. (In fact, allergies may not be responsible for the symptoms your child displays.)

Allergic symptoms are grouped in three categories: behavioral problems, sleep disturbances, and physical symptoms.

BEHAVIORAL PROBLEMS

Inability to keep still

Tendency to annoy or disrupt others

Short attention span

Failure to complete projects

Tendency to be easily distracted

Tendency to demand immediate attention

Frequent crying (often without apparent reason)

Being unhappy

Unpredictable behavior, mood swings

SLEEP DISTURBANCES

Trouble falling asleep

Waking up during the night

Getting out of bed during the night

Being hot or wet during the night even though temperatures are not warm

Irritability and fatigue in the morning, as if child has never slept

Bed-wetting, even after toilet training has been achieved

PHYSICAL SYMPTOMS

Bad breath

Stuffy, runny nose (without having a common cold)

Headaches

Excessive sweating

Swelling of hands, feet, face, tongue, lips

Nosebleeds

Rashes (eczema)

Difficulty breathing

Excessive mucus in the throat (clears throat frequently)

Darkness or puffiness (bags) under the eyes

Bloated stomach (abdomen)

Excessively large bowel movements

Very foul-smelling bowel movements

> *Excessive gas*
> *Diarrhea or very loose stools*
> *Constipation*
> *Intense itching, redness (particularly around the genitals or anus)*

MAKING THE DIAGNOSIS

If your child experiences any of the symptoms listed above on a regular basis, observe them carefully and then inform your family doctor or your child's pediatrician. The doctor will first eliminate any nonallergy causes of the reactions.

He or she may then suggest a preliminary trial diet as an early screen before going on to further testing. This trial will exclude the most common allergens from your child's diet. You will be asked to keep a diary of what your child eats and drinks, as well as any over-the-counter medications he takes. Your doctor will tell you to watch for symptoms such as eczema, asthma, runny nose, itching, and swelling.

Depending on the outcome, the doctor may then refer your child to an allergist for specific diagnosis and treatment. Treatment must be tailored to fit the needs of your child. The first step is to confirm the allergies.

Scratch tests are most frequently used. The allergist places a measured amount of a common allergen on the skin, then scratches the skin with a needle. If the skin reddens or swells, the test indicates an allergic response.

Some physicians prefer not to administer scratch tests to infants and very young children because they irritate the skin. Moreover, these tests are not always accurate. For these reasons, the scratch test is usually used in conjunction with a food-elimination diet.

Food-elimination diets are more formal and restrictive than trial diets and must be followed to the letter. They should always be planned and carried out under an allergist's supervision in case a severe reaction occurs.

WORKING WITH AN ALLERGIST

Once your child's allergist provides you with a list of items to be monitored, you are ready to begin. A food-elimination diet begins by keeping your child away from the following for three weeks: milk and all other dairy products, corn, luncheon meats, citrus fruits; all breads, starches, and cereals (especially those made with wheat and corn); foods with added sugar, corn, cottonseed oil; foods with artificial colors, flavors, and additives; and carbonated beverages.

The most important part of the treatment plan is to identify changes in physical symptoms or any changes in behavior on a daily basis and write them in your diary. If your child is old enough to keep a diary herself during the school day, by all means, let her be involved, too.

When certain items are initially eliminated, your child may immediately feel better. On the other hand, some improvements take weeks to be noticed. Be patient—this is only phase one.

After three weeks, you can begin to add foods back, one at a time, in a precise sequence. Carefully monitor your child for possible reactions to each one. The more careful you are in following the instructions, the better the information obtained will be. Your child's allergist will give you an exact list to follow. Your doctor will advise what to do should a severe reaction occur.

Also note any change in your child's behavior whenever his environment changes—a new pet, new clothing, new foods, or unusual activities. Various reactions will continue to occur until all elements are identified and all offending products are eliminated.

OTHER TESTS

There are other, less conventional tests for food allergies. In the *intracutaneous* test, a number of common allergens are injected under the skin, and reactions to each one are observed. In the *sublingual* test, a small amount of a suspected allergen is placed under the tongue. It enters the bloodstream and may cause a reaction. A blood test, or chemistry panel, can also be used to detect antibodies associated with some specific substances.

Most doctors use the traditional food-elimination diet as a first-line approach because it yields the most information. Once the allergy is identified, the allergist may bring in a registered dietitian to help plan your child's diet.

FOOD INTOLERANCES

In addition to true allergies, which are immune-system responses, some children may experience food intolerances. For example, caffeine jitters is an intolerance associated with the use of caffeine. Headaches brought on by foods containing monosodium glutamate (MSG) or migraine headaches that result from eating foods that contain histamines are also intolerances. Another common example is stomachache and diarrhea associated with lactose (milk sugar) intolerance. In this case, the problem often can be solved simply by reducing or eliminating the amount of milk or dairy products the child consumes.

Some food intolerances are psychological. For instance, if a child becomes ill after eating a particular food, he's likely to remember that experience the next time he is served the same food and become sick again. Or, if a child is eating an ice cream cone and sees a hair in the food, his stomach may revolt, and every time he sees an ice cream cone, he may have the same feeling. Children remember unpleasant eating experiences, and they continue to associate them with particular foods throughout adulthood.

One particular seven-year-old comes to mind. Her parents brought her in for an evaluation because they were convinced she was allergic to papayas. Every time she even came close to this fruit, she began to gag and vomit. After a lot of questioning, it turned out that her negative response had first occurred on a family vacation in the Caribbean. The child was offered a new fruit, unlike any she had ever seen or eaten at home. She was immediately repelled by the smell and she gagged. The gagging made her vomit. After that, every time she saw a papaya, she had the same response.

HYPERACTIVITY

For years, many people have believed that a hyperactive or disruptive child simply wants more attention. But Dr. Ben Feingold was not among them. Dr. Feingold believed that artificial colors, flavorings, and chemical additives in foods caused hyperactivity in children.

Dr. Feingold developed the well-known Feingold diet and wrote the book *Why Your Child Is Hyperactive*. At the time Dr. Feingold's theories were introduced, I was a young dietitian trying to assist families who had come to the end of their rope trying to find out why their child was so "bad."

I decided to try Dr. Feingold's diet with some of my patients, and I achieved some remarkably positive results. However, it was impossible to know if eliminating certain foods and additives did the trick, or if simply giving these children more attention solved the problem.

Today we are learning more and more about the many types and degrees of hyperactivity in children. Generally, sugar and additives are not believed to be the root cause of most of these behavioral problems. But the jury is still out on the relationship between certain foods, or food chemicals, and behavioral disorders in children. It's interesting, however, that the increased incidence of hyperactivity in children appears to parallel advances in food processing and the increased exposure of children to environmental chemicals.

TREATING ALLERGIES

After you and your doctor have isolated the causes of allergy or sensitivities in your child, you'll need to inform other members of your family, as well as teachers, school cafeteria personnel, the school nurse, and parents of your child's playmates so they can help prevent exposure when your child is in their care. Review your list of known allergens carefully with each person, particularly those who routinely serve your child meals or snacks. If they cannot guarantee that your child's diet will be kept free of these allergens, you will have to provide your child with food from home that you have prepared yourself.

You might also want to purchase a Medic Alert bracelet that lists the allergens and can be worn by your child at all times.

COMMON ALLERGY DIETS

MILK-FREE DIET

If your child is lactose-intolerant, here are foods you should exclude:

- All forms of milk (including dry, low-fat, evaporated, goat's, yogurt, buttermilk, skim, and powdered)
- Soups, sauces, gravies, puddings, and other foods processed with milk

- All cheeses, ice creams, sherbets, and frozen yogurt desserts
- Commercially baked breads, cakes, doughnuts, cookies, and pies (unless you bake them yourself, don't assume they are free of milk or milk solids)
- Butter or margarines containing milk (soy and corn-oil margarines are generally okay)

In place of milk and products containing milk, look for nondairy substitutes such as Coffee-mate (in liquid form), Cool Whip, Coffee Rich, and mocha mix. These products can be used as a substitute for milk in cereal, pancake batter, breads, and cookies. Many individuals who are allergic to cow's milk can tolerate soy milk. Soy milk is sold in health-food stores and many supermarkets.

EGG-FREE DIET

An egg-free diet should exclude all eggs and egg products. It's important to read labels on food packages, particularly in combination products (such as casseroles), since they may contain eggs. In addition, avoid giving your child noodles or macaroni (unless you know egg has been omitted), marshmallows, meat loaf, custards, puddings, ice creams, icings, waffles, cakes, and other foods that have been baked with eggs.

WHEAT-FREE DIET

Most breads, crackers, cereals, and cookies are prepared with wheat, so they should be avoided unless the food label states otherwise. In addition, wheat is used as filler in many other foods, including luncheon meats, hot dogs, chocolate candies, gravies, and sauces.

Crackers, cereals, and bakery goods that are made from rice and corn are acceptable.

CORN-FREE DIET

Many commercially processed foods contain corn. Read labels on food packages carefully: Products that contain corn oil, cornstarch, and corn syrup can all cause adverse reactions in children allergic to corn.

These are only a few of the most common food allergens. If several allergens affect your child, diets are more difficult to plan. That's where a registered dietitian or nutritionist can help. He or she will be able to provide you with an extensive list of food products that should be eliminated from your child's diet.

OTHER ALLERGY TREATMENTS

Your child's allergist may suggest a schedule of desensitizing injections, which are designed to introduce small amounts of the offending allergens gradually, until your child can tolerate these substances again. These injections are given in the doctor's office and the child is carefully monitored for reactions. Such injections are fairly expensive, although they are often covered by major medical insurance.

If your child goes on a strict elimination diet, you may be able to reintroduce foods very gradually under the direction of an allergist or dietitian, thereby building up your child's tolerance.

In addition to monitoring your child's diet and restricting substances that cause reactions, it's beneficial to increase the immune-supporting foods to which your child is not allergic. Foods that strengthen the immune system include the following: foods high in vitamin C and beta-carotene (carrots, cantaloupe, squash, beet greens, and broccoli); those high in B-complex vitamins (leafy green vegetables); and foods high in vitamin E (wheat germ, vegetable oils, broccoli, brussels sprouts, whole-grain cereals, spinach, enriched flour).

Some allergists also suggest calcium and vitamin D supplements for children with allergies or intolerances, particularly if they are hyperactive. Calcium calms the nervous system, and vitamin D helps the body absorb calcium.

Although childhood allergies can be annoying and difficult to diagnose and treat, they can be controlled and in some cases overcome. However, allergies can recur, even after years of nonreaction. When I was very young, I was allergic to tomatoes. I strictly avoided them until I was in college, when I started experimenting with a greater variety of foods. For a number of years, I had no reaction. Then, suddenly, after I came down with chicken pox, I had a severe reaction not only to tomatoes but to many other foods high in ascorbic acid. To some extent, the outcome of allergies is a matter of luck. The best way to protect your child is to stay alert for symptoms and report reactions to your physician. (If you are expecting a baby, chapters 11 and 13 provide some tips on preventing allergies in infants before they develop.)

18

COOKIN' WITH KIDS

Now that you know which foods make a healthy diet for young kids and adolescents, the next step is to teach them how to make healthy choices for themselves and to share good food with their friends.

Even though eating foods prepared by a restaurant saves time (and in some cases a few pennies), at least some meals should be prepared at home. Home-cooked meals are what most of us baby boomers remember from our own childhoods. Some kids today so seldom have meals at home that they may view them as special treats—just as we viewed going out to dinner when we were young.

Preparing a family meal needn't be on the shoulders of just one person—the whole family should be involved. Schedule one or more days of the week for meals at home. Then plan the menus. Plan early and get the family involved in shopping for ingredients. Teach all of your kids how to read food labels and to focus on the kinds of nutritious foods your family likes. (This has an added benefit for you personally: Pretty soon, your kids will be able to do the grocery shopping for you, and actually bring home the right things.)

Let your kids help you prepare meals. This is a great way to encourage kids to learn how to cook. I have a friend who has eight children, ages five to fifteen. She never does anything in the kitchen. She plans the menus and creates the shopping lists. The kids shop with her. She has taught the whole family to take turns doing various mealtime chores, everything from putting groceries away to cooking the meals, setting the table, and cleaning up afterward. The kids organize their own schedule and rotate chores every week; younger kids do the simpler jobs, and as they grow older, they assume more sophisticated tasks. This is a big family, and the children do their part to keep everything running smoothly. I swear this is a true story.

Alarmingly, however, many of today's young people often cannot cook at all. When I was a young girl, I was expected to learn how to cook. I learned by watching my mom through the years, and I got additional experience in home economics classes. The difference between my home training and school training was found in the recipes—or rather lack of them—employed at home. My mother never used recipes; she relied upon her memory, instincts, and taste. This is true for most African-American women. Over many generations, we were recognized as naturally great cooks—although it wasn't "natural" at all, but a skill we learned by watching our mothers, friends, or other good cooks; then we practiced by doing it ourselves. In fact, one of the few jobs African Americans were allowed to hold before the civil rights movement was in food preparation and service.

For this book, I have purposely selected recipes that children rate high on their favorite-foods lists. Family meals are times your kids can eat foods you know they especially enjoy. But you can also use them as opportunities to try new foods, as well. The truth is, family meals (and cooking them) are an important part of anyone's education about nutrition and choosing a broad range of healthy foods.

Enjoying some meals at home is also a good way to help kids learn table manners, family and cultural traditions, and social behavior. Mealtimes were fairly formal during my childhood. Everyone sat in a particular seat, a prayer was said before the meal, and you asked that foods be passed, instead of reaching for them. Mealtimes aren't nearly as formal today, but they should have some structure to them to create interest (and avoid chaos).

SHAKE THOSE POTS AND PANS

Even kids as young as three or four can lend a hand in food selection and preparation. As your child gets older and is able to avoid kitchen dangers like hot dishes and sharp knives, give him more and more things to do. Before you allow your child to do any task, you should feel confident about his ability to handle it safely.

NUTRITION EDUCATION FOR LITTLE KIDS

When you are helping a very young child find his way around the kitchen or a supermarket aisle, you can explain that food has things in it called nutrients—vitamins, minerals, protein, fats, carbohydrates, and water. Tell your child that his body uses nutrients to grow, to heal itself, and to keep his heart beating, his lungs breathing, and his mind creating. Nutrients also give him all the energy he needs to run, play, jump, and do his homework.

All of this information can be easily absorbed while your child is having fun shopping and cooking with you.

THE ABC'S OF GETTING STARTED

1. Choose recipes that are easy and quick. The entire meal should not take longer than one hour to prepare.

2. Review the recipes with your child before you get started.

3. Change into appropriate clothing for preparing foods or wear an apron to protect what you're wearing. Your young child will enjoy having her own apron to wear, especially if it's similar to yours.

4. Make sure you and your little helper have washed hands before handling foods.

5. Food-preparation areas and all utensils should be clean.

6. Safeguards should be in place in every kitchen. Emergency phone numbers (fire department, 911, hospital emergency room, and doctor) should be handy in the kitchen, near the telephone. The first-aid kit should also be handy (in its own drawer or cabinet). A fire extinguisher should be near the stove.

7. Make sure that paper towels, dish towels, and sponges are nearby to clean up spills. Have pot holders or oven mitts at the ready to handle hot cookware.

GOOD CHORES FOR KIDS

- Washing and scrubbing vegetables
- Separating vegetable pieces to be used in recipes, such as broccoli and cauliflowerets

- Tossing salad greens
- Sprinkling shredded cheese on pizza or on top of casserole
- Adding ingredients to batter for cakes, cookies, muffins, and pancakes
- Kneading cookie dough, dropping cookie dough from spoons, cutting cookie dough into shapes
- Spraying cookware with nonstick vegetable spray
- Measuring liquids such as water, milk, and cooking oil with measuring cups
- Measuring dry and solid ingredients such as flour, sugar, shredded cheese, and chopped vegetables in measuring cups
- Using measuring spoons to measure small amounts of liquids and dry ingredients
- Wiping countertops after getting ingredients ready
- Placing dishes in dishwasher or washing up cooking bowls and pans as they go along
- Helping to set the table
- Helping to dish up, serving, or placing foods on the table
- Helping to clear the table after the meal
- Helping to wash dishes or loading the dishwasher

READY, SET, GO!

When you hear the word *menu,* you might think of a special printed listing of foods, like you would order from in a restaurant. But a menu can also be a less formal listing of foods you will eat together at one meal. Here are a few ideas to help you plan your menus while at the same time considering variety and balance.

1. Try to include foods from the different food groups represented on the food pyramid. For example, you might choose baked chicken with steamed rice and broccoli as the main entrée; then add a fresh fruit compote, dinner roll, and milk or fruit juice as a beverage. You have all the food groups covered.

2. When you're teaching your children how to cook, you will want to choose easy recipes and leave the gourmet foods for later.

3. Remember to combine different colors and textures in your meal. A boring example would be a baked white fish, mashed white potatoes, steamed cauliflower, vanilla ice cream, and a glass of milk. Everything is the same color! A much more appealing combination would be spaghetti and Italian meat sauce, steamed carrots and broccoli florets, wilted spinach salad, and Red Zinger herbal iced tea.

4. Choose a variety of food flavors that complement one another.

5. Use both hot and cold foods in your meal—but not too extreme, especially for young children. This means making sure that hot foods have a chance to cool to room temperature before serving. Eating warm foods and following them with a cool bowl of fruit sorbet can be very satisfying, especially in the hot summer months.

6. Include foods that are preprepared to save time. For instance, if you don't have time to bake breads from scratch, buying store-bought rolls and breads that are ready to bake is the answer. If you plan to serve pie for dessert and you have a simple recipe for filling, save prep time by using a ready-made graham cracker or dough crust.

7. Use kitchen appliances that save preparation time. For instance, use a food processor or blender to mix or blend liquid combinations, instead of attempting to do so by hand. Use the microwave oven to bake potatoes, a steamer instead of boiling vegetables, a grill instead of panfrying meats, poultry, or fish.

KIDPROOF RECIPES

These are recipes that most kids like, and you will enjoy them, too, because they bring back your own childhood favorites. Although these are popular recipes you may be familiar with, I've made them over with low-fat ingredients to keep them heart-healthy. I've also chosen recipes that did not contain large amounts of sugar or sodium. My overall intention is to suggest low-fat foods that are familiar, tasty, and likely to be enjoyed by kids. With kids, it is always important to focus on balance, variety, and moderation.

QUICK COOKIE MAKEOVERS

To make cookie recipes healthier, try the following.

- *Substitute whole-wheat flour for white flour.*
- *Try oatmeal, peanut butter, or molasses cookies.*
- *Reduce sugar in recipes by one-third to one-half. The taste will be the same.*

TURKEY SALAD PITA

6 OUNCES COOKED TURKEY, DICED

½ CUP CELERY, DICED

4 TABLESPOONS GOLDEN RAISINS

4 TABLESPOONS FAT-FREE SOUR CREAM

2 TABLESPOONS FAT-FREE, CHOLESTEROL-FREE MAYONNAISE

2 TEASPOONS FRESHLY SQUEEZED LEMON JUICE

SALT AND PEPPER (AS DESIRED)

½ OUNCE HULLED, UNSALTED, RAW SUNFLOWER SEEDS

½ CUP ALFALFA SPROUTS

2 WHOLE-WHEAT PITA, CUT IN HALF TO OPEN POCKETS

In a small mixing bowl, combine all the ingredients except sunflower seeds, alfalfa sprouts, and pita. Mix all the ingredients until thoroughly combined. Scoop the turkey mixture into the pita half; then top with sunflower seeds and alfalfa sprouts.

Yield: 4 servings
Calories: 288 per serving
Fat: 7.4 gm per serving
Sodium: 472 mg per serving

"GO-GO" SLOPPY JOES

1 TABLESPOON VEGETABLE OIL

1 LARGE ONION, FINELY CHOPPED

1 RED, GREEN, OR YELLOW SWEET PEPPER (OR ⅓ COMBINATION
  OF EACH), FINELY CHOPPED

1¼ POUNDS OF EXTRA LEAN GROUND BEEF, TURKEY, OR
  CHICKEN

1 6-OUNCE CAN TOMATO PASTE

1 16-OUNCE CAN WHOLE TOMATOES

3 MEDIUM CARROTS, PEELED AND DICED

1 CUP WATER

HAMBURGER BUNS OR FRENCH BREAD

In a medium saucepan or iron skillet, heat the vegetable oil; then
add the onion and sweet pepper. Cook over medium heat until the
ingredients are softened or tender. Add the meat and continue to
cook over medium-high heat, stirring frequently, until it is
browned. Pour off any excess fat. Add the tomato paste, whole
tomatoes, carrots, and water; stir well. Simmer over very low heat,
stirring occasionally to prevent the mixture from sticking. If the
sauce is too thick, add more water. Serve on hamburger buns or
toasted French bread.

Yield: 6 ½-cup servings
Calories: 333 per serving
Fat: 20 gm per serving
Sodium: 304 mg per serving

ORANGY CARROTS

1/2 CUP WATER

1/2 CUP ORANGE JUICE

1 TABLESPOON MARGARINE

8 MEDIUM-SIZED CARROTS, PEELED AND DICED

1/2 TEASPOON VANILLA

1/8 TEASPOON NUTMEG

1/8 TEASPOON CINNAMON

1 1/2 TEASPOONS GRATED FRESH ORANGE RIND

In a saucepan, combine the water, orange juice, and margarine and heat over medium heat. Add the carrots. Cover tightly and reduce heat to simmer for about 20 minutes, or until the carrots are tender yet crisp. (Watch the carrots to prevent them from burning.) If all liquid is absorbed, add a little more water to keep the carrots moist. Sprinkle the top of the carrots with vanilla, nutmeg, cinnamon, and orange rind. Mix well.

Yield: 4 1/2-cup servings
Calories: 80 per serving
Fat: 3.1 gm per serving
Sodium: 21 mg per serving

CURRIED PEAS AND RICE

1 10-OUNCE PACKAGE FROZEN SWEET PEAS

2 1/4 CUPS COLD WATER

3 CHICKEN BOUILLON CUBES

1 CUP RAW (WHITE OR BROWN) RICE

1 1/2 TEASPOONS MARGARINE

1 TEASPOON CURRY POWDER

Thaw peas until they are loosened from a hard freeze. Set aside. Combine all the other ingredients in a heavy saucepan and bring to a boil, stirring with a fork until the bouillon cubes are dissolved. Add the peas, cover, reduce the heat, and simmer for 15 to 20 minutes. Remove from the heat, remove the lid, and let stand for 2 to 3 minutes, or until rice is dry and fluffy.

Yield: 6 ½-cup servings
Calories: 162 per serving
Fat: 1.4 gm per serving
Sodium: 465 mg per serving

BROCCOLI-STUFFED POTATOES

4 MEDIUM POTATOES

3 TABLESPOONS LIGHT VEGETABLE MARGARINE

⅛ CUP SKIM MILK

½ CUP PLAIN NONFAT YOGURT

1 CUP FRESH BROCCOLI FLORETS

½ CUP GREEN SWEET PEPPER, THINLY DICED

4 SCALLIONS, CHOPPED

1 CUP REDUCED-FAT CHEDDAR CHEESE, SHREDDED

PAPRIKA TO TASTE

Preheat the oven to 400° F.

Wash the potatoes thoroughly and then dry. With a thin, sharp kitchen instrument, prick the potato skins over the entire surface. Place the potatoes on an oven rack and bake at 400° F for 1 hour until the potatoes are soft when squeezed (or microwave on high heat per your oven's directions for baked potatoes). Remove the potatoes and reduce the oven temperature to 350° F. When cool enough to touch, slit the potatoes in half lengthwise. Scoop the potatoes out of the skins and place in a mixing bowl. Mash the potatoes until they are smooth and have no lumps. Then add the margarine, skim milk, and yogurt and mix well. Stir in the broccoli florets, green peppers, scallions, and cheese. Combine well. Spoon the mixture into the potato skins. Top with paprika. Bake at 350° F for 20 minutes, or until the cheese is melted and the potato mixture is well heated.

Yield: 4 servings
Calories: 489 per serving
Fat: 19.9 gm per serving
Sodium: 568 mg per serving

BARBECUED TUNA STEAKS

3 ENVELOPES DRY ITALIAN DRESSING MIX

½ CUP WHITE VINEGAR

½ CUP VEGETABLE OIL

½ CUP WATER

1 POUND FRESH TUNA (½ INCH THICK)

SALT AND PEPPER (AS DESIRED)

⅛ TEASPOON ONION POWDER

Prepare a charcoal or stovetop grill. Mix the dry Italian dressing mix with the vinegar, oil, and water. Place the tuna in the mixture and marinate for about 3 hours (or marinate on the previous day to save time).

Remove the tuna from the marinade and season it with salt, pepper, and onion powder. Grill the tuna for about 20 to 30 minutes, basting continual with the marinade until the tuna is done but not overcooked or burned. Divide tuna steak into four pieces and serve with mixed veggies and rice.

Yield: 4 4-ounce portions
Calories: 456 per serving
Fat: 34.4 gm per serving
Sodium: 350 mg per serving

SEAFOOD BROCHETTES

¾ POUND FIRM FISH (YOUR CHOICE), SKINNED, CUBED, RINSED, AND DRAINED

¾ POUND SHRIMP, SHELLED AND DEVEINED

1 LARGE ONION, CUT IN CHUNKS THAT CAN BE EASILY HELD ON SKEWER

⅔ CUP WHOLE MUSHROOMS

8 CHERRY TOMATOES

1 RED SWEET PEPPER, SEEDED AND CUT INTO 1-INCH SQUARES

BLACK PEPPER (TO TASTE)

Prepare a charcoal or stovetop grill. Alternate the fish, shrimp, and vegetables on four metal or wooden skewers. (Wooden skewers need to be thoroughly wet before use.) Squeeze lemon juice on the combination of foods as desired throughout preparation. Sprinkle with pepper and grill until the seafood is tender (but not over-cooked) and the vegetables are crisp but tender. Serve immediately. With small kids, make certain that you remove the food from the skewers. Serve the seafood and vegetables over steamed rice or tender pasta.

Yield: 6 servings
Calories: 139 per serving
Fat: 1.5 gm per serving
Sodium: 196 mg per serving

VERY VEGGIE SOUP

2 TABLESPOONS MARGARINE

1 LARGE ONION, PEELED AND CHOPPED

8 OUNCES FRESH MUSHROOMS, CHOPPED

¼ TEASPOON GROUND WHITE PEPPER

½ TEASPOON SALT (OPTIONAL)

2 MEDIUM CARROTS, PEELED AND DICED

3 14½-OUNCE CANS CHICKEN BROTH

½ CUP UNCOOKED MINIATURE SHELL PASTA

1 10-OUNCE PACKAGE FROZEN GREEN PEAS

1 CUP BROCCOLI FLORETS

1 TABLESPOON CHOPPED FRESH PARSLEY

Put the margarine into a saucepan and melt over medium-high heat. Add the chopped onion. Cover and cook (stirring occasionally to prevent burning) for 5 to 7 minutes, or until onion turns almost clear. Add the mushrooms, pepper, and salt (if desired). Lower the heat, cover, and cook for an additional 10 minutes. Add the carrots, chicken broth, and pasta. Cook uncovered for 10 more minutes; then add the green peas, broccoli, and parsley. Cook uncovered for 5 minutes more on medium heat, stirring occasionally to prevent boiling over or sticking. Use a ladle to pour the soup into a bowl. Serve hot.

Yield: 6½-cup serving
Calories: 160 per serving
Fat: 5.5 gm per serving
Sodium: 557 mg per serving

MY OWN PIZZA

8-INCH BOBOLI BREAD (ROUND), OR SUBSTITUTE LARGE PITA
  BREAD

½ CUP PREPARED PIZZA SAUCE*

¼ GREEN OR RED SWEET PEPPER, CHOPPED

¼ SMALL ONION, CHOPPED

1 CUP FRESH MUSHROOMS

⅛ TEASPOON DRIED ITALIAN SEASONING

½ OUNCE GRATED PART-SKIM MOZZARELLA CHEESE*

½ TEASPOON GRATED PARMESAN CHEESE

Preheat the oven to 400° F.

Spray a baking sheet with vegetable spray. Place the bread on the baking sheet. Spread the pizza sauce evenly on top of the bread. Sprinkle the sweet pepper, onion, mushrooms, Italian seasoning, and mozzarella cheese evenly on top of the sauce. Bake for 10 to 15 minutes. With an oven mitt, remove the baking sheet from the oven. Sprinkle Parmesan cheese on top of the pizza. Place the pizza on a cutting board. Cut into slices with pizza cutter. Serve hot (but comfortable to the touch).

Yield: 1 slice
Calories: 568 per slice
Fat: 13.5 gm per slice
Sodium: 1,391 mg* per slice

*Low-salt mozzarella and low-salt pizza sauce will reduce sodium content.

"HOT DAWGS" ON A BED

2 CUPS (WHITE OR BROWN) RAW RICE

¾ CUP CATSUP

1 TEASPOON CHILI POWDER

1 TABLESPOON WORCESTERSHIRE SAUCE

1 CUP WATER

¼ CUP GREEN SWEET PEPPER

¼ CUP DICED ONIONS

10 FULLY COOKED, LOW-FAT CHICKEN, TURKEY, OR SOY DOGS,
    SLICED (IN CIRCULAR CUTS)

Prepare the white or brown rice per the directions on the package label. Set aside. Combine the catsup, chili powder, Worcestershire sauce, water, green pepper, and onions in a 10-inch saucepan. Mix well, bringing mixture to a gentle boil. Add the sliced hot dogs to the sauce. Simmer gently for 10 to 15 minutes. Serve on a bed of rice.

Yield: 10 servings
Calories: 144 per serving
Fat: 8.8 gm per serving
Sodium: 627 mg per serving

EASY ALMOND COOKIES

¾ CUP MARGARINE

⅔ CUP SUGAR

1 EGG, LIGHTLY BEATEN

1 TEASPOON ALMOND EXTRACT

1⅓ CUPS WHOLE-WHEAT FLOUR

¼ TEASPOON BAKING SODA

½ TEASPOON BAKING POWDER

⅓ TEASPOON BLANCHED WHOLE ALMONDS

1 EGG WHITE, MIXED WITH 2 TABLESPOONS WATER

With an electric blender or food processor, combine and blend together the margarine, sugar, egg, and almond extract. Sift the flour, soda, and baking powder together and gradually mix into blended ingredients. When all the ingredients are thoroughly mixed, pour the mixture onto waxed paper or on a nonstick surface. Knead briefly and chill for at least 20 minutes. Preheat oven to 350° F. Roll the chilled dough into one-inch balls and arrange on a cookie sheet coated with nonstick spray. Flatten the dough with the palm of your hand or a spatula and top each cookie with an almond. Then brush each cookie with the egg-white mixture. Bake until lightly browned, about 15 minutes. Place on a rack to cool.

Yield: 24 cookies
Calories: 100 per cookie
Fat: 5.9 gm per cookie
Sodium: 15 mg per cookie

TROPICAL FRUIT–POPPY SEED COMPOTE

Fruit Mixture:

  ¼ HONEYDEW MELON, CUBED

  ¼ CANTALOUPE, CUBED

  ½ CUP WATERMELON, CUBED

  ½ CUP SEEDLESS GRAPES, HALVED

  1 PEAR, CORED AND DICED

  1 MEDIUM BANANA, SLICED

Mix all fruits in a large bowl.

Poppy Seed Dressing:

  ⅔ CUP SUGAR (OR ⅛ CUP GRANULATED NUTRASWEET)

  1 TEASPOON DRY MUSTARD

  ⅔ CUP CIDER VINEGAR

  ⅔ CUP CANOLA OIL

  4 TEASPOONS POPPY SEEDS

Combine the sugar (or sugar substitute), mustard, and vinegar in a blender and mix for a few minutes. While continuing to blend, add the oil and blend until the mixture thickens. Add the poppy seeds and blend for three minutes. Store in a covered jar in the refrigerator. Makes about 2 cups.

Place the fruit mixture in individual dessert cups and add 1 tablespoon of the poppy seed dressing over the fruit in each cup.

Yield: 6 1-cup servings
Calories: 374 per serving
Fat: 5 gm per serving
Sodium: 5 mg per serving

OATMEAL-RAISIN COOKIES

⅓ CUP PLUS 2 TEASPOONS ALL-PURPOSE OR WHOLE-WHEAT FLOUR

1½ OUNCES UNCOOKED "QUICK" OATS

2 TABLESPOONS DARK RAISINS

⅛ TEASPOON BAKING SODA

⅛ TEASPOON GROUND CINNAMON

2 TABLESPOONS LIGHT BROWN SUGAR

2 TABLESPOONS SOFT (TUB) MARGARINE

1 EGG

2 TABLESPOONS APPLESAUCE

1 TEASPOON VANILLA EXTRACT

Preheat the oven to 350° F.

In a mixing bowl, combine the flour, oats, raisins, baking soda, and cinnamon. Set aside. Using an electric mixer on medium speed, beat together in a medium-sized mixing bowl the brown sugar and margarine until light and fluffy; add the egg, applesauce, and vanilla extract and continue beating until well blended. Add the dry mixture and mix until well blended. Spray a nonstick cookie sheet with vegetable spray. Drop cookie dough with a tablespoon onto the sprayed cookie sheet. Space 2 inches apart (sheet should hold 12 cookies). Bake for about 8 to 10 minutes, or until cookies are lightly browned and crisp.

Yield: 12 cookies
Calories: 61 per cookie
Fat: 2.5 gm per cookie
Sodium: 40 mg per cookie

SWEET POTATO MUFFINS

1½ CUPS SIFTED WHOLE-WHEAT FLOUR

½ CUP ENRICHED WHITE FLOUR

2 TEASPOONS BAKING POWDER

1 TEASPOON FINELY GROUND CINNAMON

½ TEASPOON GROUND NUTMEG

½ TEASPOON GROUND GINGER

¼ TEASPOON SALT

1 CUP LOW-FAT MILK

2 TABLESPOONS CORN OR CANOLA OIL

2 EGGS

1 TABLESPOON VANILLA

½ CUP BROWN SUGAR

1¼ CUPS CANNED PUREED SWEET POTATO

Preheat the oven to 375° F.

Spray minimuffin or regular-sized muffin cups with vegetable spray. In a large mixing bowl, mix the flour, baking powder, cinnamon, nutmeg, ginger, and salt. In a medium-sized bowl, mix the milk, oil, eggs, vanilla, and sugar. Add this to the dry mixture and then stir until blended. Add the pureed sweet potatoes and then stir until blended. Fill the muffin cups to ¾ full with batter. Bake for 20 to 25 minutes or until a cake tester comes out clean.

Yield: 36 minimuffins
Calories: 52 per minimuffin
Fat: 1.2 gm per minimuffin
Sodium: 24 mg per minimuffin

Part Three

———

YOUR CHILD'S LIFESTYLE

19

R E D U C I N G   C H I L D H O O D   S T R E S S

P arents divorcing, money problems in the family, peer pressure at school, violence in the neighborhood—all are well-known situations that can cause emotional stress in children. Children growing up in stressful environments are at a greater risk of developing emotional and behavioral problems than children growing up in relatively stress-free environments. And like a pebble thrown in a pond, childhood stress has a ripple effect throughout one's life. Emotional and behavioral problems in children are connected to destructive behavior in adults. Stressed-out kids are also more prone to develop stress-related illnesses in adult life.

For African-American children, stress begins early. Whether an African-American child lives in a ghetto or a mansion, the perpetual stress of racism is harmful to his health. Many turn the stress inward, into a silent anger or even self-hatred. A few even wind up wishing they were not black. Suppressing anger leads to higher blood pressure in everyone. Imagine how vulnerable African-American children are!

Many of our neighborhoods are plagued by violence, which is another major cause of stress. Your kids might be the best kids in the world, filled with confidence, strength, and goodwill. They might use good judgment, work hard in school, and avoid trouble after school. Most of their friends may have similar qualities. But if they live in violent neighborhoods, they have either witnessed violence firsthand or have been victims of violence. They may have been pressured to become violent themselves. Gangs are more prevalent than ever, and guns are everywhere.

For a child, stress-related anxiety shows up as excessive worry about the future, about past behavior, about competence in sports or academics, or about popularity at school. These kids may be unable to sleep at night, and they may feel self-conscious around other people. Black adolescents are known to experience stress-related anxiety more frequently and with greater intensity than white teenagers. And they are more likely to suppress their feelings.

REDUCING STRESS

Despite racial prejudice and an array of other adverse conditions, most African-American children and families make healthy psychological adjustments to the environments in which they live and cope with racism to the best of their abilities. A strong self-image is a mirror that can't be broken. However, because many black kids are not getting affirmation in school or on the playground, parents have to double up their praise and encouragement. Always find time to let your child know how smart he is, how good-looking, how funny, how accomplished. No child ever gets too much of this kind of parental approval. At the same time, be honest with kids. Let them know that racism exists; *it's not their imagination—and it's not their fault*.

My sister and I grew up in a military environment, where skin color was less of an issue than it was for many of our friends growing up in civilian environments. But I still vividly remember being rejected for the all-white cheerleading squad in high school and being denied a part in the school play. I remember winning a first-place award for a state chemistry competition in the mid-1960s— and being handed my award behind the stage curtain, while the other senior award winners received theirs in front of the audience. It was the most devastating experience of my life. I was crying so hard that my father took me home before the program ended. That night, for the first time, he talked to me about what it meant to be black in America. He said we'd always be different and that somehow we were going to have to deal with that difference for the rest of our lives. At the same time, he gave me a positive, forward-looking platform on which to stand. He told me that I was just as special as anyone else but that life experiences for blacks meant overachievement and excelling to compete with whites. We can't change our skin color, but we can prepare ourselves to make important contributions in this society. Overall, the positive experiences of my childhood outweighed the negative, and every day my parents gave me hope that I could achieve whatever I desired.

HANDLING RACIAL INCIDENTS

Color consciousness can begin as early as age four, according to two of America's leading child-care experts, psychiatrists Dr. James P. Comer and Dr. Alvin F. Poussaint, who are themselves African Americans. Color awareness can be a negative experience for black children—at school, in the neighborhood, or even in their own homes (if light-skinned children are favored over dark-skinned ones, for example).

Covert racism in school and society makes our jobs as parents especially hard. Research shows that the way in which parents help children cope can make a big difference in the outcome of any potentially damaging incident. If your child is on the receiving end of racial injustice, particularly if it is on the part of school authorities, you may be forced into the role of activist, whether you want this role or not.

If your child comes home from school or an after-school program complaining of being discriminated against due to color, take a few moments first to find out what happened. Not all incidents are as serious or as race-based as they might initially seem. Remember, in situations like this, your child is looking to you for information, as well as help.

In the real event of a racially induced incident, Drs. Comer and Poussaint recommend confronting the other party soon after an incident occurs—not belligerently, but not meekly, either. The person involved may not even be aware that his attitude is wrong; if you retain your own dignity and give him a chance to retain his, the outcome can be positive all around. This is particularly important if your child's teacher is involved. It won't help your child if his teacher feels humiliated.

However, if you find you're dealing with an out-and-out racist, that person can be harmful to your child. Contact school authorities. If you can find no redress in your local school system, get in touch with the local chapter of the NAACP, or another African-

American organization that offers support and rights counseling for those who have been discriminated against. They may intervene on your child's behalf.

One good way parents can help to make a child's school experience a more positive one is to be personally involved. A friend who has four kids and a full-time job tells me that she invites each of her children's teachers to dinner at least once a year. "My mother did it, and it helped me," she says, "so I do it, too."

Another mother told me that she volunteers in her children's school library about four hours a week. "Classes are big in that school and it's hard for kids to get one-on-one attention. I think my children may be getting a little bit more attention from their teachers because they know I'm there every week."

Your child may also experience pressure from other African-American students, who may tell him that any black student who works in class, does his homework, answers questions, and is interested in the world outside the neighborhood is somehow "trying to be white."

Education has been the key to progress for all oppressed peoples. Make sure your child knows how much his ancestors valued schooling, and how they were forcibly denied education in order to keep them in inferior positions. Black students who accuse other black students of "acting white" when they're trying to learn are to be pitied. A child with an educated mind knows how to think, can evaluate options, and can outmaneuver racism, without a knife or a gun.

FAIR DISCIPLINE RELIEVES CHILDHOOD STRESS

Harsh discipline, erratic discipline, and no discipline at all generate anxiety in children. Parents who fly off the handle or blame children for family problems degrade everyone, especially if the outburst turns into physical abuse. Children become fearful, anxious, and edgy, and they usually end up blaming themselves.

Conversely, fair and reasonable limits and consistent enforcement help relieve childhood stress. Children feel secure when they can recognize the boundaries of behavior. The aim of setting limits is to teach children self-control. It's not a crime to lose your temper with kids, but it's also not a crime to apologize when you do.

To protect themselves emotionally, many African-American

children are taught to be tough and assertive in the outside world, but they are also raised to follow a strict code of respect and caring within the family. When I was a child, talking back to parents, grandparents, aunts, and uncles was a serious offense. This "tough in the world, polite in the family" concept is understandable, but in some children it creates an "us against them" attitude that can lead to discipline and behavioral problems.

If your child has a problem following a particular rule, whether it's inside or outside the home, listen to his opinion and give him a chance to argue for his side. This gives him a voice in the family, which in turn helps build his sense of responsibility and increases his sense of self-worth. It also teaches him how to think logically and find a nonviolent way to stand up for himself. None of this means you (or other authority figures in his life) have to change the rule, but you may have to explain its purpose better. You have the option to agree to a time limit for certain rules—for example: "When you're ten years old, we'll rethink the rule."

CONFLICT RESOLUTION AMONG CHILDREN

Many children growing up in rough environments learn that violence is the quickest way to solve problems. Looking at someone the wrong way warrants a fistfight, and sometimes even a gunfight. To reverse this trend, schools in some areas have started "Conflict Resolution" programs to show kids nonviolent ways to settle disputes and lower the heat in their lives. Parents can employ similar methods to help children learn positive ways to solve problems.

The state of Illinois, among others, has mandated Conflict Resolution workshops in all public schools. Illinois uses this four-part guideline. (This scenario works for two or more kids, with an adult mediating.)

Part I: Getting Started

1. Ask the warring factions to introduce themselves. Even kids who have known each other for years need an opportunity to start over and see the other person in a different way. Just really looking at the other person can be a terrific icebreaker.

2. Ask if they really want to solve the problem. Try to get them to agree. (There is no specific guideline on what to do if the answer is no. Just keep trying.)
3. When they have agreed to try, take them where they can have uninterrupted privacy and where no one else can overhear.
4. Before starting, ask them to agree to four rules:
   • Do not interrupt when someone is talking.
   • Do not indulge in name-calling or put-downs.
   • Be as honest as you can.
   • Agree to stick with it until the problem is resolved.

Part II: Defining the Problem

1. Decide who will talk first.
2. Ask that child what happened.
3. Restate what the child said and then ask him how he feels about it, and why.
4. Repeat these last two steps with the second child (and so on around the room, if there are more than two children involved).

Part III: The Solution

1. Ask the first child what he can do to resolve the part(s) of the problem for which he is responsible.
2. Get the second child to agree that these are okay.
3. Ask the second child what he can do to resolve the part(s) of the problem for which he is responsible.
4. And get the first child to agree that these are okay. (Make sure that the kids come up with a solution for each part of the problem.)

Part IV: The Resolution

1. Ask each child what he could do differently if the problem happened again.
2. Ask them if the problem is solved.
3. If it is, ask them both to tell their friends that the conflict has been solved (to prevent rumors from spreading).
4. Congratulate the kids for their hard work.

BUILDING A CHILD'S SELF-IMAGE

Many black children and adolescents—especially those who live in violent, impoverished neighborhoods—see no way out and no hope for a better future. This kind of despair and anger can lead to learning problems and poor self-image and also to violent and risky behavior, drug and alcohol use, suicide, and health-compromising sexual activity.

To grow and develop into healthy adults, all young people need to feel they have an opportunity to achieve their goals. African-American children can become what psychologist J. H. Block calls "ego-resilient."

Teach your child about his African heritage and its cultural traditions. And remind him that he also has a proud heritage right here in the United States. The achievements of our ancestors in overcoming their awful burden are unprecedented in the history of any country. African Americans have always found a way to look up, no matter how bad things are, and to anticipate a better future. Our ancestors cultivated a muddy field, and they outlived the pain and humiliation of slavery and entrenched discrimination by keeping their eye on a higher purpose. The sacrifices they made—and that we are still making—are initiatives that any child can be proud of. In their struggle to achieve equality, they created new music, dance, and humor that eventually touched every aspect of American life. Our children are the result of this blending of African and African-American cultures; they are the heirs to a strong and joyful tradition.

WHAT YOU CAN DO TO HELP

EXERCISE STRESS AWAY

Under stress, muscles tense and blood pressure and heart rate increase. This is sometimes called the "fight or flight" response, because the body is preparing to take immediate action—either to stand and fight or to run away. When a child can neither fight nor run, stress builds up in the body. Exercise helps relieve this biological dilemma by releasing muscle tension and burning off stress hormones. Exercise relieves immediate stress, and with a strengthened physical system, a child can better handle future stress. (See chapter 21.)

STRESS BUSTERS FOR KIDS

- *Exercise*
- *Singing*
- *Dancing*
- *Talking*
- *Laughing*
- *Learning*
- *Positive action*

STRESS RELIEF: A FAMILY ACTION PLAN

The best thing parents can do for children is to embrace a positive spirit themselves. Make it a habit to think and speak in a positive way to your children. Remember that ordinary daily hassles can cause even more stress than major life crises, and children feel their parents' stress, as well as their own.

- Help your child identify the source of his stress. Just knowing where the stress is coming from can help.

- If the trigger is racism, acknowledge it; then encourage a productive response, instead of focusing on racial put-downs. Explain to your child that racists are ignorant people who need to make themselves feel superior by putting someone else down.

- Encourage your child to turn her positive thinking into *positive action*.

- Always *reaffirm* your child's positive actions by reminding her of all the productive things she's doing and why she is doing them. And tell her how proud you are of her.

- Let your child talk to you and encourage her to express her feelings—whatever they are. Ask your child what's going on at school. Be patient. Most children need a little time to put their feelings into words. Sometimes you just have to wait for an answer.

- Look for specific, small ways to reduce the pressure in your child's life by replacing it with fun. Singing around the house can have good and contagious effects. Bring home a stupid joke from work—the sillier, the better. Laughter is the best stress medicine in the world.

- Give your child responsibilities around the house. He may think he already has too much to do, but tasks make kids feel helpful and can actually reduce their stress load.

- Help your child learn to recognize his own personal quirks that create stress. Is he oversensitive to criticism? Does he panic if someone doesn't like him? If so, why?

- Tackle any health negatives in your child's life that might be adding to stress. If you suspect your child is smoking, drinking, or using drugs, you will have to take measures. (See chapter 22.)

- Encourage your child to shine up his Sunday shoes and get involved in church activities.

- Help your child find ways to help others. Being a good friend and neighbor helps refocus worries away from oneself.

- Ask your child to write down all the subjects that interest him, no matter how outrageous. What are his favorite animals, countries, games, sports? He can name any subject that has sparked his curiosity, even if he knows nothing about it. This list will change and grow with time.

- Encourage your child to join in activities that connect to the topics on his list. He can read more about them, join youth organizations, seek out people who know something about the subject and interview them, and participate in field trips.

- If she wants one, let your child have a pet and teach her how to take care of it. Caring for pets and receiving love and loyalty in return is a sure antistress practice that can last a lifetime.

QUICK FIXES FOR STRESS OVERLOAD

- Count to ten (or twenty, or even thirty). Show your child how to "take a break" when she feels frustrated or angry. Help her cool off, and consider immediate positive actions.

- Take several deep breaths: Go limp and get loose.

- Stretch. (A physical response to a mental strain helps relieve stress.)

- Wash hands with warm water (or take a warm bath). Tension reduces circulation, and warm water helps restore it.

- Use progressive relaxation. Show your child how to tense up his feet for a few seconds, then slowly let them relax. Go on to the legs, chest, arms, and hands.
- Massage his temples and ask him to roll his jaw around. (This relieves the strain from clenched teeth.)
- Take a walk outside together.
- Divert his attention from an anxiety-provoking problem—with a game, a song, a story. Explain what you're doing, and tell him he can go back to the problem later (with a fresh viewpoint).

WHEN TO SEEK MEDICAL HELP

Relentless, unrelieved stress *can* make your child sick. If none of the methods you try help, you should seek professional counseling.

In general, the mental health of African Americans has been seriously neglected, partly due to the medical stereotype that we are not readily susceptible to depression and related disorders. Rather, we are more likely to be diagnosed with a serious mental illness. (For example, blacks are more often classified as schizophrenics, while whites are more often classified as having depressive disorders. Whether the diagnoses are accurate is unknown.) Research also shows that when we do seek help, we also receive less-than-adequate treatment in most community mental-health programs.

As a result of this kind of stereotyping and also our own cultural practices, we are more likely to seek help from a minister or a family doctor or friend than from a psychologist or other mental-health professional. Obviously, a lot of new work needs to be done in the area of mental health to make African Americans feel more comfortable using such services.

I believe that if your child is suffering from severe stress or emotional and behavioral problems, the important thing is to reach out and to try to get some good help as soon as possible. Start where you feel you can get valuable information. You can discuss the problem with your family doctor or pediatrician, and ask for a recommendation to a mental health professional (see pages 398–399). If you can find a black psychiatrist, psychologist, or social worker, so much the better; it may be difficult in some parts of the country, however, since the overall number of such professionals is still low.

POSTTRAUMATIC STRESS DISORDER

When stress builds up in young children, the effects on their emotional and physical well-being may not show up for several years. Children who experience cumulative traumatic experiences may display delayed reactions, called posttraumatic stress disorder (PTSD). Two groups particularly at risk are children who are repeatedly exposed to violence and children who have been abused.

Symptoms, when they do appear, include panic attacks, recurring nightmares, depression, and feelings of powerlessness. While PTSD is relatively uncommon, black children are more than twice as likely as white children to suffer from it. The most reported symptoms are nightmares about violence in their neighborhoods.

20

―――――

OVERWEIGHT KIDS

Nationwide, childhood obesity has grown dramatically in recent years. In less than twenty years—from 1963 to 1980—obesity rose 54 percent among six- to eleven-year-olds and 39 percent among twelve- to seventeen-year-olds. Today, surveys estimate that one in five American children is obese. It's estimated that 40 percent of obese children and 70 percent of obese adolescents will also be obese adults.

A child's weight *at birth* does not necessarily determine his or her future weight. Yet obesity may begin in early childhood, as early as age two in girls and age three in boys. (Fat comprises a greater percent of body weight in females than in males.)

Obesity can result from an increase in the *size* of fat cells, or an increase in the *number* of fat cells, or a combination of both. There are two periods when a person is most likely to add to their number of fat cells—early childhood and early adolescence. Once fat cells have been formed, their number cannot be reduced, which is one reason why children who are overweight may have lifelong weight problems. (It's also the reason why it's so hard for overweight adults to lose weight permanently.)

Obesity can contribute to a number of health problems in children. There are also many social and psychological ramifications of being overweight in childhood. Overweight kids are often teased and ridiculed by classmates, as well as left out of games and social activities. They often have a poor self-image, a sense of failure, and express feelings of inferiority and rejection.

The earlier weight is brought under control, the better. As adults, overweight people often struggle and fail with one diet after another. Yet you can make adjustments to a child's diet that are virtually unnoticeable, and this improved eating behavior can become a permanent part of his or her life. There are literally millions of Americans today, including me, who wish someone had done the same thing for them.

The older your kids are, the harder it's going to be. One way teenagers practice independence is by making their own food choices. But there are still steps you can take to help them make better choices, so read on.

WHY SOME PEOPLE ARE OVERWEIGHT

Research conducted at the federal Centers for Disease Control and Prevention shows that black women between the ages of twenty-five and thirty-four are the segment of the American population most likely to gain weight. This is one of the more mysterious health statistics to emerge from a decade's worth of research. Overall, researchers blame a diet high in fatty and fried foods and surmise that better education about nutrition might solve the problem.

I believe that social pressures and cultural influences on African Americans also play a big role, as well as the lack of consistent exercise. Using large quantities of fat for cooking everything from biscuits to greens, fruit cobblers to fried fish, is such an entrenched cultural habit that we don't even think about it. This was certainly true in my own family.

Many of us also eat inexpensive processed carbohydrates— French fried potatoes, baked beans, cakes, chips, candy, and bologna on white bread with mayo, and other fatty foods—because of their appeal to the brain's comfort zone. When it comes to quieting dull emotional aches, these foods seem to fill the bill. For many people, fullness equates with feeling safe.

This "comfort" eating is quickly habit-forming and extremely hard to overcome in adult life. If you suspect that your child is overeating for emotional reasons, the best thing you can do is help him learn how to express his feelings. The earlier you intervene, the easier it will be. Encourage your child to talk about how he feels and let him know that emotions are normal and needn't be shut down. Using food to feel better cannot solve a problem, because once the food is gone, the problem is still there.

Obesity does tend to run in families. A child with no obese parent has only a 3 to 7 percent risk of becoming obese. The risk increases to 40 percent if one parent is obese; and if both parents are obese, the risk rises to 70 to 80 percent. The causes of a family tendency may be genetic or environmental, or both.

Environmental factors that promote excessive weight include family eating habits, being an only child, the absence of one parent, excessive television watching, being poor, and living in a frustrating family or school situation.

Beyond all of that, a child can simply inherit a tendency to be fat. Twins raised by adoptive parents will both grow up to have the body shape and weight of their biological parents—even if they're raised in separate adoptive families. (Body *shape* cannot be changed, but excessive weight gain can.)

Despite hereditary influences, kids aren't doomed to be fat. Only their weight *potential* is predetermined. A thin child can become an obese adult if she continual makes unwise food choices. And a fat child can grow into a healthy weight and maintain it for the rest of her life.

People gain weight for many different reasons, but the best way to *control* weight is the same for everyone, regardless of age, color, or weight predisposition: Lasting weight control results from a permanent eating and exercise-management plan.

YOUR CHILD'S "IDEAL" WEIGHT

Let me say right out: There is no "ideal" or "right" weight for kids at any given age. But three important factors can help you evaluate your child's present eating habits and predict future weight problems.

- Is there a history of obesity in your family?
- Does your child have poor eating habits? Is she in love with desserts and high-fat foods? Does she always take second or third helpings? Eat heavily before going to bed? Snack constantly? Even if your child's weight seems normal, these eating habits should be changed—now.

- Is your child getting enough physical exercise? Think about it. What can you do to help your child become more active? (See chapter 21.)

For the vast majority of kids, excess weight comes from eating too many calories relative to their energy requirements. Less than 5 percent of obese children have an underlying medical problem.

Keep in mind that there are times in life when it is normal for some kids to be a little chubby, particularly as they approach puberty. This normal plumpness, referred to as "prepubescent growth," usually occurs by age eight for girls and by age ten for boys. (Not every child is chubby when puberty approaches. In fact, some are very skinny, which worries parents as much as obesity, but this, too, is usually normal.)

Many children lose this extra fat when they hit their next growth spurt, which may start as early as nine years old. About half of all children start the growth spurt by age eleven. Rapid growth continues over a period from eighteen to twenty-four months, and energy requirements are increased, which is why diets and weight loss are not recommended for children.

KIDS SHOULD NEVER DIET

The evidence is rolling in that diets simply don't work for adults, and they certainly don't work for kids. Diets are especially harmful for children and adolescents, because growing bodies need a wide variety of nutrients to develop fully.

PREVENTION STRATEGIES

The best way to keep your child from becoming obese is prevention, and the best prevention is to let your child respond to his natural hunger signals. Children are born with a biological mechanism that lets them know how much food they need for normal growth.

Feeding infants on demand, instead of at designated time periods, is by far the best way to prevent obesity. Obesity is also minimized by breast-feeding and by delaying the introduction of solid foods until four to six months of age.

Continuing to feed growing children on demand keeps them in

touch with their hungry/full signals. Granting children this self-directed freedom maintains their inborn eating control.

If your child has lost touch with this mechanism, you can help him reestablish it.

WEIGHT-REDUCTION STRATEGIES

As a general rule, children should not be put on weight-loss diets, and never on fad diets. Restrictive diets are perceived by children as punishment. (Therefore, they will overeat whenever they get the chance, and they may become "secret" eaters.) Instead, children should be given time to grow into their present weight. This means slowing down the rate at which they gain weight, so that as they grow taller, they will become slimmer.

The nutritional weight-control plan I recommend for over-weight kids is the same one I use myself:

- Eat a variety of foods in moderate amounts.
- Watch the amount of fat, sugar, salt, and high-calorie foods.
- Increase the level of exercise.

I believe this approach works for most people, regardless of their age. Deprivation and self-denial are unnecessary, even harmful, for kids. A child's diet should always provide enough protein, carbohydrates, fat, minerals, and vitamins to meet the needs of lean tissue growth, and it should be composed of foods the child is familiar with.

If you keep after your child to diet and exercise more, he'll get one message only: Something is wrong with me. Putting your child on a restrictive diet sends the message that you don't like the way he looks and you will like him better when he is thinner. You should not encourage a short-term, numbers-oriented way of eating. You're looking to transform your child's eating patterns into healthful lifetime habits.

Your attitude makes all the difference. If you feel your child is attractive and competent, he will feel the same way about himself. Kids usually know who is thin and who is overweight. Perhaps your child is teased at school. Maybe he doesn't do well in sports and is usually chosen last for teams. Maybe he's embarrassed because he has trouble fitting into clothes or buying new ones. These are frustrating and painful issues for overweight children.

Encourage your child to talk about how she feels. Acknowledge that her feelings are real, and even painful. Then explain to her that people come in all different sizes and shapes. Remind her that she is still growing and that as she gets taller, she will also be slimmer. Reassure her that you love her and think she's wonderful no matter what her size.

Help your child choose clothing that's flattering on a chubby body until he has trimmed down. Everyone who looks good has put time and effort into finding attractive clothes that fit well, and your child deserves the same caring attention. Be patient and encouraging when you take kids shopping for clothes. If your child tries on something and you see a sad look come on his face, or possibly tears in his eyes, say something positive and move on to another item immediately.

CHANGING FAMILY EATING HABITS

You cannot change your child's eating habits without changing your own. A double standard at the family table undermines the child's efforts and makes her feel that she is being punished. The best way to help your overweight child is by establishing some changes in your *whole family's* style of eating and activities.

FAMILY LIFESTYLE QUIZ

Use the following quiz to evaluate your family's present eating habits, make necessary changes, and find ways to reinforce the changes so they become a permanent part of your child's life. This quiz is adapted from the Family Lifestyle Quiz recommended by The American Dietetic Association.

Do you and your family:	No	Yes
1. Have regularly scheduled mealtimes?	___	___
2. Eat meals together?	___	___
3. Eat planned snacks only?	___	___
4. Eat portions that meet your needs?	___	___

5. Plan and prepare meals together?   ____   ____
6. Avoid skipping meals?   ____   ____
7. Try to make mealtimes conversational?   ____   ____
8. Avoid being members of the   ____   ____
   "clean plate club"?
9. Make meals last more than fifteen minutes?____   ____
10. Eat only in the kitchen or dining area?   ____   ____
11. Store food out of sight?   ____   ____
12. Eat only when you're hungry?   ____   ____
13. Avoid using food to punish or reward?   ____   ____
14. Enjoy physical activities together regularly? ____   ____

If Your Child Is Overweight. Copyright © 1993 by The American Dietetic Association, used with permission.

If you answered yes to most of these questions, you're probably doing fine. If not, you can see some ways to improve the situation immediately. The suggestions below will help you change a no answer to a yes.

- *Mealtimes.* When the family eats together, children tend to eat more nutritious and more varied foods. They also learn more social skills. Establish a daily routine for meals and snacks.

- Sit down for meals in the kitchen or dining area. (Never let your kids see you eating standing up or lying down in bed, and don't let them do it, either.) Turn off the television during meals, and enjoy conversations instead.

- Put food away until mealtime or snacktime. Food left on counters, especially cookies and snacks, is easy to grab and eat without thinking about it.

- *Snacks.* Kids need snacks to get the extra nutrition they require. Two or three snacks a day are fine for most children. Make sure the right snacks are available. Eliminate cookies and candy, and substitute fresh fruit, fruit canned in its own juice, yogurt, cereal with skim milk, or even half a sandwich.

- Make snacktime a regular time in the day, in a specific place—at the kitchen table or on the back porch, for example (not in front of the TV or lying in bed, or while playing). Serve snacks at least one hour before meals. If your child isn't hungry at mealtimes, make the snacks smaller or serve them even earlier.

When you first start to structure meals and snacks, it may seem that your child is eating more than ever. It's more likely that you've simply started to notice what and when he's eating. Eventually, you will both get used to the new structure and make adjustments.

- *Portions.* Start with smaller portions (on smaller dishes). Dish up individual servings in the kitchen and don't leave excess food on the table to tempt. And don't insist that your child clean his plate.

- *Speed limit.* Encourage everyone to slow down and take their time over meals. Overweight children tend to eat faster than do thinner children. The slower a child eats, the more satisfied she is with less food, because the brain has more time to get the message that the body is filling up. Set a good example. Put your own fork down between mouthfuls. Wait five minutes before asking for a second helping. Make second helpings smaller.

- *Plan together.* Get kids involved in planning and cooking meals. This gives them a healthy measure of control over what they eat. (See chapter 18.)

- *"But I hate spinach!"* Every child should be allowed to single out one or two foods that he hates and never has to eat—as long as the list doesn't get too long. Foods you prepare should complement his food preferences.

  A lot of "kid-friendly" food can easily be adapted into lower-fat versions. If your child has many foods that he doesn't like (like *all* green vegetables), or rejects foods he has never tried, don't turn it into a struggle. Ask him to sample a small amount. You decide what the minimum is—perhaps two tablespoons—and stick to it.

- Pay special attention to the amount of fat your child is eating. High-fat foods are high in calories. Kids need a certain amount of fat for healthy growth, but often simply reducing the number of fat grams a child consumes in everyday foods will achieve slimming results.

- Concentrate on the complex carbohydrates—whole grains, cereals, vegetables, and fruit—which offer many vitamins, minerals, and nutrients and also help your child feel fuller longer. Remind your child that this kind of diet is closer to our eating patterns in Africa, which were far more beneficial than those we've adopted here in the United States. The rural African diet is still based on grains, fruits, and vegetables, with a minimum of sugar and salt.

- *Are you hungry?* It's not necessary for kids to feel full every minute of the day. And it's normal for growing kids, particularly adolescents, to be hungry several times a day. Teach your child to distinguish real hunger signals. When he says, "I'm hungry," ask him to rate his hunger on a scale of one to ten. One means he's not really hungry at all. Ten indicates he is extremely hungry. If he puts his hunger level at four or less, he may be eating out of habit, or because he's bored, or because he's anxious. If he is at five or more, he's probably hungry.

- *Food is not a reward.* Using food to punish or reward a child only leads to bad eating habits.

- *The family that plays together is one that loses weight.* Overweight kids may be able to control their weight simply by playing more. Physical activity burns calories and controls appetite. The following chapter describes the importance of exercise in maintaining a healthy weight and overall good health.

Remember, the goal is not to lose weight, but to slow the rate of weight gain. Depending on how old your child is, it may take six months, a year, or even longer for your child to grow into his weight. It takes time to change eating habits that have developed over the course of years. Set your sights on what is possible, not on what you think is perfect.

Gradual changes are more likely to become permanent. If you've been serving hot dogs and french fries three nights a week, don't go cold turkey by serving your family a bowl of salad with no dressing for three nights the next week. Instead, work in one less fatty option to your usual menu: Serve broiled fish with the french fries, or plain corn on the cob with the hot dogs. You've already gone from high-fat foods to medium-fat foods three nights a week. Give everyone a chance to get used to one adjustment before making another. In following weeks, change one of these medium-fat nights to a low-fat one by serving fish with vegetables.

TEENAGE GIRLS

Girls judge and label themselves according to current fashion trends. Fear of getting "fat" often interferes with the normal weight gain that is a part of their maturation. Girls who practice gymnastics, figure skating, and dance are even more fearful of gaining weight. Some diet with such dedication that growth stops and puberty is delayed.

Parents may unwittingly contribute to this problem by becoming alarmed by the sudden development of their young girl's hips and breasts. The growth spurt is so rapid that it sometimes frightens parents who aren't ready to accept their child becoming an adult.

Your attitude can make all the difference to a young girl. If you hear her complaining about "getting fat" or saying she wants to start dieting, remind her that she is only developing hips and breasts, which is perfectly normal. Even if your child *is* fat, don't promote, or even support, dieting until she gets through puberty. You can't judge what is normal growth, and you can't know yet how it will all turn out. If your child is still overweight after the rapid growth of puberty, dieting might be useful, but this is unlikely. The best course *at any age* is to make healthy changes in both eating habits and exercise that can last a lifetime.

EATING DISORDERS

Teenagers of both sexes, particularly children of better-off families, are under a lot of pressure to be smart, successful, athletic, attractive, understanding, competitive, career-oriented—and thin! Because kids tend to be extremists in everything they do, the pursuit of thinness can become a serious concern.

Current estimates show that about half of all nine- to fifteen-year-old girls see themselves as overweight (about 23 percent of boys the same age see themselves as overweight). Only about one-quarter of these self-diagnosed "fat" kids are actually overweight. The rest suffer from a distorted body image. They see themselves as fatter than they really are. If this misconception is allowed to affect their eating habits, serious problems can result.

Until recently, eating disorders such as anorexia and bulimia were associated primarily with upper-class white girls. However, from talking and working with high school kids of various ethnic groups around the country, I've noticed changes in this pattern, particularly as schools have become integrated and role models in school are magazine-model thin.

DIURETICS AND LAXATIVES

A recent study has found that laxatives and diuretics are a popular form of attempted weight control for African-American girls. A survey of 1,269 high school students (tabulated by the American Dietetic Association in 1992) reported that 61 percent of the black girls and 77 percent of the white girls dieted. A significant number of black girls purged with laxatives and diuretics ("water" pills), and a significant number of white girls purged by vomiting. (By contrast, 41 to 42 percent of all boys dieted, mostly by simply reducing their food intake.)

Continual use of diuretics and laxatives is dangerous: The careful balance of body salts and minerals (electrolytes) may be destroyed, placing stress on the heart. These products have virtually no effect on weight. (Most of the calories in food are absorbed by the body *before* the laxative or diuretic goes to work.) Prolonged use of laxatives also creates a dependency; after a while, the colon loses its ability to contract and cannot function properly without drugs or enemas.

Why black girls and white girls choose distinctively different ways of trying to control their weight is a mystery. This is pure speculation on my part, but I hear many of my black patients say that their mothers and grandmothers recommended "cleaning the system" from time to time. My own mother used to insist that we use mineral oil or castor oil several times a year for this purpose. Laxatives fit right in with this idea. Diuretics are also familiar to African-American girls, because many of their parents take them to get rid of excess fluid associated with high blood pressure.

We need to educate our daughters about the dangers of using laxatives and diuretics. We also need to get them started on paying positive attention to their weight by improving their nutrition.

Parents may be unknowingly contributing to a child's eating disorder. Be careful not to transfer your own fears and concept of ideal weight and body shape to your child. This dangerous dynamic is known to occur frequently between white mothers and daughters, although it has never been explored exclusively among black mothers and daughters. The important thing for every parent to remember, regardless of race or ethnic identity, is that every child is an individual, not an extension of her mom or dad.

Anorexia (a result of not eating enough to sustain health), binging and purging (vomiting, and the use of laxatives and diuretics), and compulsive overeating reflect underlying problems related to self-image and self-esteem. Eating—or *not* eating—frequently involves issues of control. Food may be used to smother or soothe emotional upsets or to reward by creating a false sensation of being loved. If the underlying cause of the eating disorder is not addressed, a teenager may embark upon a lifetime of yo-yoing from one weight to another.

WARNING SIGNS

- Rapid weight loss or great fluctuations in body weight
- Excessive exercise and/or hyperactivity
- Preoccupation with dieting and weight loss
- Dissatisfaction with body image—feels fat even when thin
- Consumption of large quantities of food
- Disappearing after eating, usually to the bathroom
- Diarrhea, constipation, bloating, or frequent stomachaches
- Eating only a few types of foods
- Indications of frequent depression, moodiness, or insecurity

WHAT TO DO IF THERE'S A PROBLEM

If you believe your child has an eating disorder, get professional help as soon as possible. Start by calling your family doctor or pediatrician and describing your observations based on the above list. Then schedule a medical examination *and* a psychological evaluation. Start with the medical exam so the psychotherapist will have your child's medical status to use as a frame of reference.

Next, you must tell your child that she is going to the doctor. Find a calm setting in which to talk to her. Your child has been trying to hide the eating behavior from you, so opening it up for discussion can be difficult. Make it clear that it is the behavior you're

---

KEYS TO SUCCESSFUL WEIGHT CONTROL
FOR CHILDREN

- *Help your child to set realistic goals that take into account the family's lifestyle, his personality, and family history.*
- *Encourage your child to play sports, run, ride a bike, or jump rope.*
- *Forget about being perfect.*
- *Forget about dieting. Focus instead on the good health and bolstered self-esteem your child will derive from good eating habits.*
- *Try creative menus. Find menus that let your child eat well and feel satisfied.*
- *Avoid drastic measures, such as fad diets, laxatives, herbs, or diuretics.*
- *Do it together. These changes are permanent. What is good for your overweight child is good for you and the rest of the family, too.*
- *Encourage your child's efforts to manage her weight. And make sure other family members and friends offer encouragement, too.*

---

rejecting, not the child. The idea is to show love and support. Be direct and honest in describing the behavior you have noticed. Always tell it from your point of view—what you're concerned about and what you have noticed. Don't fall into the trap of blaming or accusing the child, and do not try to label her feelings for her. Do not harp on her eating behaviors or her weight.

But be absolutely firm and clear that she has no choice in this particular matter: She is going to see the doctor for a medical checkup because you are concerned about her overall health. (The doctor may want to talk to your daughter, or son, alone to get her view.)

If your family doctor or pediatrician cannot recommend a psychotherapist who specializes in eating disorders, check your phone book for a local chapter of the American Anorexia/Bulimia Association, which can provide a list of professionals. Or contact the association's national office in New York City (see page 393).

21

FITNESS

"Stand on one foot, like a stork. Place your hands on your hips. Now, close your eyes and try to hold this position while counting to fifteen." If your child can do this without falling over, he is in at least fair physical condition.

A child between the ages of eight and ten should be able to jump rope thirty to fifty times, feet together, without missing a turn. (Between the ages of eleven to fourteen the figure should be 75 to 100 times; between the ages of fifteen and eighteen, 150 times.)

A child over twelve years old should be able to crawl on his stomach at least forty feet, using only the elbows to propel him, and no leg movements whatsoever.

Exercise is good for kids, and it feels good, too. Yet every year since 1954, the government has warned that American children are getting too fat and sitting around too much. At first, this may not seem to match with your own experience. "*My* kids sitting around too much? They must be talking about someone else's kids."

But every major study of children's weight confirms that in the mid-1990s American children are heavier than they've ever been. And when we look at physical fitness, we find fewer and fewer fit kids, even among those who aren't fat. Researchers who recently studied four- and five-year-olds during their free-play time at school found that most of them used the time just to sit!

When I was in school, we had very active physical workouts every day. We ran, participated in sports, and did push-ups, sit-ups, and we looked forward to it! Even if we didn't, we had no choice. Gym class was a daily requirement for everyone, from seventh to twelfth grade.

Today, gym class is required in only one state. A recent study of physical education in one state showed that gym classes averaged only half an hour, and kids actively exercised for about three minutes! Moreover, the 97 percent participation rate in elementary and junior high gym classes slides down to 52 percent by the end of high school.

This drop in school gym requirements is serious because exercise is a learned behavior, and one that is less likely to be acquired as kids get older.

Only about 29 percent of all African-American high school students say they exercise regularly. That's 10 percent less than whites and 5.5 percent less than Hispanics. Only 17 percent of African-American girls say they exercise. (Surveys also show that girls are continuing to smoke at high rates and are using drugs as frequently as boys do—habits that make them even less likely to be active.)

Teenage girls continue to drop away from sports and exercise activities steadily as they age. In 1990, researchers at the Centers for Disease Control and Prevention surveyed eleven thousand students and found that 35 percent of ninth-grade girls participated in twenty minutes of what was called "vigorous activity" three times a week. Four years later, they followed the students again, and they found that by the time the girls reached their senior year, that number had decreased to 25 percent. (The number of boys who exercised stayed approximately the same: 53 percent in 1990 and 50 percent in 1994.)

Children who lived in poor neighborhoods reported the lowest activity. Lack of access to sports facilities, including swimming pools and tennis courts, and safe parks contributes to the disparity, particularly among girls. Helping around the house, caring for younger siblings, and trying to do homework and meet school expectations also prevent many girls from finding time to exercise.

Lack of exercise contributes greatly to the battle with unwanted weight gain in teenage girls, which in turn sets them up for diabetes, obesity, and heart disease in later life. Let's look at some of the ways exercise helps kids.

THE GOOD EFFECTS

Exercise does the following:

- Helps build stronger, denser bones.

- Increases the size and strength of muscles, which protects against unexpected strains.

- Promotes an active life. Once your child is in the habit of exercising regularly, you'll notice he or she has more energy for everything.

- Improves physical stamina by increasing the work capacity of the heart and lungs.

- Acts as a natural tranquilizer, which helps relieve stress, anxiety, and depression.

- Provides a natural high and helps prevent use of alcohol and drugs.

- Boosts the immune system, making the body more resistant to disease and infection.

- Helps prevent obesity. If there were only one positive benefit to exercise, this would be it. Exercise, combined with a healthy diet, is the most effective way to help kids maintain ideal body weight.

- Reduces the risk of developing heart disease later in life. Studies show that regular exercise increases the amount of "good," or HDL, cholesterol, which protects against fat deposits accumulating in the arteries.

WHAT TO DO ABOUT TOO MUCH TV

Bikes, sleds, roller skates, and balls—all sit in the corner, untouched. It's Sunday, the sun is shining, and it's a perfect day to play. Where are the children? They're playing Street Fighter II on Sega Genesis. At least their fingers are getting a workout.

Many parents depend on television to keep children amused. TV is not necessarily hazardous to good health. But too much television watching discourages activity. TV does carry some exercise programs, but by and large, it's a passive, sedentary activity.

Video games can promote hand-eye coordination, and can also train young memories. But some children become obsessed by video games. Studies suggest that playing video games may contribute to stress and hyperactivity.

You can check on just how much time your kids are watching television and playing video games by keeping a television viewing log for a week. Most parents are shocked to discover that their children are watching more than twenty hours of television a week on a regular basis.

It's not so easy just to turn off the television. Parents need to establish a few rules about watching television and be firm about them. For example, you might tell kids that they can watch television or play video games for an hour and a half immediately after school—*period*. Or you might say that homework comes first, then a limited amount of television before or after dinner. You might allow some leeway on Friday nights and over the weekend, but set limits there, too. Discourage the entire family from eating meals or snacks while watching television.

Be selective about what your children do watch, and watch with them whenever you can. This will give you an opportunity to talk about the shows, and *talk about the advertising* (which might be giving your kids the impression that eating chips and drinking beer is a dandy meal).

GROWING, GROWING, GROWN

Biologically, children are not smaller versions of grown-ups. They produce less power, relative to their size, than adults, and their bodies get hotter during exercise and take longer to cool down afterward. Compared with adults, their hearts pump faster and their breathing comes heavier when they're running around, so they tire more easily. They also burn off more calories and are ready to run around again a lot sooner than exhausted adults.

Emotionally, though, children are often miniature versions of the adults they will become. A child who develops a habit of regular exercise is more likely to become an adult who exercises.

WHAT KIND OF EXERCISE IS BEST?

Children need three kinds of exercise:

- Strength (to develop and maintain muscles): push-ups, pull-ups; free weights
- Flexibility (good tone and litheness, particularly in lower back and abdomen): gymnastics and simple stretching exercises
- Endurance (to maintain physical activity for a reasonable period of time): running, skipping rope, or any other aerobic activity that sustains an elevated heart rate for at least twenty minutes

HOW MUCH EXERCISE?

For children over six years old, most fitness experts recommend a *minimum* of twenty minutes of endurance activity (aerobics) three times a week.

CAUTION

Always pursue any exercise program slowly and build up. If your child complains of pain, shortness of breath, or any other significant physical symptom, stop immediately and call a doctor.

EXERCISE PROGRAMS AND ACTIVITIES

FREE-PLAY SUGGESTIONS

Walking, running, basketball, and dancing are about as good as it gets, and they're all free. But it's sometimes hard to find places outside the house for kids to play. City kids playing on the sidewalk have to look out for cars and dangerous people. And playgrounds, whether city or suburban, are not always reliable.

Some parents have developed neighborhood "kids watch" committees to ensure that kids are protected in the places where they play. If this doesn't work for your children, think about activities they can do inside the house.

Dancing is one thing they can do at home.

Bending over and touching toes doesn't make any noise that might disturb the neighbors and it doesn't take a lot of time. You can do toe touches with your children for about five minutes, and everyone benefits.

Some apartment dwellers opt for minitrampolines for young children.

Weights are okay for older children, but any lifting program should be checked out carefully—not too much too fast. You can buy free weights at a sports store (or use cans of vegetables), gradually increasing size and weight.

Young boys who lift weights to get big muscles will probably be disappointed. Before puberty, their bodies just don't produce enough hormones to make their muscles big. But rhythmically lifting weights will help make a young boy or girl fit.

For busy parents who can't get to a gym or playground, experts recommend a good brisk walk. Think about all the times you could choose walking rather than driving. It will be good for both you and your child.

LOW-COST ATHLETIC PROGRAMS

Many nonprofit organizations have advantages similar to high-priced health clubs, without the high price. The following are oriented especially to children or families.

Boys' Club and Girls' Club. These clubs charge a nominal fee for a membership. They are open to children ranging in age from four to seventeen. Most have gyms and supervised play, as well as other programs.

YMCA and YWCA. Although not high-priced, membership can definitely be a tug on your pocketbook. Family membership can run $280 a year or more in some cities, with extra charges for special facilities and special programs. A bonus of belonging to the Y is that children can get swimming lessons.

Martial-arts schools. Most emphasize a nonaggressive philosophy and the importance of a strong mind and strong body. Children can begin as young as age four. Because of TV shows like *Mighty Morphin Power Rangers,* most kids have some passing knowledge of martial arts. There are many different types: judo, jujitsu, tae kwon do, tai chi, karate, kung fu, and others. The key thing to look for is a program stressing discipline, respect, and restraint. Self-defense programs are sometimes offered at the Y.

Group dancing. All different kinds of music and dance are offered by a variety of community and church groups. With rap, disco, African, and Caribbean music to dance to, kids get a surprisingly good workout and have fun, too. Many classes perform for special parents' evenings and community and school events, which gives kids the added benefit of a chance to build self-confidence and poise.

Boy Scouts and Girl Scouts; Cub Scouts and Brownies; the 4-H Club. Many scout troops go on hikes and camping trips and encourage physical activity and group participation. 4-H clubs have an enormous number of fitness- and health-related programs for kids. Local chapters exist across the country.

Youth organizations. Look for any that feature athletics as part of their program. In New York, for example, RBI (an acronym for reviving baseball in inner cities) enrolls over two hundred members between the ages of eight and sixteen. The kids play ball all summer, and they also attend special after-school programs and participate in special events and trips. The Police Athletic League (PAL) also sponsors sports activities for kids. Look them up in your White Pages, or check your Yellow Pages under "Youth Organizations and Centers" and "Social and Human Services" to see which programs are offered in your area.

FAMILY FUN

The best way to encourage children to be active is to participate actively with them. If your child is overweight, she or he may feel awkward or uncomfortable about working out. Start off with activities that are fun, even if they're not aerobic.

- Emphasize enjoyment rather than competition and strenuous bodybuilding workouts.
- Run in the park, walk through a zoo or museum, ride bikes, go swimming. Volunteer for community projects in which

your child can help, also. If you live in the city, community gardening can be fun, educational, and physical.

- Look into the activities offered at local parks and recreation centers.

- Take a look at community pools and programs at the Y or other community centers where children can swim inexpensively.

- If you have a dog, make dog walking one of your child's responsibilities.

- Provide age-appropriate toys that encourage physical activity— skates, balls, bats, jump ropes, kites—particularly equipment involved in any activity your child seems to be interested in.

PLAYING SPORTS

Competitive sports are not necessarily appropriate for all kids and at all ages. Younger children should choose sports with less physical impact and less potential for injury. As a child develops more strength and muscle mass, contact sports can be enjoyed. For example:

> *Ages six to eight: baseball, swimming, skating, and tennis*
> *Ages eight to ten: basketball, soccer, wrestling*
> *Ages eleven and older: football and hockey*

Schools require medical examinations for children who play on school teams. These examinations are important to spot any physical or health conditions that could make playing that sport harmful to your child. If your child's school does not offer these important routine physical examinations, take the initiative to have your child's doctor perform the examination, anyway.

Not every child enjoys team sports. If your boys or girls don't respond well to team sports, don't pressure them—especially not to get involved in sports for which they have no particular aptitude.

Certain social situations can discourage kids from participating. For example, girls may be told that playing certain sports isn't feminine. Alternatively, boys may have their masculinity challenged on account of their sports choice (or nonchoice). A child playing in the wrong position (for him) in a sport he otherwise enjoys can also get turned off sports.

The important thing is for kids to try a variety of activities.

Sometimes body changes that come with normal growth can cause a kid to outgrow or become awkward at a sport he's enjoyed in the past. The smooth transition into other sports or activities can be encouraged so that normal growth doesn't hold your child back.

There are also plenty of sports that can be played alone or with a friend. For example, shooting hoops is fun anytime. Fantasy baseball (throwing a ball against a wall and catching it) and handball can be played alone or with a friend. Soccer is great exercise and doesn't require much in the way of equipment, although it does require plenty of running room. Soccer balls are available in most sports shops, but almost any ball of similar size can be used to practice the footwork.

Hockey, on ice or roller skates, is not as popular in the black community as other sports. For one thing, skating rinks are uncommon in most of our neighborhoods, and professional hockey teams are mostly composed of white players. However, this is a great sport and African-American children enjoy playing it when given the opportunity.

Roller skating is sensational for kids. Skating gives them a sense of balance. The moves are excellent for lower-body strength, agility, and fitness. It also provides great cardiovascular and respiratory benefits. However, the potential for injury with Rollerblades is very high. Knee and elbow padding and a helmet are musts.

NUTRITION FOR THE SPORTS-ACTIVE CHILD

Physically active children need more fuel to keep from burning themselves out. Active kids need between five hundred and fifteen hundred extra calories each day, from a variety of nutrition-rich foods. Carbohydrates are the best fuel for quick and sustained energy. Pasta, beans, whole-grain bread and cereals, rice and potatoes, and all kinds of vegetables and fruits are great sources of carbs. Low-fat milk and yogurt are also good workout foods because they provide protein and calcium for bone and muscle development.

Dried apricots and raisins are carbs with extra iron. Of course, cookies and Ding Dongs are also carbs; while they provide extra calories and quick energy, the energy is short-lived. Simple sugar is absorbed rapidly and initially increases blood sugar, but levels quickly drop, and so does the energy.

Protein is important in a healthy diet, but its main function is to build and repair body tissues. In recent years, more emphasis has been placed on protein than other nutrients. However, getting too much protein can actually be more stressful on the body in the long run.

The most important part of any child athlete's diet is fluids. Children do not tolerate temperature extremes well. They get hotter during exercise and are more susceptible to dehydration. Kids should wear light clothing during workouts (as light as possible, depending on the coldness of the air), and in hot climates they should try to exercise in the cool part of the day or evening. All child athletes should drink plenty of plain cool water before, during, and after exercise. Room-temperature or cool fluids are absorbed faster than extremely cold or extremely hot ones. Drinking water is the easiest way to rehydrate the body. Sports drinks are unnecessary, unless your child is working out in an extremely hot climate or for extended periods of time, where children lose lots of fluid in perspiration (and electrolytes along with it). In general, sports drinks should be reserved for continuous endurance events lasting ninety minutes or more.

If your child insists on drinking fruit juice, dilute it with at least two parts water. Soft drinks and undiluted fruit juice are rich in carbohydrates, which can cause stomach cramps, nausea, and diarrhea if taken during exercise. Also, fluids rich in carbohydrates may satisfy an appetite before adequately replacing fluid losses. Caffeinated beverages will dehydrate the body even more. *Salt tablets should never be taken.*

Parents, coaches, and teachers should know the signs of heat illnesses, which can progress rapidly from one stage to the next.

Heat Cramps: Signs of thirst, chills, clammy skin, throbbing heart, muscle pain, spasms, nausea.

Move the child into the shade and have him take off any excess clothing. Have him drink about one cup of cold water every ten to fifteen minutes.

Heat Exhaustion: Signs are reduced sweating, dizziness, headache, shortness of breath (sucking wind), weakness, fast pulse, dry mouth, extreme fatigue.

Move the child to a cool place and remove wet clothes. Place an ice bag on his head. If possible, weigh your child and have him drink two cups of water for every pound he's lost while exercising. If you can't do that, have him drink one cup of cold water every ten to fifteen minutes.

Heatstroke: Signs are lack of sweat, lack of urine, dry, hot skin, swollen tongue, seeing spots, hallucinations, rapid pulse, unsteady gait, fainting, low blood pressure, loss of consciousness, shock.

Heatstroke is an emergency. Call 911 or get the child promptly to an emergency room. While waiting for help to arrive, remove the child's wet clothing and place an ice bag on the back of the child's head. If the child is conscious, help him or her take a cold shower. If the child is in shock, elevate his or her feet, and keep people from gathering around.

In general, most of us assume our children are getting enough exercise because they always seem so busy and energetic. It's true that young children usually get plenty of exercise simply by jumping up and down and running around. But as they grow older, many African-American children encounter barriers that prevent them from exercising regularly, unless they can become involved in school sports. As a result, our kids are not developing good exercise habits in childhood that will last them a lifetime. Even if your child has good muscle tone, even if he or she looks perfect from head to toe, regular exercise can improve his stamina, coordination, and heart and lung function as well as control weight. Learning to exercise in childhood makes it easier to continue exercising in adult life, when results pay off in a big way.

22

TALKING ABOUT SMOKING, ALCOHOL, AND DRUGS

According to L. Perez of the Office of Substance Abuse Prevention (OSAP), recent surveys show that African-American youth drink less alcohol than other groups and have lower levels of drug use in general. Heroin use, particularly, which was a plague in our cities for thirty years, is down.

Although this good news is very welcome, it may not be as good as it sounds. The OSAP surveyed high school students but not dropouts. Therefore, it is not necessarily an indication of the actual society-wide prevalence of substance abuse among blacks.

The fact is that drugs hurt African Americans more than anyone else. The trade in illegal drugs, and the violence that goes along with it, is still centered in our communities. Even legal drugs, such as alcohol and cigarettes, kill African Americans at a rate far higher than whites: We suffer higher rates of lung cancer, heart disease, and stroke from smoking. African-American males are ten times more likely to develop cancer of the esophagus. We're much more likely to die from alcohol-related liver disease. In other words, we may be abusing these substances less than others, but we're abused *by* them a lot more.

Smoking, alcohol, and drug use most often begin during adolescence. Once established, the damage accumulates quickly, and the addictions are extremely difficult to give up. The first line of defense is prevention.

You can help your child lay the groundwork against smoking,

alcohol, and drugs as early as the age of seven. It may seem that seven is too young, and you might even be afraid you'll spark an interest that wasn't there. But today, your seven-year-old has already heard about or witnessed the use of drugs and alcohol.

Be honest when you talk to children about these behaviors. "Some people smoke to fit in"; "Some people drink because it helps to relax them"; "Some people like drugs as an escape" are all true statements. Parents can be truthful about the allure without underemphasizing the negatives.

It may help to remind kids that all drugs, including tobacco, fit the concept of diminishing returns: Whatever their benefit might seem to be at first, they quickly become destructive. You forget the things that made you happy, and the drug itself stops making you feel better.

The pervasiveness of teenage substance abuse may convince your child that everyone smokes and uses drugs. While talking to children, remind them that less than 50 percent of all adolescents smoke, drink, or use drugs. It is entirely possible that with a dose of prevention, your child will remain among the lucky ones.

If you suspect or know that your teenager is already using any substance, the earlier you act, the greater his or her chance of stopping before serious damage is done. Let's look more closely at the three groups of addictive substances.

TOBACCO

Ninety percent of all smokers pick up the habit in their teens, and their reasons for doing so are the same now as they were fifty years ago: Their friends smoke. A cigarette is a cool accessory. They think cigarettes keep them thin. (Girls use this reason more than boys, and girls are also less likely to quit smoking once they start.) The use of cigarettes as a weight-control tool is insidious because it seems to work.

Teen smokers will not know until the day they try to quit that they are exposing themselves to a substance, nicotine, that the National Institutes of Health says is as addictive as heroin and five to ten times more potent than cocaine or morphine in producing effects on mood and behavior.

Dr. David A. Kessler, the head of the Food and Drug Administration, recently called smoking "a pediatric disease." While the adult quit rate is increasing, the teenage start rate stays the same. During the past ten years, there has been a decrease in smoking among all age groups *except* adolescents, and the number of young female smokers has actually gone up.

Dr. Kessler has asked for a comprehensive program that would involve not just educating youngsters about the danger of nicotine but making it harder for them to buy cigarettes. He also wants to eliminate the powerful imagery in tobacco advertising and promotion that is so attractive to kids. Studies have shown that old Joe and Josephine Camel are as familiar to six-year-olds as Mickey Mouse. Marlboro gives away free combination flashlight-radios if you send in coupons from packs of cigarettes. Tobacco companies even sponsor big sporting events that kids often attend.

Dr. Kessler thinks that cigarettes should be sold in plain black-and-white packages, and that vending machines should be banned from public places.

Every year more than 400,000 Americans die from illnesses related to this "pediatric disease." Surely a country that has erased so many other diseases associated with childhood can rid itself of this one, as well.

A lot of children try their first cigarette at the age of eight or nine. Sixty percent of all current smokers began by age fourteen, and 88 percent start before they reach the age of eighteen.

Of the 3,000 adolescents who begin to use tobacco *each day,* nearly 750 will die prematurely from a smoking-related disease. Cigarette smoking is bad news all by itself, but researchers over the past couple of years have described a "gateway effect" to alcohol, marijuana, and other illicit drugs that begins with tobacco. One study reports that cigarette-smoking kids are ten to thirty times more likely to use illegal drugs, and other studies bear out that connection. Smoking is certainly a behavior that's worth trying to head off at the pass.

TALKING ABOUT SMOKING

Catching it early. Younger children between the ages of five and twelve are usually receptive to a discussion about the negative effects of smoking: tobacco odors on clothes and hair, stained teeth and fingers, bad breath, decreased stamina and athletic performance, and addiction.

Ask your child if he believes there is any harm in trying smoking.

Ask if he or she has tried tobacco or whether any friends use it.

Observe how your child is doing in school. Poor academic performance increases the risk of cigarette smoking and other addictive habits, particularly for girls. Ask if smoking is discussed in the classroom.

Make sure your child knows that most adults and adolescents do not smoke.

Do not let your child "smoke" candy cigarettes. Candy cigarettes make smoking seem acceptable, and young children who use them may be more likely to smoke.

Ask your child to practice refusing cigarettes out loud. You act the part of a friend and offer him a cigarette. Then ask your child how he might refuse it. If your child finds a way to refuse, compliment him to reinforce his skill. If he can't think what to say, help him out: "No thanks, it makes my clothes smell," or "It's bad for your health."

Show your child magazine ads and point out how smoking is falsely portrayed as glamorous, healthy, and mature. Children who understand the misleading nature of these advertisements have power to resist them.

If you or other members of the family smoke, the chances of your child taking it up rise dramatically. The best thing you can do is quit. But even if you haven't been able to quit, you can still strongly disapprove of your child smoking, and, by doing so, greatly improve her chances of not becoming a smoker. Take this tactic early, because by the time your child reaches thirteen, there's a good chance it won't make much of a difference. (Making a big stand against smoking at that age can even make the problem worse.)

Teenagers. Cigarette smoking is often a part of adolescent rebellion, and lectures on the negative effects of smoking probably won't work. Conversation is always better than a lecture at any age. Acknowledge that you recognize the "appeal" of smoking, before moving on to the negatives. Help your child to decide for herself. Always congratulate a young person who does not smoke.

If your child has started experimenting with cigarettes, you may be able to catch it near the beginning of the habit. It's not easy to start smoking. The first cigarettes are harsh on the throat, and most people have to learn how to inhale.

Warning signs include smoky smell on hair and clothes; nicotine stains on the fingers and teeth; coughing a lot, but not from a cold.

Give her the "talk," and make sure you mention the hazards associated with smoking: reduced athletic capability, expense, body odors, cigarette burns, and fire hazards. (If your teenager is using smokeless tobacco, make sure he knows that even adolescents have died from oral forms of cancer.)

If your child is nutrition-conscious, it may interest her to know that tobacco use seriously depletes the body of calcium, vitamin C, and other essential vitamins and minerals. Moreover, smokers are generally careless about nutrition. Some who just enjoy foods thoughtlessly overeat; others less interested don't eat enough for proper growth and development.

Most kids don't realize how hard it is to quit once the habit is established. Try to get her to quit now, while it's still relatively easy.

HOW YOU CAN HELP YOUR CHILD QUIT

- Set a quit date together.
- Consider signing a stop-smoking contract.
- Help adolescents think of ways to say no to peers.
- Encourage your child to get involved in school programs designed to help kids set goals, make decisions, solve problems, and resist peer pressure.
- Encourage your child to join in sports, exercise, and social activities that are incompatible with smoking. Swimming and singing both require good breath control.
- School prevention programs can help delay the onset of smoking. Ideally, prevention programs should be offered in all grades. At the very least, they should begin in the sixth grade and continue through the ninth grade, the age group when young people are most likely to take up smoking. Booster sessions in subsequent years help to sustain the program's effectiveness.

We all can work to oppose advertising of tobacco products, especially ads that target young people. Advertising is the primary reason kids think that everyone smokes. Parents can get involved in community organizations that encourage merchants to stop cigarette sales to minors, and mandate the removal of vending machines from places where kids have easy access.

ALCOHOL

A few years ago, there was a billboard advertising Canadian whiskey; it featured Wilt Chamberlain standing tall beside an equally tall liquor bottle. The slogan was, "Up Where You Belong." I know a powerful message when I see one, and so did the kids in black neighborhoods who saw the billboard fifty times a day.

Wilt Chamberlain is not the only celebrity who has endorsed alcohol products. But alcohol is marketed very aggressively and very publicly in black neighborhoods. Your children can learn to be advertising-savvy at an early age. Ads are slick and manipulative, but even children as young as three or four can see through them if someone helps point out the half-truths (and outright lies) contained within them.

Make sure to educate your child about the dangerous misconception that beer and wine are "refreshing beverages" and harmless alternatives to hard liquor. Some teenagers who would never dream of getting into their parents' liquor cabinet and drinking some vodka think it's okay to split a six-pack with a friend. In fact, sixteen ounces of beer or five ounces of wine pack the same alcoholic punch as one and a half ounces of 80-proof liquor. Wine coolers also contain alcohol, and in some cases lots of it. Fruity coolers go down easily, but the results are just as devastating as hard liquors.

Adolescence is a time of trials and experimentation. Adolescents look for ways to express themselves as adults. Many adults use alcohol and teenagers want to see for themselves what it's like. Most teenagers who experiment don't ever get to the point where alcohol rules their lives. However, children whose parents have drinking problems and children who have emotional problems before they reach puberty are the ones most likely to have substance-abuse problems later on.

Over three-fourths of eighth graders have been initiated into drinking. Some parents introduce their children to alcohol themselves, figuring that they're going to try it anyway and may as well try it at home. My own parents took this approach. My sister and I were allowed to have spiked eggnog on New Year's and a hot toddy when we had colds. We both hated the taste of alcohol, and as adults, neither of us drinks more than an occasional glass of wine. Today, however, experts on alcohol abuse say home initiation is usually not a good idea because it sends a message of acceptance on your part and also helps a child begin to acquire a taste for alcohol.

If a teenager tests the limits and shows up drunk one night, it's probably best not to overreact. Overreacting may make her feel as if you don't trust her, which may lead her to doing it again. But looking the other way may lead her to believe that it's okay. Take the middle path and, whatever you do, keep the lines of communication open. Explain that 10 percent of all deaths in the United States are linked to alcohol. Teens who drink are instantly exposed to a multitude of potential disasters—from drunk-driving accidents, which kill 22,000 people each year, to unplanned sexual episodes.

Some of the longer-term health problems associated with alcohol include damage to the brain, nervous system, stomach, and the whole length of the gastrointestinal tract. Because alcohol is cleared by the liver, the toxic effect on this organ is very serious. Complications from liver disease are the ninth-leading cause of death in the United States; and the mortality rate for black Americans is nearly twice that of whites.

Women of all ages are especially sensitive to the toxic effects of alcohol because they have lower amounts of the enzyme that breaks down alcohol in their stomachs; therefore, their bodies absorb more alcohol. This may be the reason that female alcoholics suffer greater degree of liver damage sooner than do males.

Nutrition and alcohol. Alcohol also has a devastating effect on nutrition. Alcohol impairs the body's ability to absorb proteins and fats, as well as vitamins A, D, E, and K.

Alcohol also lowers blood sugar, which can lead to volatile emotions. People who drink also tend to take in large quantities of caffeine, nicotine, and sugar, which causes blood-sugar levels to rise and fall unpredictably, creating wide swings in mood.

DRUGS

In a study that tracked approximately one hundred children from the time they were three until they reached eighteen, all the seven-year-olds whose moms were consistently angry and negative toward them had problems with drugs later on. Other studies that focused solely on adolescents found that those who didn't use drugs had strong emotional ties to both parents, and their fathers were more involved with the family than the fathers of drug-using teens.

All drugs weaken the immune system, making the body vulnerable to degenerative diseases, including cancer, and viruses that can kill. Beyond that, behaviors associated with drug use can directly cause HIV infection and AIDS—unprotected sex and using needles that are contaminated with the blood of a person with the AIDS virus.

Any addiction—alcohol, crack, marijuana, or a host of other drugs—produces a wide range of mental and emotional disturbances,

---

GENERAL WARNING SIGNS OF DRUG USE IN CHILDREN

Here are some of the most frequently observed signs of drug use reported by the Partnership for a Drug-Free America:

- *Red eyes*
- *Being overly defensive about privacy*
- *Chronic cough*
- *Odd hours coming and going*
- *Declining grades*
- *Cutting school*
- *Constant lying*
- *Constant fatigue*
- *Hostility*
- *Stealing*
- *Long periods of "the silent treatment"*
- *Mood swings*
- *New friends*

including acute anxiety, paranoia, poor concentration, frequent mood swings, and hallucinations. Those addicted to drugs lose their temper easily, experience crying spells, and have slow, slurred speech.

ILLEGAL STREET DRUGS

The illegal drug industry is the top employer in some of our neighborhoods. I know a fourteen-year-old boy, whom I will call William, who made one hundred dollars for every four-hour shift that he worked as a lookout for a drug-selling operation. Customers came to his block from all over, and they were from every race and income group. All William had to do was to stand outside the burned-out building and guide the customers inside. If a police car turned onto the block, he was responsible for alerting the sellers. When anyone suggested that he was hurting himself and others, he would look around the nearly abandoned block and say, "Hurting this? If I quit, where am I ever going to make this kind of money?"

William saw no options in his neighborhood. But even better-off teenagers may be attracted to the drug life because they think it's part of the black experience.

For many black teenagers, addictions are nurtured by peer pressure and compounded by a reluctance to seek help from parents or the medical establishment. A description of common street drugs follows.

Marijuana. Marijuana can be dark brown to light yellowish green. It can be powdery, thick, or leafy. Different kinds of marijuana have different smells—there's no single accurate description of marijuana's odor, except that it is distinctive. It comes in all different strengths and at a wide variety of prices. Marijuana produces euphoria or a quick high, and paranoia often follows. Smoking marijuana causes increased heart rate, impaired brain function, and lung cancer. These days, marijuana use among teenagers is on the rise once again, and new varieties are stronger than before.

Heroin. In the early 1960s, heroin was the common drug bought on the street. Heroin use subsided during the 1980s, but according to latest estimates, there are still between 2 and 2.5 million heroin addicts in the United States. Of these, some 70 to 75 percent are African Americans.

Many heroin users vomit after taking it, but they don't care. Heroin can cause psychological dependence, and fast. The drug produces a calm, untouchable feeling. The "nod" is a trancelike state that could almost be mistaken for sleep, except it can happen while someone is standing up. Heroin calmness easily turns into extreme irritability.

Heroin is a white or brown powder, or brown gummy substance. It is snorted, injected, and sometimes smoked. Heroin that is injected intravenously is the most dangerous, because sharing dirty needles with partners and partygoers can transmit life-threatening diseases, including hepatitis B and hepatitis non-A and non-B, as well as syphilis and bacterial and fungal infections. The worst scenario: The AIDS virus is often transmitted by heroin needles.

LSD. This is not an especially popular or physically addictive drug, but recent reports show that LSD is making a resurgence and is especially popular on the West Coast. LSD can produce effects that make the user appear insane. Moreover, LSD trips can have lasting effects, including hallucinations and flashbacks. LSD may look like a liquid, a pill, or a dot on a piece of paper.

PCP and angel dust. PCP is a dangerous cheap drug that can be smoked, snorted, injected, or taken in pill form. The user looks and acts drunk but actually feels even more whacked-out. Effects include possible hallucinations and acting and feeling stupid. It can cause coma or death.

Angel dust is PCP sprinkled on marijuana or tobacco. The effect of one joint can last twelve hours and is stronger than that of a joint of the strongest marijuana.

Cocaine. Feelings of euphoric self-confidence can easily crumble into paranoia and violent mood swings. A cocaine high lasts only a few minutes, and the low that comes when the high wears off can be very low. Some users try to drink themselves past the low, others take pills, and others just keep doing more cocaine, until they collapse. Among its many health dangers, cocaine may cause increased blood pressure, heart attack, coronary artery spasm, and life-threatening damage to the heart muscle.

Cocaine used to be expensive and reserved for people with money, but that is not true anymore. It is a white powder that can be snorted, injected, or crystallized into a hard rocklike substance and smoked. The smokable, crystallized version used to be known as freebase and is now known as crack.

Crack cocaine. The cheaper, highly addictive crack form of cocaine has devastated black neighborhoods all over the country. Crack has all the high points and low points of cocaine, only much higher and much, much lower: great pleasure followed by unbearable pain. Crack is extremely dangerous and extremely addictive. This drug has ruined more lives than we can ever count. Most sadly, hundreds of thousands of infants born to crack-addicted mothers will never know what it is to have a normal life.

ADDICTIVE MEDICATIONS

Many mind- and body-altering medications are made of chemicals that are just as dangerous as illegal drugs. Kids can get their hands on legal prescription drugs just as easily as they can get illegal drugs. These pills come in all shapes and sizes. They can cause addiction or serious health consequences, even death.

If you see your child or adolescent with pills (or cough medicine) that are not prescribed for an ailment you are aware of, confront your child with them. You can also take the pills to your pharmacist or family doctor for identification.

Here is a short list of prescription drugs that are sold on the street. All are addictive and all are dangerous.

- Percodan; Percocet: These contain chemicals extracted for morphine. (Percocet is twice the strength of Percodan.)
- Dilaudid: Comes in pills and liquid. Dilaudid (hydromorphine hydrochloride) is a derivative of morphine. It is used for pain relief.
- Thorazine: Used for treatment of severe mental illness.
- Valium; Demerol; Librium: These are tranquilizers. All are addictive, and they may have irreversible side effects. Increased doses become necessary with continued use.
- Codeine (pills, cough syrups): Codeine is a very addictive painkiller.
- Darvon; Darvoset; Demerol: These are painkillers.

- Methadone: Used as replacement therapy for heroin addicts; it is extremely dangerous. Methadone is usually sold by addicts to get the money to buy "the real thing."

In addition to these, also watch out for downers (depressants)—quaaludes, Placidyl; Amytal, Ativan, phenobarbital, Nembutal, Restoril, Seconal, Pentothal, Halcion, Dalmane, Xanax, and Tranxene—and uppers (stimulants)—Dexedrine, Equanil, Talwin.

TALKING ABOUT ALCOHOL AND DRUGS

If your child's friends are into alcohol or drugs, he's four times more likely to do it, too. Once a child is part of the drug society, it's very difficult to break free. He not only must deal with drug withdrawal but he also has to withdraw from his circle of friends, who will call him a traitor. Quitting is hard, especially if it seems as if it will mean losing friends.

Some schools are offering new social skills and refusal-skills workshops that teach teenagers how to avoid or get away from the drug world. Teenagers learn how to set goals and stick to them, how to stand up for their rights, and how to turn down something they don't want to do. They also learn better ways to deal with their stress.

Schools that have implemented refusal-skills workshops usually focus on seventh and eighth graders. The workshops report a decline in beginning (or "gateway") drug use of between 20 and 40 percent. These programs cost money, and budgets are getting tighter every day. Parents should go to the local board of education and encourage schools to adopt such programs.

Experts also recommend that parents get involved in more after-school activities, help kids with homework, and set explicit rules against alcohol and drug use at home. The more explicit the rules, and the more open parents are in presenting, discussing, and enforcing them, the more likely adolescents are to avoid substance abuse. Writing in *Raising Black Children,* Drs. Comer and Poussaint say that it's important to talk with your child, even if you just point out what seems obvious.

Self-esteem and confidence are necessary for independent thought, which in turn is essential for your child to resist the sales pitch from other kids who are abusing drugs. Junior high and high school can seem like the whole world to adolescents.

Teenagers need to know that they are valuable and that the world is bigger and more expansive than their school or the neighborhood. They especially need to be reminded that they can count on their parents' listening in times of stress.

If your teenager is already a substance abuser, don't give up hope. Patience and restraint may not be enough, but love and hope should never be left behind.

ALCOHOL AND DRUG TREATMENT PROGRAMS

If your child has an alcohol or drug dependency, you must help him find treatment as soon as possible. Dr. Al J. Mooney, along with co-authors Arlene and Howard Eisenberg, wrote the valuable resource *The Recovery Book*. They say that different treatments work for different people; which one will work for your child depends on his personality, the nature of his addiction, and his life experience. If one program doesn't work, encourage him to try another. Treatment isn't supposed to be easy, so teens shouldn't expect a smooth ride, but most people can tell whether a program is working.

Most kids and parents need a helping hand to help sort through the treatment options and get started. Ask someone to help you, perhaps a family member, a trusted friend, your doctor, or your minister (if he or she is savvy about alcohol and drug problems). Perhaps you know someone who goes to AA or another self-help program. Here is a brief description of treatment options.

AA AND OTHER SELF-HELP PROGRAMS

AA meetings, or a similar type of twelve-step support group, are a key element of most successful treatments. (The term *twelve-step* refers to the series of steps devised by the founders of AA as they turned away from alcohol. The term is now used by many other recovery groups.) AA looks upon addiction as a disease that can be stopped but not cured. The heart of the program is lifetime abstinence from alcohol and other drugs—one day at a time.

The only requirement to join AA is a desire to stop drinking or using drugs. A teenager doesn't need an appointment to go to an AA meeting; all he has to do is show up and recognize that he needs help. (There is no charge; a hat is passed for contributions to cover rent, coffee, and cookies.)

At meetings, people talk about their past experiences with alcohol and drugs, and they talk about their fears and their hopes. Listening to others and sharing experiences help to relieve the compulsion to drink or use drugs. These discussions remind addicts that they're not alone, which is especially comforting to teenagers.

AA has many mixed-aged or teen-only groups. Counselors can be adults or teens, as long as they are alcoholics in recovery. AA meetings take place in many kinds of places—church basements, cafeterias, hospitals, in people's homes—at all hours of the day and night, everywhere in the world. Most people have a "home" meeting they attend regularly, but they may also attend other meetings wherever they happen to be. If a teenager feels uncomfortable in a particular group, one of his counselors should help him find another meeting.

One of the twelve steps involves recognizing that there is a "higher power" that can help you overcome your addiction. The idea of this makes some people uncomfortable. But don't let your teenager throw this up as a roadblock to treatment. Many nonbelievers belong to AA. And many others discover their own spirituality after they join.

Alateen is a special support group for children of alcoholics. A parent's alcoholism affects children in ways they find difficult to talk about. Alateen helps teenagers express their feelings among a group of their peers. Alateen is helpful whether or not a teenager has a substance abuse problem himself. Parents who attend AA meetings can also ask about family meetings, which are especially important if a child has already begun experimenting with alcohol or drugs.

Black teens and self-help programs. When African-American teens look around the room and see only unfamiliar white faces, their defenses immediately go up. Many of us, at any age, hesitate trusting our private feelings to strangers. Black teens often feel that other groups cannot appreciate African-American cultural issues.

Color or culture was never intended to be a factor in these programs. AA does not believe that ethnic background or environment causes alcoholism or drug addiction. It's true that the people in AA and other recovery groups, no matter what their background, age, or color, have much in common. Yet it's also true that many, and perhaps most, self-help programs are primarily white groups, and minorities can sometimes feel out of place. It may help to remind your teen that everyone going to self-help meetings, regardless of background, feels out of place at first. It feels weird to talk about experiences and feelings in front of others.

Encourage your child to give it a fair trial. Although AA believes strongly that alcoholism is a disease, it has become more willing than before to discuss cultural and environmental issues. Also, more blacks are joining. If your child continues to feel uncomfortable talking in front of the group, Dr. Mooney recommends getting together separately with any other black members in her group, in addition to attending the regular meetings. Once teens get the hang of talking among a few brothers and sisters, it is usually easier to talk in front of a larger group.

Some all-black self-help groups are starting up. Many neighborhood black churches are getting their own programs going, so you should check. These programs are similar to AA meetings, but they also include black issues and community problems. Whatever the case, don't let your child use "it's too white" as an excuse not to go.

PRIVATE PHYSICIANS AND PSYCHIATRISTS

An experienced physician can help your child get through withdrawal and work through an alcohol or drug problem. Make sure the doctor is certified by the American Society of Addiction Medicine (ASAM) or the American Academy of Psychiatrists in Alcoholism and Addiction (AAPAA). If your child receives addiction therapy from a doctor, she will also be urged to go to a self-help support program such as AA.

ADDICTION COUNSELORS

Many counselors and therapists treat chemically dependent people, but look for someone who puts the addiction issue first, the psychology second. Counselors should meet the standards for a certified addiction counselor or credentialed alcoholism counselor. Most use a similar approach, which usually includes individual and group therapy, as well as AA meetings.

OUTPATIENT TREATMENT PROGRAMS

Outpatient treatment consists of regularly scheduled counseling sessions, including individual, group, and sometimes family therapy. It may also include evaluation interviews, a complete physical exam, periodic drug screening, and signed attendance at AA meetings. Treatment may begin before withdrawal, or after sobriety has already been achieved.

INPATIENT PROGRAMS

Some people start with outpatient programs, then find they need a more intense inpatient or residential facility. Many others do the reverse.

Private inpatient programs offer drug and alcohol users around-the-clock support, individual counseling, and group sessions. Private clinics are very expensive. They treat their clients carefully, paying extra attention to health and nutrition. Some use drug therapy; that is, they wean the user off one drug by giving him another. Eventually, they wean the user off the substitute, too.

Public treatment programs are usually underfunded and understaffed. Waiting lists are long. Many users are there on court orders, rather than from personal motivation. They often complain that they were treated "like a kid," or "like I wasn't human." Despite these problems, some people attending public clinics successfully beat their addictions. While these programs haven't eliminated heroin use, they have at least lowered it.

Methadone-maintenance clinics raise other questions. Black critics say that the only difference between methadone and heroin is that methadone is legal. In other words, the prime reason for methadone maintenance is not treatment, but lowering crime associated with the illegal drug trade. Some experts consider methadone a Band-Aid approach to treatment, and methadone-controlled addicts often return to their former habits.

THERAPEUTIC COMMUNITIES

Independent therapeutic communities such as Phoenix House or Gateway offer multiracial programs that have had a lot of success in turning around the lives of both young and adult addicts. These communities, staffed mostly by former addicts and graduates of the program, stress a self-help approach. Their goal is to change all aspects of the drug user's life. They use encounter and confrontational therapy techniques based on peer pressure, thus helping to reinforce change. These programs also provide some job training. Residence can last from three months to two years, though most people stay less than six months. Once a user has joined a therapeutic community, he or she is always considered a member, even after graduation.

Independent communities are set up mostly for hard-core users. They are supported by private donations and public funding, so most are usually free.

Counselors and family should support the teenager who is complying with the methods used in the community. It's important for parents to maintain open communication with a child in treatment. Help your child understand the rules and encourage him to become an active participant in the community. After your child graduates from a program, reward him and offer positive reinforcement as he follows postprogram instructions.

At the same time, parents need to be aware that noncompliance can occur. Avoid judging noncompliance too harshly, and encourage your child to get back on track.

Another type of residential help is called Toughlove. Its methods have been successful with some teenagers, but devastating to others. Toughlove focuses on encouraging the addict to help himself, become more responsible for his actions, and regain his self-esteem. It works best when family and friends work with qualified mental-health providers to plan the course of action and help set boundaries and limitations.

Recovery strategies are evolving, and more community-based organizations are developing treatment programs. These range from counseling services offered by African-American organizations to halfway houses administered and run by blacks. If you live in or near a black community of any size, you probably have access to at least one of these programs. There are people and organizations around that will help. Use them. If you want to find a self-help group or treatment center in your community, look in the Blue Pages under "City Government Offices, Health Department."

Remember, too, that teenagers (unlike many adults) are not trying to recover so they can resume careers or family life, but, rather, so that they can *begin to build*. A teenager in recovery may never even have held a job in his life. A teenager has fewer resources than an adult to fall back on once he becomes clean and sober. Any recovery program you choose should encourage and/or provide skills, training, and education—so that your child will have the tools to start making a life for himself.

23

TALKING ABOUT SEX

We all know that kids today are being initiated into sex at a much earlier age than we were. Fifty percent of adolescents have experienced their sexual debut by their sixteenth birthday and more than 70 percent by their nineteenth birthday.

Overall, adolescents and young adults under the age of twenty-five comprise more than half of the 20 million STD cases reported annually. Twenty-five percent are expected to become infected with an STD before graduating from high school. Two recent surveys show that the rate of syphilis is rising more among African-American adolescents than among any other group. And while the incidence of gonorrhea fell among white teenagers, it remained stable among black teenagers.

The problems that black teenagers are having with disease and unwanted pregnancies aren't because they're having sex more than anyone else. In poor neighborhoods, lack of money leads to poor health services. Poverty without hope leads to risk-taking behavior. Lack of reliable information is another factor. Peer pressure and youthful bravado (thinking that bad things only happen to other people) also play a part. Children with problems at home are more likely to seek substitutes for the love they're missing. Finally, drug and alcohol use increases everyone's risk-taking behavior; someone who's high is more likely to have unprotected sex.

Some teenagers are saying publicly that they intend to remain virgins until they are twenty-one or until they get married. Good for them. But many other young people feel pressured into experimenting with sex, often without taking simple precautions against pregnancy and disease. They have gone through a sudden growth spurt and may look like adults, but their life experience and emotions haven't caught up with their bodies yet.

Despite sex-education programs in schools, the task of helping young boys and girls sort out their feelings and make intelligent, mature choices falls largely to parents. For most parents, this is not an easy assignment, partly because sex is a private matter for everyone, including teenagers, and partly because there is a natural barrier between parents and teens. Adults and children feel uncomfortable when face-to-face in a discussion about sex.

Nevertheless, the dangers of modern society require that parents at least make sure their children are well informed. In this day and age, *all* parents should be prepared to confront the subject head-on and to talk frankly with their children.

The best time to start is when children are young. Young children who feel they can ask questions freely about sex and other sensitive matters acquire better information and can make better decisions about sexual activities as they mature. When they become teenagers, they will have positive, accurate information, allowing them to cope better with peer pressure. They are more likely to postpone sexual behavior; and if and when they do become sexually active, they are more likely to use contraceptives and protect themselves, and their partners, against unwanted pregnancy and sexually transmitted diseases.

In their book *Different and Wonderful,* Drs. Darlene Powell Hopson and Derek S. Hopson relate an anecdote of a child whose mother had spoken openly with her about aspects of sexuality from an early age. When the child became a teenager, a boy she was dating began to pressure her to have sex. She felt secure enough to discuss this problem with her mother. In talking it over, the girl admitted that she wasn't ready, and she chose not to see the boy anymore.

AGES THREE THROUGH SEVEN

Most educators believe that good sex education should start *before* the first stirrings of sexual change are felt. (If you wait until a child is ten or older, hormones are beginning to be active, and talk about sex can be difficult.) To a seven-year-old, talk about sex and reproduction is no more alarming than talking about why the sky is up and the ground is down.

Children start learning about sex at about the same time they start learning anything at all. Even in their cribs, they're checking themselves out; as early as three or four years old, they're checking out others. A three-year-old notices that her mommy and daddy, or her brother and sister, are different, even without anyone explaining it.

The key to understanding any subject is education. Children can learn about hot and cold without burning their hands or freezing their toes. They can learn about reproduction without actually reproducing.

EARLY QUESTIONS

Very young children usually ask specific questions. In *Raising Black Children,* Drs. Comer and Poussaint point out that the first questions about sex may come at the age of three or four. Children's questions often come out of the blue and can catch you off guard. At this age, they aren't looking for lengthy explanations, and they handle information best if it is simple and truthful.

Planned Parenthood recommends answering truthfully and using the proper names. To any "What is that?" questions, they suggest answers like, "This is a penis," or "These are breasts." "How come I [or you] don't have one?" "Boys have penises, girls have vaginas, and women have larger breasts than men." Most psychologists agree with this approach.

Say you and your child are visiting the zoo. If your child sees animals mating and asks what they are doing, answer, "They are having sex." If the child asks why, answer, "To have babies."

Sexual abuse. Sexual abuse is an event more common than we believed possible in the past. Such acts against children are usually kept secret. The child victim may feel shame and guilt, and he or she almost never speaks of the crime.

Many public cases have involved day-care centers, but studies have shown that child abuse most frequently occurs in the home, and the abuser is usually a friend of the family or relative. (Day-care centers are actually one of the least likely places for abuse to happen, because there are so many potential witnesses.)

None of this means that abusers are lurking on every corner. Despite the reports, chances are that it probably won't happen to your child. And no statistics suggest that sexual abuse is any more or less likely to occur in black families than in other families. Some of the figures released (30 percent and up) during the height of media attention to this issue were inflated. This is somewhat understandable: There was a kind of overcompensation for all the years of painful silence on the issue. Nonetheless, all parents need to be alert and young children need to know how to protect themselves.

When your children are four or five years old, you can prepare them without using scare tactics. Tell your child never to go anywhere with a stranger—not to the store, not into a car, not to the corner. Make a pact with your child. Tell her, "I will *never* send anyone you don't know to pick you up from school. If someone you don't know comes to school to pick you up, run to other kids, or get an adult supervisor as quickly as you can."

Prepare your child by asking what he would do in certain situations. For example, ask him, "What if you get separated from me at the store, or the amusement park? What would you do?"

Then help him come up with good answers that he can easily remember: "I would go to someone who works at the store and wait for the boss to find you," or "In the park, I would go to a policeman or security guard or to a restaurant and ask the boss to take me to a policeman so he could help me find you."

With preschool children, four and up, Drs. Comer and Poussaint counsel that they should be told never to play a game an adult says is a secret, or any game in which someone touches them in private areas. Make sure they know what the areas are: anus, vagina, penis.

Tell kids that these rules apply to parents and other relatives, too. Tell them that if anything like this occurs, they should try to get away if they can. And emphasize that they should always tell you about it, and that you will always believe them.

If your child has been sexually abused, the way you deal with it at the time can help minimize problems later on. One of the worst things about this crime is that children often feel as if it happened as a result of something they did. Reassure your child that she is absolutely loved, that she did the right thing by telling you, and that anything that happened is not her fault. No child ever asked to be sexually abused.

Planned Parenthood recommends that you arrange a visit to the doctor for your child. Then call the cops on the abuser. (Any calls you make or any investigation you do with an accused abuser should be done out of your child's earshot.)

Fortunately, most young children today are learning to recognize behavior that is dangerous to them, thanks to careful and appropriate preparation by their parents and teachers.

AGES EIGHT AND UP

When children reach seven or eight years of age, they begin asking more questions. Parents who can talk about sex simply and realistically are usually able to prepare children to look at it in the same way. Romance may be full of mystery, but sex is mostly nuts and bolts.

Don't worry that you might be pushing sex on a child by explaining matters. Most kids have already heard about it in bits and pieces. That's why they're asking. You're merely increasing the probability that your child will have the information she will need *when* the time comes.

As children get older, they need more detailed information about sexual function. Both boys and girls need to be prepared for the changes they will encounter in puberty.

PREPARING A GIRL FOR PUBERTY

Somewhere between the ages of nine and twelve, most girls get their first period. In describing this natural process to your daughter, you'll want to be simple, direct, and reassuring. If you are a single father, you might want to ask a female relative or friend to discuss menstruation with your daughter. Experts agree that using the proper terms for the parts of the body is best, but even an educated adult can get tripped up in names, parts, and functions. Drawing a picture might help. The following is a basic description for preteens.

Every woman has a uterus, which is shaped like a triangle and holds a baby when the mother is pregnant. Branching off from the upper corners of the uterus are two fallopian tubes. At the end of each free-floating tube is an opening that looks like petals of a flower, called the fimbria. One petal is slightly longer than the other. Two small pouches, called ovaries, are attached to either side of the uterus by short stalks. The ovaries contain thousands of eggs. These eggs have been inside the ovaries ever since the girl was born. A girl's first period is the signal that an egg, or ovum, has been released from one ovary.

The egg made its way to the surface of the ovary and then simply floated off the top. It was caught by the long petal of the fimbria and gently rolled into the fallopian tube. The inside of the tube is lined with millions of delicate hairlike cells waving like grass. The egg is gently moved through the tube, toward the uterus.

The uterus is like a nest for the egg. The body has prepared to receive the egg by lining the uterus with extra tissue. If the egg isn't fertilized by sperm, it simply falls before it even reaches the nest. Without a fertilized egg, the uterus doesn't need the extra tissue. The uterus discharges the excess blood and tissue through the cervix, a small opening between the uterus and the vagina. This is menstruation.

A woman's body goes through the same process every month of her life, usually until sometime between age forty and fifty, when her ovaries run out of eggs. Then pregnancy is no longer possible, and menstruation stops. This is called menopause.

If you would like more detailed information on female reproductive anatomy, write Planned Parenthood for their pamphlets on talking to kids about sex (see page 401).

PREPARING A BOY FOR PUBERTY

If your ten- or eleven-year-old son comes to you, asking why his penis suddenly got hard or why his testicles are larger than they used to be, he is about to enter puberty. If you are a single mom, you might want to ask a male relative or friend to talk over your son's physical development with him. The male reproductive system is complicated. Show your son a drawing or, if you can, make a sketch of this system, which includes the bladder, scrotum, testicles, seminal vesicle, urethra, vas deferens, epididymis, prostate gland, and penis.

Explain that his testicles will soon begin manufacturing millions of sperm. Each of these single-cell organisms has a whiplike tail that propels it, and each has the potential to fertilize an egg, or ovum, released by a woman's ovary.

It takes about sixty-four days for a sperm cell to mature inside the testicles. On ejaculation, sperm travel a complicated route through two long, heavy tubes, called spermatic cords (vasa deferentia), leading from the testicles and going up either side of the pelvic cavity. The cords run along the sides of the bladder, over the ureters, and then down into the prostate gland. As soon as sperm are ejaculated from the testicles, fluid pours into the tubes to transport the sperm. Most of the fluid comes from a pair of seminal vesicles and the prostate gland. Together, fluid and sperm are called semen. Each drop of semen contains millions of sperm, each with the potential to create a new life. Once a boy's reproductive system begins producing semen, he will probably be producing it for the rest of his life.

Once semen reaches the center of the prostate gland, it enters a tube called the urethra. The urethra emerges from the bladder opening and continues down through the prostate gland; there, the ducts carrying sperm empty into it. The urethra then exits the body through the penis.

The urethra is designed to carry both semen and urine, but not at the same time. During orgasm, an automatic muscle clamps shut the bladder entrance, so semen has the tube to itself. A boy can urinate through an erect penis, and he can sometimes ejaculate even if his penis is soft. But he cannot urinate and ejaculate at the same time.

Many adolescent boys get involuntary erections that seem to happen out of nowhere. This is the most common—and normal— reaction to the onset of puberty in boys. Boys might have wet dreams, and most begin masturbating.

MASTURBATION

From early childhood, children are remarkably sexual beings, and all children explore their bodies. Masturbation, during and after puberty, is simply a natural result of this exploration. Chances are that your children will feel embarrassed or guilty about masturbation and won't mention it to you. But that doesn't mean they understand what's going on. They may try to bring up the subject in oblique terms, possibly by asking questions about other aspects of sexuality. They're trying to find out—without asking you directly—if you think masturbation, or any expression of sexuality, is normal behavior.

Masturbation is normal and common behavior among young-sters, and your child will benefit from being assured that there's nothing wrong with it. This is especially important for girls to hear. Boys usually get reassurance from their friends, but girls seldom mention it to anyone, even their closest girlfriends. They are there-fore much more likely to worry that something is wrong with them if they masturbate.

Masturbation has beneficial effects for both boys and girls. It is a natural way to learn about their bodies. And releasing sexual tension can reduce the pressure to be sexually active too early. You don't have to be this specific with your teenagers. The important message to get across, even indirectly, is that they are developing normally and all of the new sexual feelings and urges they are experiencing are simply a part of growing up.

If you happen to walk in on a teenager who is masturbating, Drs. Poussaint and Comer say it's probably best simply to excuse yourself and walk away. In early puberty, boys sometimes masturbate in front of one another. This is simply experimentation and doesn't say anything about their sexual orientation. But if you walk in on a group session, you'll probably want to break it up in a straightfor-ward, "no big deal" way, explaining that masturbation is something that's done in private.

As kids pass puberty and sexual development becomes obvious, they may feel pressure to try sex with a member of the opposite sex. Young teenagers may become confused and even frightened by their growing sexuality. They are bombarded with sexual messages everywhere they turn—from the mass media to the locker room walls. Adolescents are particularly vulnerable to peer pressure, mostly because of their need and desire to fit in.

Even in the "old days," when it was rare for young people to have any privacy at all, kids found a way to have sex, and some became pregnant. Because kids have more unsupervised time now, it's much easier to find the privacy for sex.

At this point, kids need direct information about abstinence and protection. I talk with young teens all over the country. The talks are geared to health and nutrition, but when I talk to girls separately, they often find ways to bring up the subject of sexuality. That's because an adult with a listening ear may be open to discussing other subject matter. That's okay by me. All health-care professionals—in fact, all adults—should be able to discuss a variety of health-related subjects, even if they lie outside our particular area of expertise.

I've come to realize through these talks that while teens may be exposed to sex at a younger age than we were, they're often just as misinformed. One sexually active fifteen-year-old boy told me, "I only have to use a condom when I have sex with a girl I don't know. If it's someone from the neighborhood, I don't have to." Obviously, he had heard about sexually transmitted diseases, but he did not understand that he is at risk for an STD whether or not his sexual partner lives nearby. Nor did he understand how to prevent pregnancy.

GAY AND LESBIAN TEENAGERS

Being gay or lesbian can be a trying experience for adults, and for teenagers, it can be a very lonely experience indeed. Recognizing that one is homosexual in a world of predominantly heterosexuals can be stressful to a child or adolescent who doesn't understand why his sexual attractions are different from those of his peers. Estimates on how many teenagers are gay or lesbian run from 3 percent to 10 percent—about the same as the percentages in the adult population.

Because the teen years are such a time of sexual uncertainty, gay and lesbian teenagers can be objects of derision and cruelty from their peers. African-American gay and lesbian teens are a minority within a minority. They need exceptional strength to get through this time in a positive and emotionally healthy way. And they need more understanding as they try to sort through their feelings and grow to accept their sexual orientation. Gay teens really need somebody in their corner. Counseling from a mental health professional, such as a psychologist or social worker, along with support and love from parents can greatly reduce these anxieties.

TALKING ABOUT PREGNANCY

When talking about pregnancy, the same guidelines you used when your child was very young still apply. Be honest, and keep it simple. By all means talk about abstinence. But make sure your kids know what the word *abstinence* means.

The subject came up in a recent health discussion I was having with a group of junior high girls in the Midwest. The girls brought up the subject of sex. They told me that they were all virgins but that they were getting a lot of pressure to have sex from their boyfriends. They knew about condoms, but they didn't actually know how to have intercourse, and they were extremely curious. They assured me that when the time came, they would make sure to use a condom.

"What about abstinence?" I asked.

"Oh, that's okay, too," said one thirteen-year-old.

"What's that?" another asked.

I looked at the group for a response. No one responded. I realized that the girls had *heard* of abstinence but didn't know what the word meant.

I believe that young people should know that you respect their intelligence and rely on their good judgment. But no one can make good judgments without good information. Start talking to your daughter when she is ten or eleven years old. Talk openly, adult to adult. Skip the lecture. Ask conversational questions (not interrogational ones) to draw your teenager into the discussion. "What do you think about condoms? What do you think about teenagers who get pregnant? What would you do if that happened to you? What would you want to happen?"

If you find this just too difficult—and many parents do—think about giving permission for your teenager to attend a sex-education class (if one is not part of your child's school curriculum), or about asking your teen if he or she would like to talk to another older person about sex—someone who is not Mom or Dad. The goal is to make sure your teen is well informed.

I've noticed that many young teens have extremely romantic notions of what it's like to have a baby. One fourteen-year-old told me, "Oh, if I get pregnant, my boyfriend and I will get our own apartment, and he'll get a job, and we'll go to high school, and then we'll go to college, and buy a house." Another said, "If I get pregnant, my mom will take care of the baby."

At this age, they really don't get it. If you overhear these sorts of statements from your child or her friends, use them as an opportunity to point out how unrealistic these notions are. Try to go to the heart of the matter, without flying off the handle.

One conversation is not enough. Kids need to hear this information in a positive way, from many different sources and at many different ages. Adolescents remember some things and forget others, depending on their particular concerns at any given time. They may hear part of your message, yet miss the rest, like the boy who thought he needed to use a condom only if he had sex with a stranger. All of this information needs repeating—in the family, in the school, and in youth groups.

Remember, too, that although a teenage girl *can* have a baby, there are both emotional *and physical* reasons why she *shouldn't*. Her reproductive system is still immature. Teenage girls have the highest risk for giving birth to a low-birth-weight baby, which is the prime cause of infant death in the United States. (See chapter 2.)

DANGEROUS MYTHS ABOUT CONTRACEPTION

Many teenagers engage in what Planned Parenthood calls "magical thinking." Some think they can't get pregnant if they don't have an orgasm. Another myth is that if a girl douches afterward with soda, like 7-Up or Pepsi, she won't get pregnant. Drs. Hopson and Hopson, authors of *Different and Wonderful,* report that many teens think they can't get pregnant the first time they have sex; if they don't want to get pregnant; if they have sex while standing; if they stand up immediately after sex.

The perpetual popularity of the rhythm method as a means of contraception is another problem. For seven or eight days each month, a girl has an egg in position to be fertilized. No matter how regular her periods are, she can't know for sure that intercourse won't make her pregnant, because she can never be entirely sure when her monthly egg is going to drop. Also, sperm can live inside the vagina and fallopian tubes for several days. That means that when the egg drops into the fallopian tube, a sperm may already be there to meet it—even if the girl hasn't had sexual contact in a week.

CONTRACEPTION

Sex is the most natural of all the pleasures we seek, but because of unplanned pregnancies and destructive infections, abstinence, especially for kids, is the safest form of safe sex. Abstinence is the only sure way to prevent the potentially destructive side effects of sex. But whether your children practice abstinence or safe sex, education is essential to preserve their health and happiness—and perhaps even their lives. Whatever course you encourage your teenager to follow—and whatever course he or she chooses to follow—a frank discussion of contraception should not be avoided.

CONTRACEPTIVES FOR BOYS

If a teenage boy is going to be sexually active, the message must be about the proper use of condoms. In the teenage mind, many issues of performance and insecurity argue against condoms. Boys are still learning control; many have quick orgasms and are erect again two minutes later. Tell them to use a condom, anyway (they'll take longer to reach orgasm, and protect themselves and their partners at the same time). Above all, boys need to hear that they have a responsibility to their partners. Girls are not objects on which they must prove their manhood. They need to get this message from their fathers, their brothers, uncles, and all the men they come in contact with. In my own teenaged years, parents encouraged their sons to be responsible. If a boy found his partner pregnant, he was expected to show true responsibility by marrying the girl and getting a job to support the family.

Condoms are sold in a variety of styles and sizes, but they are not all the same. *Latex condoms lubricated with the spermicide nonoxynol-9* are the best defense (other than no sex at all) against pregnancy and disease. Even when used correctly and consistently, condoms are not 100 percent effective, but they do work against disease better than any other contraceptive device.

CONTRACEPTION FOR GIRLS

There are several contraception options for girls, but only two, the pill and the diaphragm, offer significant protection against pregnancy, and *none protects her against disease*. A girl's only adequate line of defense against disease is insisting that a boy use a condom.

She can add further protection against pregnancy by using some form of contraception herself. In descending order, from most to least effective, here are her options.

The pill. It is available by doctor's prescription only. Because of potential side effects, the contraceptive pill should be used only if a girl is continuously sexually active and only after she has had a thorough medical examination. Most effective protection against pregnancy; no protection against STDs.

Diaphragm. A diaphragm is available by doctor's prescription only. It is awkward for most inexperienced girls to use; girls are more likely to use one if a parent, doctor, or nurse is encouraging and explains how they work and the proper insertion technique—and if they use the device regularly.

Foams, creams, gels (spermicides). Used alone, these chemical barriers are only about 82 percent effective against pregnancy; obviously, they offer greater effectiveness when used with a diaphragm or condom and this is the preferred method of use. Spermicides also offer some (minimal) protection against STDs. However, spermicides are not very practical, because they must be reapplied immediately before sex, and when used with condoms they add another step to the contraceptive process. Some women are also sensitive to chemicals, and many find them messy to use.

IF A CHILD HAS A PROBLEM

No matter how much you may disapprove, no matter how strongly you have advocated abstinence, no matter how strong the urge to administer punishment might be—if a child gets pregnant or contracts a disease, you must put your feelings on hold and help deal with the situation. Not knowing what to do, or doing nothing, or doing the wrong thing—any of these can lead to truly terrible outcomes. Your child's life may be at stake.

ABORTION

Abortion is a legal option that all adult women have. (Most physicians who perform the procedure will not do it to someone under seventeen years old without parental consent. However, teen advocacy programs, legal aid, and local ACLU chapters can often help younger teens who do not have parental consent.) If this is a choice your daughter makes, you will feel reassured to know that a properly performed abortion does not have any known detrimental physiological effect on a young girl's future ability to become pregnant and deliver a healthy baby. However, you must prepare your daughter for the possible emotional reaction following an abortion.

Abortion is never an easy choice. Certainly no one thinks it is a viable form of contraception. But unplanned pregnancies do happen, and they happen to all kinds of women and girls in all kinds of circumstances. According to Faye Wattleton, a previous president of Planned Parenthood, minority women are twice as likely as white women to experience unplanned pregnancy and seek abortions. And black women generally do not seek the procedure until they are in the second trimester, when abortion is significantly riskier. If your teen becomes pregnant and is confused about keeping the baby, adoption or abortion counseling will help. Choosing the right counselor is important. Clergy, social workers, and mental-health professionals are the best choices. Many clinics and programs will also provide trained counselors who can answer your teenager's questions and concerns. You are in a position to offer the most caring and supportive advice. Ultimately, the final choice is up to your teen and her partner, since his opinion is important, too.

SEXUALLY TRANSMITTED DISEASES

Currently, one out of every four people who engages in sex contracts some sort of STD. Left untreated, many can have devastating results, particularly in young girls, whose natural defense mechanisms are relatively immature and not always able to ward off infection. Even minor STDs can have serious consequences, including pelvic inflammatory disease, infertility, tubal pregnancy, and adverse pregnancy outcome. Any STD requires a visit to the doctor for treatment.

Most experts agree that parents should at least try to give kids some basic preventive information, even if they say they don't want to hear it. Sometimes, just giving your son or daughter a pamphlet or a book, without comment, is the best way to go. With a pamphlet in hand, natural curiosity usually overcomes even the most rebellious teenager. And reading may lead to a private talk with you.

Here is a brief rundown on the most common STDs.

CHLAMYDIA

This is the most common STD in the United States. Doctors estimate 4 million cases a year, males and females. Left untreated, chlamydia can reach a girl's pelvic cavity and lead to undetected pelvic inflammatory disease, which can permanently damage the reproductive organs. In men, chlamydia infects the urethra and is easily passed to sex partners.

Symptoms. Chlamydia may have no symptoms at all in women, which makes it particularly dangerous. Some women have a small discharge, pain during intercourse, and a burning sensation during urination. Symptoms are more common in men, who may experience burning, as well as more frequent urination.

Treatment. The disease is often discovered by a simple test performed during a routine checkup. It is treated with antibiotics.

GONORRHEA

Gonorrhea is the most reported communicable disease in the country. Gonorrhea can lead to infections of the fallopian tubes and ovaries in women and to blockage of the urethra in men, causing problems getting an erection. For both men and women, it can cause arthritis, heart trouble, nervous disorders, and sterility.

Symptoms. Males experience a discharge that looks like pus and pain while urinating. Females most often experience no symptoms. Occasionally, there may be green or yellowish green discharge; mushroomlike odor; blood or pus in the urine; pain in the pelvis and abdomen; swelling around the opening of the vagina.

Treatment. Antibiotics. Both partners must be treated at the same time in order to prevent reinfection.

HERPES SIMPLEX VIRUS, TYPES I AND II

At first, doctors thought there were major differences between Type I and Type II, but further experience with herpes has shown that there aren't. Type I is more common and causes cold sores and fever blisters, usually in the mouth and around the lips.

For years, many African Americans viewed herpes as a "white" disease. The common saying was, "You get herpes from oral sex, and we don't do that!" Of course, African Americans engage in a variety of sexual activities. And herpes may be transmitted by vaginal, oral, or anal sex.

Symptoms and problems. There may not be any symptoms at first, but when they appear, they're inescapable. In women, blisters may show up in the vulva, inside the vagina, and on the rectum; in males, blisters usually occur on the penis or in the urethra. Blisters may go unnoticed until they break open; then they are very painful. The first time blisters appear can be the worst, often accompanied by low-grade fever, headache, and tender, swollen lymph nodes in the groin. The entire episode lasts about two weeks.

Blisters eventually disappear, but then they reappear. Type I herpes returns once or twice a year; Type II, four to six times a year. Fever, headaches, weariness, and itching are other symptoms.

Males and females who have contracted herpes should *not* have sex when they are having an outbreak. However, the virus may be active for some time before and after sores erupt, and it's possible for someone to transmit herpes unknowingly even when symptoms are inactive. Herpes in pregnant women is very serious and must be monitored by a doctor.

Some people have only mild and rare attacks, and eventually the body builds its own defenses against the virus, so for many people, the problem diminishes over time.

Treatment. Acyclovir (ointment and/or tablets) helps decrease pain and the number of blisters, but it is not a cure.

HUMAN PAPILLOMAVIRUS (HPV)

Several types of HPV are in existence, and not a whole lot is known about them. Some types of HPV show up as genital warts; others can lead to outcomes as serious as cervical cancer. In one urban clinic, 38 percent of adolescents were found with some form of HPV; in another, 16 percent. It is most frequently diagnosed by a Pap smear.

Symptoms and problems. In both males and females, warts may appear on the genitals and sometimes in the area of the anus, especially in moist places. These little fleshy lumps may grow into large bulky masses. They may grow singly or in clusters; they may itch and produce a malodorous discharge.

Condoms offer some but not total protection from sexual transmission, since the HPV may be present in areas not covered by a condom. The virus seems to be most contagious when warts first begin to appear. Several months may pass between the time of infection and the actual appearance of warts, which means that if the individual has more than one partner it is often difficult to trace the sexual contact.

Treatment. Genital warts are often treated by carefully applying a chemical called podophyllin to the surface of the warts only (it is very irritating to normal skin). Laser treatment may be suggested when the warts are numerous, are resistant to chemical treatment, or appear during pregnancy, when podophyllin should be avoided.

Like other viral infections, genital warts have a tendency to recur. If the warts persist in growing back, a biopsy may be recommend to make sure they are not cancerous. Some physicians now recommend that a female with HPV have regular Pap tests of the cervix every three to six months because of a possible link between HPV and precancerous changes in the cells of the cervix.

SYPHILIS

Syphilis is the second most dangerous STD after HIV. It can kill if it isn't treated, and even if it doesn't kill but is allowed to reach its late stage, it'll make the infected person's remaining years a living hell. (Besides this, the organism can be passed on to the fetus during pregnancy.) Syphilis is caused by a spirochete, a tiny bacterial organism, and early treatment is relatively easy and painless.

Symptoms and problems. Three weeks after infection, a single moist nodule with elevated edges appears at the spot of infection, most often the genitals, but not always. In females, the chancre is usually inside the vagina, where it can't be seen. In males, it's usually on the penis. It can also show up on the lips, in and around the mouth, and around the rectum. This blister, called a chancre, doesn't hurt, is extremely infectious (it's moist because it's oozing the spirochete), and heals by itself anywhere from one to five weeks later. That doesn't mean that the person who's had it is healed. Also, not everyone with syphilis gets the chancre.

Another symptom is a reddish brown rash that appears on the palms or soles of the feet. Other symptoms are headaches, fever, and weight loss.

Syphilis is divided into stages. The first stage is the chancre. If there is no treatment during the first stage, the second stage can occur anywhere from a month and a half to six months later; it is characterized by a rash, as well as a feeling of malaise, muscle pains, and loss of appetite. Patches of hair might fall out. An infectious gray-white rash, usually found on the lips of the vagina, shows up and develops into oozing sores. The sores are filled with the spirochete. The second stage, if it is untreated, lasts between four to twelve weeks.

Latent, or tertiary, syphilis begins when the second stage is over. There are no symptoms, but a pregnant woman can pass the spirochete to her fetus. Latent syphilis can last for years. After four years, it is called "late" syphilis, an advanced stage of the disease that involves the heart, liver, and other organs, until the individual eventually dies.

Treatment. Penicillin is the drug of choice. Doxycycline and tetracycline are also used.

HIV/AIDS

The incidence of HIV infection is rising rapidly among teenagers, particularly African-American and Hispanic youth, who for various reasons are not getting, or absorbing, vital AIDS-prevention information. See chapter 24 for a full discussion of HIV and AIDS in children and adolescents.

CONFIDENTIALITY

If you suspect that your teenager is sexually active, it is especially important that he or she have some knowledge of the diseases discussed in the previous section. He or she should also get a regular checkup that includes testing for STDs. Most adolescents do inform their parents when they suspect they are pregnant or have contracted an STD, but many don't. A teenager suspecting any of these outcomes *must* see a doctor. The earlier treatment is initiated, the better the outcome, and the less chance of passing a disease to another partner.

Ideally, your teenager has developed a relationship with a pediatrician or family doctor over the years, or even has a doctor of his own. But most teens do not know a doctor they feel they can trust. It's difficult for adolescents to believe that they'll get confidential medical care from any doctor, yet confidential medical care is just what they need. In a situation where a teenager is afraid of parental reprisal, confidentiality is crucial.

In general, minors cannot give legal consent for their own health care. But there are important exceptions: Unless specific state law mandates against it, adolescents may give legal consent for pregnancy diagnosis and care, abortion, contraceptive services, treatment of STDs, and counseling and management of substance abuse. Some states have free clinics where teenagers can be examined and treated for disease (Planned Parenthood has clinics in forty-nine states and in Washington, D.C.).

Youngsters whose parents have given them a strong sense of self-worth since the day they were born won't need premature sex and pregnancy to make them feel loved and wanted. The best way to discourage your adolescent from experimenting with sex before he or she is ready is to lay down a positive foundation early. Teach them respect for themselves. Teach them that their bodies are private and that they should share themselves only with someone whom they truly love and who loves them.

Part Four

Your Child's Health

24

CHILDHOOD HIV AND AIDS

HIV/AIDS is spreading rapidly among African-American and Hispanic populations, particularly among children and teenagers. In fact, African-American infants are the single fastest growing group of patients with AIDS, which is transmitted from mother to child during pregnancy. Currently, the numbers look like this: An estimated 240,000 Americans have AIDS; 10,000 are children. Of these, 53 percent are African American and 25 percent are Hispanic. It is estimated that every year eighteen hundred American infants will be born with HIV.

WHAT PARENTS NEED TO KNOW ABOUT HIV/AIDS

Roughly 25 to 30 percent of infants born to HIV-positive mothers are also infected, either during pregnancy or during birth. Relatively few infants become infected through breast-feeding, but it can happen. The late Elizabeth Glazer passed the disease to her infant daughter this way.

Children can contract HIV by being sexually abused by someone infected with the virus. Teenagers can become infected if they are sexually active in any way. They can also become infected by contaminated needles during intravenous drug use.

Children can also become infected through a transfusion of infected blood; however, new screening methods are believed to have eliminated HIV from the blood supply. Organ transplants are also generally safe, although somewhat riskier than transfusions.

Knowing how the virus *cannot* be transmitted is also important. The HIV virus is fragile and cannot live long outside the body. It cannot be transmitted through casual acts such as kissing and hugging, sharing eating utensils, using a public toilet seat, or other ordinary activities. Nor is it transmitted by mosquitoes or other insects.

WHAT YOU NEED TO TEACH YOUR CHILD

Many schools begin to educate students about HIV and AIDS in elementary school. It's the rare American child who hasn't at least heard of this disease. Despite these efforts, many children remain misinformed and confused. A 1990 study surveyed Georgia teens about their knowledge of the causes and transmission of HIV/ AIDS. Most teens knew the rudiments of transmission but were confused about the actual course of the disease. Minority teens who participated in the study—especially those admitting to IV drug use—were more afraid of catching AIDS than whites were. At the same time, they were also the least well informed.

The facts point dramatically to the need for better sex and contraceptive education among children and adolescents. Parents cannot rely on schools to provide all the answers. Experts agree that the AIDS-prevention message is most powerful when it comes from parents. This is not a one-time-only message. Children absorb different facts at different ages, and in between a lot of mythology can seep in. Children can become confused by information they get from other kids and from television. The information parents give needs to be repeated and updated periodically as children grow older.

When you talk to your children, try to find out what they already know, correct any misinformation, and offer calm, clear explanations appropriate for their age.

YOUNGER CHILDREN

Children as young as age four or five have heard of AIDS, and they know you can die from it. If asked, they may admit it is scary to them.

Tell them that AIDS is a disease that causes some people to get very sick but that they should not worry, because there is little danger either they or their parents will become infected.

By late elementary and junior high school age, children need to know how HIV, the virus believed to cause AIDS, is transmitted. Tell them that people get AIDS primarily through sexual contact with someone who is infected with the virus or by using contaminated ("dirty") needles while doing drugs. Explain that any needle can be dirty, especially a needle that is shared.

Make sure you tell children how HIV is *not* transmitted. They will not get HIV by touching an infected person or by using water fountains. Children with AIDS pose no risk to other children or adults. They do not spread the virus through toys, spoons, bottles, dishes, hugging, or playing.

OLDER KIDS

By junior high and high school age, teenagers should be told that the only safe sex is no sex. The next best choice, if they do decide to become sexually active, is always to use a latex condom with a spermicide (nonoxynol-9).

Teens contract HIV through sexual activity or drug use. African-American teens are the group hardest hit and so far least responsive to prevention methods. The reason may be that teenagers simply cannot fathom the possibility of dying and consequently they indulge in high-risk behavior with little regard for the outcome. Some psychologists theorize that minority youths are already so despairing about their future that they take even greater risks than other teens. I have observed that kids of all ethnic and economic backgrounds have a lot of information that they appear to understand, but it's as if they're suffering from information overload. And when teenagers are confused, they don't want to look dumb by asking questions.

Ask your kids what they know about HIV and AIDS. If they say they know "all about it," ask them to tell you what they know. Clarify their information, or misinformation. Always ask if there's anything they're not sure about that they would like to ask you. Encourage kids of all ages to ask questions about HIV/AIDS.

Ask a few questions of your own and probe for their answers. The point to keep in mind is that information your child says back to you in his own words is more likely to be remembered.

It's likely that your child will not want to admit to you or a physician, even confidentially, if he's having sex or using drugs. Realistically, however, statistics show that nearly one-third of all teens have had sexual intercourse by the age of fifteen.

Keep open the channels of communication to let your child know it's critical to think about whether they want to have sex, and with whom. Explain the importance of using latex condoms. Teenagers must know how to ensure that their partners always use condoms and practice safe sex. They are also old enough to comprehend the moral issues involved in potentially spreading a deadly disease.

Adolescents have a lot of misinformation about condoms. Ask your kids what they've heard about condoms, and correct any myths. Condoms do not eliminate sensation. Nor are they solely for use with prostitutes. "Nice" girls do buy and carry condoms. Carrying condoms doesn't imply an individual, male or female, is having sex with a lot of different people or doesn't trust a partner.

Some kids are worried that they may have been exposed but are afraid to tell their parents. HIV testing can help relieve their worries (if they are negative), or put them on the road to early treatment and prevent further transmission of the infection (if they are positive). Make sure that your child knows that he or she can be anonymously tested for HIV.

RISKS FOR WOMEN AND BABIES

Women at risk for transmitting HIV to their babies are those who have had unprotected sex with someone who is HIV-positive, have shared syringes during intravenous drug use, or have had other sexually transmitted diseases.

In New York, all newborns are routinely screened for HIV in order to keep track of the epidemic. Yet the state is caught on the horns of an ethical dilemma. Unless the mother has given her permission, the infant who tests positive remains unidentified—even to the family.

The New York State legislature is considering mandating the identification of newborns' HIV status. Such a requirement sounds reasonable, but in reality, testing a newborn does not reveal the infant's HIV status, because a newborn who tests positive may later prove to be HIV-negative. But it does reveal the HIV status of the mother. Newborn testing amounts to mandatory AIDS testing for pregnant women, which would make them the only class of Americans tested without their consent (except for federal prisoners). All infants born to mothers who are HIV-positive initially test positive themselves because of the in utero exchange of antibodies. But at least three out of every four of those babies shed the antibodies; perhaps 80 percent eventually will be HIV-negative.

Proponents of mandatory testing say that only special-interest groups obsessed with privacy are against it. They say any mother would want to know the truth. And even babies who test negative at fifteen months may still be HIV-positive.

Ideally, HIV-positive babies should have immediate access to preventive health care. However, as stated, tests of newborns are inconclusive.

The urgency of newborn testing is being pressed home with new medical findings that support the earliest possible drug therapy to protect infants against opportunistic infections. PCP, or *Pneumocystis carinii* pneumonia, is the leading opportunistic infection in HIV-infected children and adults and a major cause of death from AIDS. The risk of PCP is highest in young infants, with more than half of such cases occurring in children aged three to six months.

New 1995 guidelines from the federal Centers for Disease Control and Prevention stress the need to diagnose HIV infection in pregnant women during pregnancy and to start all infants born to infected mothers on prophylactic therapy between four and six weeks of age. Drug therapy would be stopped if a child is later found not to be infected. Beyond age one, infected children would continue to receive drug therapy based on laboratory and clinical information.

New studies indicating that AZT taken during pregnancy may deter transmission of the AIDS virus to the baby have made the issue of voluntary testing among pregnant women even more urgent.

The question now is, Should HIV testing of pregnant women be mandatory or voluntary? No other group in the United States has to submit to mandatory testing. Why should pregnant women have to relinquish their rights to someone else? Many health professionals and AIDS activists working on the front lines with AIDS patients strongly disagree with mandatory testing. The vast majority of babies born with the HIV virus are born to poor women of color who do drugs or sleep with people who do. These are the patients who most fear recrimination by police or medical authorities. The concern is that mandatory testing will drive some women to have their babies delivered outside the hospital and would even scare many away from prenatal clinics, at the time when they need care the most.

Where is a viable, useful approach that will help our most vulnerable and most helpless? It should be obvious to everyone that every woman, regardless of her circumstances, wants to protect her child. Doctors at New York's Harlem Hospital believe that when pregnant women understand what kind of help is available to them and their babies, they will agree to be tested on a voluntary, confidential basis. Dr. Janet Mitchell, who runs the pregnancy clinic at Harlem Hospital, put the theory to the test. Clinic doctors talked to pregnant patients at every visit about the dangers of HIV transmission and the potential benefits of testing, just as they talked about nutrition, smoking, drugs, and other prenatal health issues. Nearly 90 percent of the pregnant women agreed to be tested voluntarily. The babies of mothers who tested positive were born in the hospital, where they could be immediately placed in comprehensive treatment programs.

Newborn testing is still a hotly debated issue, and each state will make its own decision as AIDS statistics continue to increase among infants. Most African Americans do not like the idea of mandatory testing. However, regardless of your opinion, it's important to make your voice heard. You can call any AIDS activist organization in your community to get more information, assistance, or to participate in activities.

HELPING CHILDREN LIVE WITH HIV

For many babies, HIV first manifests itself through symptoms of illness, including recurrent fever, bacterial infection, chronic diarrhea, recurrent oral thrush, or failure to thrive. Some HIV-positive kids simply grow more slowly than their peers.

Early high-quality medical management means that children and adults who are HIV-positive are living longer, healthier lives. As in adults, management of HIV in children depends upon five elements:

- Identification
- Antiretroviral treatment

- Preventive medication against opportunistic diseases
- Treatment of opportunistic diseases
- Supportive care

IDENTIFICATION

A newborn who tests HIV-positive should have a blood analysis every three to six months for two years to prove or disprove the diagnosis.

ANTIRETROVIRAL TREATMENT

AZT (zidovudine) and ddI (didanosine) are the most commonly used antiretroviral medications in adults. Antiretroviral medications slow the progression of AIDS by temporarily blocking production of the HIV virus. Until very recently, AZT was considered the drug of choice in treating HIV-infected children. However, in February of 1995, federal health officials halted the AZT part of a comparison trial of AZT and ddI in children because of severe side effects. Children receiving AZT alone had more rapid rates of disease progression as measured by failure to grow, myriad infections, deterioration, and death.

The second drug, ddI, continues to be tested alone and in combination with AZT in this long-term study. The study, sponsored by the National Institute of Child Health and Human Development and the National Institute of Allergy and Infectious Diseases, began in August of 1991 and involves 839 children initially aged three months to eighteen years. Until the results are in, the new findings leave doctors uncertain about how to treat children with HIV infection. Whatever drug choice is made—ddI or ddI combined with AZT—antiviral drugs are themselves toxic to the body. The potential benefit—slowing the period between HIV-positive status and full-blown AIDS—must be weighed against damaging side effects that also have the potential to shorten life.

PREVENTIVE MEDICATION (PROPHYLAXIS) AGAINST OPPORTUNISTIC DISEASE

Drugs that prevent opportunistic infections are considered first-line therapy by most experienced physicians. Bactrim, Dapsone, or pentamidine are used to combat PCP (*Pneumocystis carinii* pneumonia), the most common HIV-related infection in the United States. Another drug, intravenous immunoglobulin (IVIG), provides more general, blanket, protection from infections.

IMMUNIZATION

Childhood diseases such as chicken pox and measles are potentially devastating to HIV-positive children. Thus, it is very important that they receive routine childhood immunizations. However, some modification of the schedules is required, depending on the status of the child's immune system. In general HIV-infected children should not receive live viral vaccines. MMR (measles/mumps/rubella) is the only live viral vaccine recommended for routine administration since the benefits of vaccination outweigh the possible risks of a child getting a vaccine-related illness. The new chicken pox vaccine is not currently recommended for HIV-positive children.

TREATMENT OF OPPORTUNISTIC DISEASES

Learning the early signs of infection in HIV-positive children and getting immediate medical attention are essential steps for parents to take. The HIV-positive child's immune system may not be strong enough to fight off even the most ordinary illness. Early treatment, often with drug therapy and possibly hospitalization, can save a child's life.

SUPPORTIVE CARE

The current emphasis in HIV treatment is long-term management. Many children infected with HIV are living longer and entering the public school system. It is your child's legal right to attend school, unless his doctor does not approve. The school principal should be informed of your child's health status, and you may also decide to alert some of the teaching staff and/or the school nurse.

Every HIV-positive child should have a health-care team working on his or her behalf. Your child may need the services of a nutritionist, physical therapist, pain-management specialist, and dentist in addition to a pediatrician. As well as receiving antiviral and/or preventive medications, an older child can also participate in maintaining his own health by eating a nutritious, balanced diet and by exercising.

More than anything else, the HIV-positive child needs love, attention, and nurturing to make the most of his or her life. Although many of these children have already lost their mothers, all members of the extended family can fill this supportive, caring, loving role.

25

ASTHMA

Roughly 12 million Americans have asthma, a number that's on the rise, especially among African-American children. The illness is rarely fatal, but the poorer the neighborhood, the higher the risk of dying from asthma. Ten years ago, African Americans were about twice as likely to die of asthma as whites; today, we are three times as likely to die of asthma; and among those aged fifteen to forty-four, African Americans are five times as likely to die of asthma.

Researchers have found few reasons to explain why African-American children are so vulnerable to asthma, or why the incidence of asthma is increasing among them. Exactly why poverty increases the risk is unknown. Increased exposure to substances that set off asthma attacks and poor access to health care may be factors. Another possible catalyst is greater use of aerosol inhalers, called beta-agonists, which may mask a worsening of the disease.

Asthma attacks occur when the bronchial tubes and air sacs responsible for circulating oxygen through the lungs become inflamed and clogged with mucus. Inflamed tissues swell, constricting the airways and causing muscles to spasm. The victim makes wheezing sounds as he tries to push air through smaller and smaller bronchial channels. Asthma sufferers often cannot expel air in the lungs—during an attack, it's tough even to extinguish a candle.

Asthma attacks are accompanied by sweating, rapid pulse, and dizziness, which tend to make them look like panic attacks. If the air supply is compromised for too long, toes and fingers can turn blue—a dangerous sign of oxygen deprivation. For days after a bad attack, an asthma sufferer's chest may be sore from the sheer effort of breathing during the crisis.

Asthma tends to occur in families where other members have either asthma, hay fever, or eczema. Asthma is often due to an allergic response. Exposure to allergens, such as cat and dog dander, mold and dust mites, freshly painted rooms, or particular foods can trigger an attack. Asthma can worsen during cold weather, when windows are likely to be shut; poor air circulation causes allergens to be trapped in building materials, upholstered furnishings, bedding, and carpets. Often, however, there is no clear reason for any particular asthmatic attack.

Once asthma is established, the airways become hypersensitive and it takes less and less irritation to trigger an attack. A cold or cough, infections, changes in weather, or emotional stress can trigger an attack. Although many children grow out of asthma, about 10 percent are troubled by it all their lives.

TREATMENT

The treatment of asthma varies according to the severity of the problem. Some children have only rare episodes of asthma; others have daily attacks, which severely compromise their growth and ability to function in school and at home.

MEDICAL THERAPY

When your child has an asthma attack, the primary goal is to curtail it quickly, either with medications or by taking the child to the hospital. Doctors rely on medications that open the airways and break up mucus, which can then be coughed up and spit out. These drugs, called beta-agonist bronchodilators, can be injected, inhaled, or taken as pills.

During a severe attack, a doctor may give your child a shot of epinephrine to ease his breathing. One temporary side effect of this treatment is an elevated pulse, so it's customary to keep a patient under observation until heartbeat returns to normal.

Medical therapy provides relief of symptoms, often dramatically so. The newest, fastest-working inhalants include terbutaline, metaproterenol (Alupent), albuterol (Ventolin), isoproterenol (Isuprel,

Medihaler-Iso), and salmeterol (Serevent), which is a sustained-release inhalant.

It's important that you monitor your child's asthma treatment in order to avoid harmful side effects, which include increased blood pressure, irregular or rapid heartbeat, difficulty in urination, nervousness, and dry mouth.

Inhalants work quickly and effectively. However, scientists are worried that bronchodilators may be contributing to the worsening of the disease. Possibly, by opening up the airways with drugs, asthma patients are exposing their lungs to more of what's harmful. Dr. Albert Sheffer, an allergist at Harvard Medical School, says bronchodilating inhalers should not be used more than twice a day; the medication in one inhaler should last for a month. If your child finds it more and more necessary to resort to an inhaler, it's probably a signal that something is going wrong internally and it's time to reevaluate his medications. Your child also may be instructed to use a "peak flow" meter several times daily, in order to monitor the amount of air he expels. If the level drops too low, a trip to the doctor for a change in medications is required.

A more advanced line of attack is to prevent attacks by using corticosteroid drugs to reduce inflammation in the lungs and airways and keep lungs in good working order. Although these are not the same as the steroids used by bodybuilders and other athletes to build muscle, they do have their own negative side effects. Long-term use can delay growth, cause thinning of bones, and cause stomach ulcers. These corticosteroids can also be expensive, making them problematic for anyone with limited funds or without health insurance.

Another important medication that has been used for prevention is cromolyn sodium (Intal). This drug is often used as an inhaler. It is more expensive than inhaled corticosteroids but acts to stabilize elements in the immune system that ordinarily result in asthma attacks.

PREVENTING ATTACKS THE NATURAL WAY

Because of the side effects associated with drug therapy, asthma treatment is turning more toward preventing attacks by reducing allergens in the child's environment. Here are important techniques you can use to reduce allergens in your home.

- Remove rugs and pillows from your child's environment.
- Change bedding frequently.
- Avoid plants and foods that cause reactions.
- Dust and vacuum often.
- Wash or vacuum plush toys frequently and only buy stuffed toys labeled "nonallergenic."
- Store out-of-season clothes in airtight bags.
- Change heating, air-conditioner, and humidifier filters often.
- Keep your child's environment free of secondhand smoke.

PETS

As a general rule, asthmatic kids should not be around pets. Your child may be allergic to cats but not dogs, or vice versa. In either case, if you have pets in the house, don't let them sleep with your child or even in your child's room.

MAINTAINING A SMOKE-FREE ENVIRONMENT

A study conducted for the National Health Interview Survey found that children whose mothers smoked had more than double the risk of asthma. The importance of a smoke-free environment is most critical from conception through age three.

HUMIDITY

Good hydration lubricates the airways and loosens mucus clogging the air passages, making it easier to breathe. Asthmatics should drink lots of water and other liquids, since dehydration aggravates breathing problems. Some physicians recommend tea with honey to help break up phlegm. Steam treatments, including standing in a steamy bathroom several times a day, are another good way to promote hydration.

EXERCISE

Asthmatic children may find that being in good physical shape helps them manage their disease better. Asthma needn't keep your child on the bench. Plenty of top-level athletes are asthmatic, including Olympian Jackie Joyner-Kersee. In fact, forty-one medals went home with asthmatic Americans competing in the 1984 L.A. Olympics.

Sports activities that call for sudden bursts of energy can be tough on asthmatics, however. Teach children to warm up slowly when beginning an exercise session. Swimming is highly recommended, partly because it's a long, steady effort and partly because water is largely allergen-free. Some doctors recommend using an inhaler fifteen minutes prior to exercising to guard against an attack.

Hopefully, increased communication among medical researchers around the world will help the American medical community expand its outlook for treatments of this increasingly dangerous disease that affects so many of the children in our community.

26

DIABETES

Diabetes means that the body doesn't properly use—or does not make—insulin. Insulin is a hormone that lets cells absorb glucose from carbohydrates you eat; without it, cells starve. There are two distinct types of diabetes: Type II (adult-onset), the most common form, and Type I (juvenile).

TYPE II DIABETES

In this kind of diabetes, the pancreas may actually produce normal levels of insulin, but for some reason the body is unable to use it. Sometimes insulin levels are insufficient and the pancreas gradually loses its capacity to produce any hormone at all.

Before 1940, Type II diabetes, which accounts for 90 percent of all cases of diabetes, was thought to be relatively rare among African Americans, but today, all minorities in the United States have higher rates of diabetes than whites. Native Americans have the highest prevalence of diabetes in the world—more than ten times that of whites. Hispanics and African Americans are next, 3.1 and 1.5 times higher, respectively. Among African-American women, the rate is two times higher. The gap between whites and minorities continues to increase as individuals grow older. African Americans also have a greater risk of complications and premature death from diabetes than do whites. The increasing incidence may be partly due to better screening and reporting methods, but other factors are also involved.

Type II diabetes overwhelmingly occurs in people who are overweight. The disease usually develops slowly over time, and it is seldom diagnosed until the individual is an adult. Sometimes it is discovered only after complications such as heart, eye, kidney, or nerve damage are discovered. This makes it extremely dangerous.

Although researchers don't yet know exactly what triggers diabetes, we know that the disease often runs in families. If parents, grandparents, aunts, or uncles have diabetes, a child's risk is immediately greater. Researchers suspect a genetic predisposition that is expressed only when people are exposed to certain environmental factors, such as excess weight, high stress, and poor nutrition.

We know that obesity—the most common risk factor for diabetes—is significantly higher among black women. The *types* of foods we eat also contribute. African Americans typically consume less fiber, which is thought to help control levels of glucose in the blood. Black women and men also have an exceptionally high rate of hypertension, which worsens the impact of diabetes on target organs. Finally, we have less access to consistent health care and self-help education, which are the hallmarks of diabetes management. All of these factors may be present in childhood and increase the risk of our children developing diabetes in adult life.

PREVENTION

Type II diabetes is now being diagnosed at younger ages, even before adulthood. Certainly we know that the template for diabetes is set up in childhood. Whether or not diabetes runs in your family, weight control in children is paramount when it comes to prevention. Here's where parents can be a great help. About one in every four American kids is obese—a tendency that has increased 54 percent in two decades.

The best way to avoid this disease is to teach your child the importance of a well-balanced, low-fat diet combined with regular exercise. This not only ensures good nutrition, but helps a child maintain an appropriate weight and cholesterol level. If you have a family history of diabetes, be sure your child's blood-glucose levels are regularly screened.

Children's eating patterns are primarily learned at home, and children learn by your example. You can't coast by with a "Do as I say, not as I do" attitude and expect them to acquire good habits. (Part Two of this book should be read carefully.)

TYPE I DIABETES

Juvenile diabetes occurs when beta cells in the pancreas are completely destroyed and the body abruptly halts insulin production. Glucose from digested food is dumped directly into the bloodstream and excreted through urine. The body, forced to seek other sources of fuel, starts to convert fat and protein into energy. This drain of nutrients can cause the individual to lose weight rapidly. The heart, lungs, eyes, and other organs can be severely damaged. Without prompt treatment, coma and even death can result.

Symptoms of juvenile diabetes include frequent urination, unquenchable thirst, unexplained weight loss, muscle weakness, irritability, nausea, and vomiting.

About 10 percent of the 11 million diabetics in the United States have this type of diabetes, which usually begins abruptly in childhood or adolescence, although it sometimes appears in young adults. Juvenile diabetes appears to be caused by a genetic predisposition that causes the immune system to malfunction. Environmental stresses may tip the balance, determining who will become ill.

A 1992 study at the University of Toronto's Hospital for Sick Children found that this immune response may be triggered by consumption of cow's milk and other dairy products in childhood. Breast-feeding for as long as possible appears to reduce the risks of predisposed children developing the illness. For now, there is no known way to prevent juvenile diabetes. Its onset is sudden, and treatment must be lifelong.

To survive, children with juvenile diabetes must be able to inject themselves daily with insulin, and also follow ongoing exercise programs and nutritional monitoring. Although the incidence of juvenile diabetes among African-American children is slightly less than among white children, the condition presents serious management problems for them.

MANAGEMENT OF JUVENILE DIABETES

At present, there is no cure for juvenile diabetes, but it is possible to control the disease with daily insulin treatment, a special diet, exercise, and, equally important, consistent medical supervision.

Children with juvenile diabetes must see their doctors frequently, and every visit should include blood and urine tests for sugar levels, ketones, and protein. Because diabetes predisposes them to heart disease and stroke, their cholesterol levels must also be routinely checked. Doctors are striving to improve the quality of life for young diabetics. The result is that countless new and improved syringes, lancets for blood tests, and blood-glucose monitors are now available.

Your child's physician will also help you devise a family plan to help care for your child at home.

INSULIN INJECTIONS

Insulin must be given at the same time each day. Your doctor will show you how to rotate the locations of your child's injections, since insulin causes fat to build up in a little lump at the site, slowing its absorption. Remember, too, that different parts of the body absorb the drug at different rates. Abdominal shots absorb fastest, buttocks shots the slowest. Massaging the spot speeds absorption. Consult with your doctor about the best locations to use.

Meals and exercise must be coordinated with injections; naps and bedtime also must be consistent. Granted, this can be difficult. Children's eating patterns may be sporadic, subject to sudden, seemingly arbitrary changes as they cycle through food preferences.

When a diabetic child is ill, it may be difficult to regulate blood sugars. A child who is eating less needs less insulin, theoretically; however, fever and illness increase the body's insulin requirements. Sometimes these warring factions balance themselves out. Under any circumstances, never stop giving your child insulin.

MEALS

It's unrealistic to try to keep a very young child on a restrictive diet. And as kids get older, monitoring their diets can be tough, since they often eat away from home.

Since a diabetic's risk of heart disease and high cholesterol is increased, a good rule of thumb is to avoid foods high in fats and concentrated sugars, as well as salt, which can cause water retention and aggravate the potential for hypertension.

The typical diabetic diet is low in fat and cholesterol, with increased amounts of protein, and only moderate amounts of carbohydrates, which should be largely composed of whole-grain breads and cereals. Growing children fare best with three main meals and three between-meal snacks. Good snacks for diabetic children are crackers and peanut butter, low-salt cheese, rice cakes, low-fat or skim milk and yogurt, nuts and sunflower seeds, and soy nuts.

Your child may naturally want to eat candy and other sugary snacks with his friends. Teens, especially, are readily influenced by the dietary habits of their friends, which may have severe consequences on their diabetes. Most diabetic children don't have to say "never" to birthday cakes, but they have to learn how to account for them, either through dietary modifications or medication. For special occasions, your child's dietitian or nutritionist can easily calculate plain cake into her diet.

ALCOHOL AND TEENAGERS

Diabetic teenagers should not drink alcohol. The symptoms of a blood-sugar change may be mistaken for drunkenness and he or she may not get proper medical attention. If you know that your diabetic teenager is drinking, do everything you can to stop him. Make sure he sits down with his doctor and understands how alcohol can affect his medical condition.

HOME TESTING

Frequent at-home blood-sugar testing is another vital part of disease management; this allows you and your child to observe how different foods affect blood-sugar levels. You can coordinate a child's diet to make the most of these differences, serving a food that makes blood sugar high when he will be engaged in vigorous activity and exercise.

EMERGENCIES

A child with juvenile diabetes should wear a Medic Alert bracelet or necklace. An emergency supply kit with medication and items such as orange juice and insulin should be kept at his school and the school informed about his disease.

If your child has to go to the emergency room for any reason, be sure the staff understands they are dealing with a diabetic. Be certain to educate any baby-sitters you hire on how to recognize and cope with a blood-sugar reaction. "Emergency snacks" include hard candy, gum drops, fruits, and fruit juices. Equip the sitter with numbers for the child's doctor, the local hospital, and an ambulance service.

Scientists are working on a way to identify people likely to develop diabetes before they evince symptoms of the disease; in addition, they are trying to develop immunity-boosting drugs to counteract the deficiency causing diabetes.

Someday, an implanted insulin pump may take over for a diabetic's faulty pancreas. Scientists in Boston are experimenting with a nasal insulin spray. Elsewhere, researchers are looking for an effective way to manage beta-cell transplants.

For the present, managing diabetes is a family affair—it's hard for a child to eat right and exercise alone. You can empower your child by actively involving him in managing the disease himself. Children with high self-esteem and control over their own bodies are more likely to adhere to the lifelong habits that enhance good health.

27

THE HEALTHY HEART

Although coronary heart disease (CHD) primarily affects middle-aged and older adults, its foundations are laid early in life, and many American children are on their way to developing it before they reach school age. This has been confirmed by the Bogalusa Heart Study, which is tracking risk factors for CHD in individuals from birth through age twenty-six in a biracial community in Louisiana. Every three years, each person is evaluated for blood pressure, cholesterol levels, growth and development, dietary patterns, stress, alcohol, cigarette, and oral contraceptive use. Scientists now believe damage to the arteries can occur by age five, and even in infancy, leaving these children at risk for CHD in their adulthood.

More than 60 percent of children between the ages of seven and twelve who were part of another study done at the University of Michigan had at least one risk factor for heart disease. In other words, the first doctor to worry about CHD should be a pediatrician.

These new findings are vitally important, since heart disease is the number-one killer of all Americans. The death rate for African Americans from heart attack and stroke remains one of the highest in the world.

CHD is caused by a narrowing and hardening of the arteries that carry blood to the heart muscle. This can happen when cholesterol levels climb too high, since the excess cholesterol winds up in the bloodstream, where it is deposited like paste, or plaque, along arterial walls. The deposits harden and arteries become rigid, unable to transport adequate blood and oxygen to the heart and other organs. This clogging and hardening, called atherosclerosis, begins early in life and progresses slowly. It grows steadily worse, until symptoms of pain (angina) or heart attack occur in middle age.

In the early stages, CHD produces no symptoms; thus, without screening, the individual doesn't know CHD is present until an artery becomes thoroughly blocked, leading to a heart attack.

RISK FACTORS

FAMILY HISTORY

Scientists recognize that heart disease runs in families, but they do not yet understand all the reasons why. We know that blacks have higher rates of diabetes and hypertension, which may be inherited, and both conditions can lead to heart disease. Some people also appear to inherit high blood-cholesterol levels (called familial hypercholesterolemia), which contributes to coronary heart disease.

The American Heart Association reports that children's cholesterol levels cluster with those of their relatives. Children with elevated cholesterol tend to have relatives with CHD.

CHOLESTEROL

There are two kinds of cholesterol, HDL (described as "good") and LDL ("bad"). Both contribute to the total cholesterol count, but only LDL causes artery-damaging plaque. Even people with normal total cholesterol are at risk for CHD if their HDL cholesterol is also low. The ultimate goal for cholesterol management is to improve the ratio between HDL and LDL.

High LDL cholesterol is common among kids. The researchers involved with the Bogalusa Heart Study performed autopsies on eighty-eight children who died as a result of accidents or suicide. Fatty streaks were present in the aortas of all children over the age of three, and fatty plaque clogged coronary arteries of some fifteen-year-old children.

Cholesterol levels are affected by diet, exercise, and stress. Experts believe that reducing cholesterol early would help to prevent heart disease later in life.

STRESS

In the Bogalusa study children are being tracked for type A personality, which is marked by an intense, impatient type of behavior associated with increased risk of heart disease. Children deemed to be type A in this study were found to have higher cholesterol levels than those deemed to be type B personalities. Type A behavior has also been linked to higher blood pressure.

Type A personality in adults is characterized as aggressive, competitive, hurried, unsatisfied, hostile, and anxious. These traits are present in a somewhat milder form in type A children, and they tend to increase as a child grows older. Therefore, it is a wise parent who teaches a type A child to slow down, cultivate a more relaxed view of the world and its problems, and find effective methods of stress reduction. (See chapter 19 for useful stress-reduction techniques for children.)

CIGARETTE SMOKE

Active and passive cigarette smoke promotes the buildup of fatty deposits around the arteries. Smoke also raises levels of fibrinogen, a clotting component of the blood that can leave one prone to blood clots if it gets too high, as well as increase the risk for heart attack or stroke.

SCREENING CHILDREN FOR CHOLESTEROL

Many CHD experts believe that a child's cholesterol levels have little bearing on levels later in life. Cholesterol levels rise from around 70 mg/dl at birth to 150 mg/dl by age two. They usually fall again as the child reaches puberty. Whether cholesterol levels rise again later in life seems to depend on genetics and lifestyle factors.

Based on this information, the National Heart, Lung, and Blood Institute and the National Cholesterol Education Program have called for cholesterol screening only in children whose parents or grandparents have a history of heart disease and/or high cholesterol. The guidelines recommend that children aged two and up should be screened for cholesterol if any of the following circumstances apply.

- At least one parent has had high blood cholesterol (over 240)
- One parent or grandparent had heart disease before age fifty-five
- Their parents' health status is unknown

Cholesterol levels in children are classified this way:

Acceptable: 140–170 mg/dl

Borderline: 170–199 mg/dl

High cholesterol: 200-plus mg/dl

The National Cholesterol Education Program recommends that a child found to have very high cholesterol levels should receive dietary intervention and counseling about exercise and other health-related factors such as smoking and salt restriction. The members of his immediate family should also have their cholesterol levels checked.

Dr. Gerald S. Berenson, director of the Bogalusa Heart Study, does not agree with these screening guidelines. He believes that *all* children should be screened for high blood cholesterol. Those found to have high blood-cholesterol levels could then receive early intervention in the form of dietary makeover, as well as counseling about exercise, smoking, and salt restriction. Such a universal screening program would encourage the whole family to live more healthy lives by pointing out the very real risk each and every one of us faces. Ultimately, Dr. Berenson believes, the cost of implementing a screening program would be more than offset by the huge savings in medical bills for coronary bypass surgery.

PREVENTION

The primary method of preventing heart disease is by preventing obesity. In addition to maintaining a healthy weight, blood-cholesterol levels can be controlled with diet, exercise, and lifestyle practices. Reducing stress, particularly by maintaining an exercise regimen, also keeps cholesterol levels in check.

There are two ways to control cholesterol levels: reducing foods that contain cholesterol and reducing foods that contain large amounts of saturated fats. Saturated fat is found in meat, dairy products, eggs, coconuts, avocados, and tropical oils.

Children should be encouraged to eat high-fiber foods, such as fruits, vegetables, whole-grain breads, and legumes. These are highly nutritious, and fiber helps move cholesterol out of the body.

Certain foods, such as egg yolks, organ meats, and some shellfish, are relatively high in cholesterol but low in fat, so they can be enjoyed in moderation. The American Academy of Pediatrics recommends children under two years old be allowed to eat whatever they like—including whole-milk dairy products—to ensure appropriate growth.

Over the age of two, children benefit from a diet that derives less than 30 percent of total daily calories from fat. Switching to low-fat dairy products at this age has no adverse effects on a child's mental, physical, and sexual maturation.

Steer children toward low-fat, low-cholesterol snacks as much as possible. Even kids unwilling to give up high-calorie, high-fat, high-cholesterol food can be induced to try low-fat or nonfat products, which are baked instead of fried and may be prepared without salt.

Good choices include unsalted pretzels, fresh fruit, fresh vegetables, rice cakes, cereals, and unfrosted angel food cake, which is made only with egg whites and contains no fat.

LOWERING BLOOD-CHOLESTEROL LEVELS

It's important for everyone to reduce their fat and cholesterol intake. Follow these simple guidelines for your child.

- No more than 30 percent of daily calories from fat
- Less than 10 percent of calories from saturated fat
- Less than 300 milligrams of dietary cholesterol

If your child's cholesterol is already borderline or high or if he is seriously overweight, you can further reduce the intake as follows. (There is also the later option of using cholesterol-lowering drugs in extreme situations.)

- Less than 7 percent of daily calories from saturated fat
- Less than 200 mg of dietary cholesterol

Though obesity, poor nutrition, stress, and inadequate exercise set up children for later CHD, the good news is that altering these habits early, in addition to maintaining a healthy lifestyle, can dramatically reduce that risk.

28

HIGH BLOOD PRESSURE

Fifty million Americans have hypertension—one out of every five people. In our community, however, one out of three African Americans has the disease, and we also suffer its severest consequences. Most people who have hypertension, or high blood pressure, first show signs of the disease in their thirties. However, African Americans tend to get the disease at a younger age. The Bogalusa Heart Study found that blood pressure was substantially higher among African-American children than among white children and that this difference appeared quite early, before the age of ten.

Hypertension often produces no symptoms. In fact, individuals may never know that hypertension is present until years after it has done its worst damage. Untreated hypertension can increase an individual's risk for heart disease, stroke, and kidney failure. Heart disease and stroke are the first- and third-leading causes of death, respectively, in the United States.

On the other hand, the deadly effects of hypertension can be avoided if blood pressure is properly controlled. Even a relatively small drop in blood pressure results in significant health benefits and longer life. For this reason, the National Heart, Lung, and Blood Institute now recommends that screening begin early in life.

Blood pressure is the force exerted by blood on the walls of the arteries. Systolic pressure (the higher number) registers the pressure of your heart pumping. Diastolic pressure (the lower number) registers the amount of pressure exerted as your heart relaxes between beats. It's normal for blood pressure to vary throughout the day in response to activity, but it should always stay within an average range. When blood pressure is consistently higher than this range, it is called hypertension.

Nearly all hypertension is primary, or essential, meaning that in most instances it is not caused by an illness or injury. (Only 5 percent of hypertension is caused by an abnormality such as a tumor or obstruction. In these rare situations, correcting the problem eliminates the hypertension.) Hypertension can be modified by lifestyle changes or medication. But the tendency to be hypertensive *always* exists.

Because it is unknown what causes essential hypertension, it's impossible to know why blacks are more likely than other groups to develop the disease. We know that hypertension runs in families. Regardless of your skin color, income, or education, if your parents or grandparents had high blood pressure, you are likely to have it as well. Hypertension and strokes factor prominently in my family history. My mother and grandmother had hypertension. My sister was diagnosed with hypertension when she was in her early thirties. I have not developed the disease, but I continue to have my blood pressure monitored on a regular basis and I long ago eliminated risk factors associated with the disease.

One genetic theory about hypertension is based on the observation that some individuals retain vital body salts under stress. Bonita Falkner and Harvey Kushner tested the effect of giving extra salt (sodium loading) to a group of black children and a group of white children while they played a video game. The blood pressure in black children went up.

Dr. Clarence E. Grim, professor of medicine and director of the Charles R. Drew UCLA Hypertension Renal Clinic in Los Angeles, believes that salt sensitivity in black Americans is a survival mechanism, or "rapid evolutionary" adaptation, that originated during the slave trade. Many Africans sweated to death during the long marches from their villages to the underground holding dungeons, and many more died of massive fluid loss during the ocean crossing.

Those who survived were those naturally disposed to retain salt and fluids, a trait that is now a health risk for their descendants.

Roughly 75 percent of African-American hypertensives are salt-sensitive—about twice the rate of whites. Salt is retained because of a low level of renin in the kidneys.

Salt sensitivity makes a strong case for a genetic predisposition to hypertension. However, the form of hypertension that does not respond to salt also tends to run in families. And blacks in the Caribbean, whose ancestors were subject to the same brutal passage, do not have as high rates of hypertension as blacks in the United States.

There may be more than one hereditary factor involved in hypertension. And it is also probable that heredity works hand in hand with environment to determine who develops high blood pressure. The impact of environmental factors on the disease may also override heredity.

The environmental components known to exacerbate hypertension include high-fat diets, sodium, obesity, and stress.

By contrast, when these environmental factors are not present, high blood pressure is less likely to develop.

Despite the many intriguing clues, we still have no definite answer for what causes hypertension. Fortunately, we do have several ways to control the disease; these methods can reduce and even eliminate its negative consequences. The same methods may also prevent the disease from ever developing.

PREVENTION AND TREATMENT

From as early as two years of age, a child's blood pressure increases as his or her weight increases. Ninety percent of four-year-olds will have blood pressure below 170/69. Most eight-year-olds' blood pressure is below 177/75. By age ten to fifteen, blood pressure has usually reached adult levels, 120-130/80-90.

If a child's blood pressure is out of the average range, early intervention can slow or possibly stop hypertension from developing. Optimally, every African-American child over the age of three should have his blood pressure checked on each routine visit to the doctor, or at least once a year. There are standard graphs that physicians use to determine normal values for the age and sex.

(Note: Hypertension may not produce any symptoms in adults or children. However, severe headaches and dizziness may be signals of high blood pressure in children. Pay special attention to pain in the back of the head that occurs when your child first wakes up.)

Here are the best self-help methods to prevent or treat hypertension in children and teens.

REDUCE CHILDHOOD STRESS

We know from studies carried out in various neighborhoods throughout Detroit that the higher the stress level in a person's environment—things like overcrowding, high crime rates, and broken families—the greater the risk of that person developing hypertension.

In adults, finding a healthy channel for anger and developing effective methods for stress management (biofeedback, meditation, yoga) are known to lower blood pressure. Children are at least as susceptible to stress as adults, and possibly more so. Read chapter 19 carefully for advice on reducing stress in your child's life.

REDUCE SALT IN YOUR CHILD'S DIET

In people who are salt-sensitive, reducing sodium in the diet can lower blood pressure. Though the effects of salt retention aren't obvious in childhood, some researchers believe that a lifelong habit of loading up on salt will eventually produce higher blood pressure in anyone who does so. Therefore, reducing sodium in the diet is good for all children.

Salt affects blood pressure like helium affects a balloon: The more you have, the higher it goes. Salt is processed through the kidneys, and most people get rid of the excess salt through their sweat or urine. But a significant number of African Americans process salt in the opposite order: Salt is retained by their kidneys. Their bodies are literally "salting it away" until they'll need it. The more they sweat, the more it hangs in there.

The solution seems obvious: Remove the salt shaker from the dining room table and reduce the amount of salty foods you provide for your kids. The next step is to begin using salt sparingly in cooking. Sodium is naturally present in most foods, and your child will not suffer sodium deprivation if you reduce the amount of salt you add to foods.

Children don't miss salt if it isn't there to begin with. If your kids are already habituated to salt, reduce more gradually the amount you add to foods.

Some physicians suggest it's not only excess salt that causes problems but also lack of potassium and calcium. Adding potassium-rich foods to diets is easy to do and part of every healthy diet. Give your kids bananas, oranges, and cantaloupes. Calcium is another nutrient that may help control blood pressure. If lactose in fresh dairy products causes digestive problems for your child, substitute yogurt, cheese, dark green leafy vegetables, and both canned sardines and salmon (with bones).

PREVENT CHILDHOOD OBESITY

Blood pressure is affected by excess weight, which increases the volume of blood flowing through the body. Not every person who is overweight develops hypertension, but many do. About 20 to 30 percent of adult hypertensives can lower their blood pressure by losing weight. High levels of blood cholesterol also contribute to high blood pressure.

We also know the greatest number of strokes occurs in the southern states, where African Americans account for a large section of the population. This is also a part of the country where the term *southern fried* characterizes the cooking practices. People who are overweight are also more likely to develop diabetes, which can increase blood pressure.

The easiest and best time to establish permanent weight control is in childhood. If your child is already overweight, read chapter 20 carefully.

EXERCISE

Aerobic exercise poses little risk for hypertensive youths and is known to help reduce blood pressure in adolescents. Weight training may be problematic because the sustained isometric motion momentarily increases diastolic blood pressure. Daily exercise is better than infrequent bursts of activity; exercising at a low or moderate level is extremely effective.

DISCOURAGE ALCOHOL USE

More than two drinks daily may increase susceptibility to hypertension, and a small percentage of hypertension cases (5 to 7 percent) are attributed to excessive alcohol consumption. This is one more important reason to control drinking among teenagers.

MEDICATION FOR CHILDREN

Drug therapy for hypertension in children and teens differs from therapy used for adults. As a rule, high blood pressure in African Americans seems to respond better to diuretics and calcium channel blockers than to beta blockers, but these are not necessarily the right course of treatment for every black person. When prescribing antihypertensive medication for children, doctors usually begin with the smallest dose of one antihypertensive drug and elevate dosages in stages, or experiment with a combination of drugs, to achieve control.

If your child is hypertensive, there are certain common medicines sold over the counter that he should *not* use. Many cold and flu medicines, for example, should not be used by people with high blood pressure because they constrict blood vessels. Some medications also interact with antihypertensive drugs, causing a negative reaction in the body. Before giving your child any medication, read all package labels carefully; when in doubt, consult with your pharmacist or pediatrician.

29

SICKLE-CELL DISEASE

Sickle-cell disease (SCD) is one of the most prevalent genetic diseases in the United States. About 2.5 million African Americans carry the sickle-cell trait and roughly 80,000 have the disease. Each year, roughly 1 in every 375 black infants is born with SCD and sometime between the ages of six to twelve months will start to display symptoms of the disease. However, *SCD is not solely a "black" disease.* It is also found to a lesser degree among southern Italians, Greeks, East Indians, and many Hispanics.

One of the most disabling symptoms of SCD is a deep, agonizing pain that feels as if it is radiating out from the bones. Some African people call the disease "body chewing" or "body biting." The Fanti tribe of Ghana call it *nwiiwii,* a word that sounds like the moans of its victims.

SCD is transmitted genetically. Because the gene is recessive, a child must inherit it from both parents in order to develop the full-blown illness. At least 8 to 10 percent of African Americans carry the sickle-cell trait and can pass it along to their children without ever becoming ill themselves.

When both parents are carriers, their child has a 25 percent chance of inheriting the disease, a 25 percent chance of eluding both trait and disease, and a 50 percent chance of inheriting the trait but escaping the disease.

If only one parent has the trait, a child has a fifty-fifty chance of inheriting the trait.

Not long ago it was rare for a person with SCD to live past the age of forty. But in the past twenty years, thanks largely to improved treatment of complications, SCD sufferers live longer, healthier lives. A recent study at Children's Hospital in Boston, published in June of 1994, found that 85 percent of infants with SCD survived until at least the age of twenty, and 50 percent lived into their fifties and beyond. Nevertheless, 10 percent of children with SCD die within the first five years, and survivors are robbed of roughly twenty-five to thirty years of life. In 1995, however, promising developments now provide hope for treatment. That hope has been a very long time coming.

WHAT IS SICKLE-CELL DISEASE?

It's probable that sickle-cell disease arose as an evolutionary muta-tion—in areas such as Africa, the Mediterranean, East India—as a self-protection against malaria. Children born with the trait for sickle-cell are actually immune to the severest form of malaria.

SCD is characterized by crescent-shaped, or sickle-shaped, red blood cells. Sickling is caused by a defect in hemoglobin, the spe-cial pigment found in red blood cells that transports oxygen all over the body.

Some of the most common problems caused by SCD are ane-mia, infections, pain, and damage to body organs. Sickled cells have a much shorter life span (from ten to twenty days) than normal red blood cells (120 days). The cells die so quickly that bone marrow cannot keep up with production, and anemia is the result. Mild anemia often can be corrected by diet and vitamin/mineral supple-ments. Severe anemia, however, is life-threatening and requires hos-pitalization and transfusions to prevent death.

The shape of the sickled cell also causes problems: Normal red blood cells are round and soft, able to squeeze through the tiniest blood vessels and reach every part of the body. By contrast, sickled red blood cells are rigid and elongated, snagging on one another and building up until they clog small vessels. As a result, the flow of oxygen to major organs is blocked.

Pain in the abdomen, chest, and back is the most common symptom, but the whole body may be affected, particularly the joints and spine. As the hard, sticky sickle red blood cells pile up and block blood vessels, diminishing the flow of oxygen to nearby tis-sues, the whole area starts to hurt. "Hand-and-foot syndrome," in which a clot forms in the hands or feet, causing fever and painful swelling in fingers and toes, is one common complication in children between the ages of six months and two years.

Pain episodes are almost never fatal, but they can be terrifying. Some children experience painful episodes only once a year, while others may have fifteen to twenty episodes a year, many so severe that hospitalization is needed to give intravenous fluids and painkillers.

Sickle-cell clots can also be life-threatening, depending on where they occur. For example, blockage in the lungs causes respiratory complications. A blockage in the brain can cause seizures or stroke. Other clots may damage the heart, kidney, liver, or eyes. Brain clots occur in about 10 percent of children with SCD. Treatment is usually with chronic transfusions to prevent recurrences.

SCD children are especially susceptible to pneumonia, sepsis, shock, and meningitis. Urinary and bone infections are also common. Organisms such as pneumococcus, h. influenza, and salmonella can pose special threats. In infants and small children, infections can go from fever to death in as short a time as nine hours.

As children mature, the blood supply to the long bones of the arms and legs, the spinal column, and the hips is often inadequate, and pain can be severe. Growth is often slow and sexual maturity is usually late. Roughly one-third of all teens experience recurrent attacks of gallstones, and many need to have the gallbladder removed.

Sickle-cell complications are swift and unpredictable; they may last a few hours or several days. A child may have several crises one year, followed by a period relatively free of illness and pain. Not all children experience every complication, and even two children in the same family can be affected in dramatically different ways.

As the disease progresses, major organs begin to sustain damage. Older patients continue to be vulnerable to infection, and they are susceptible to pneumonia and chronic lung disease. Eyes often look yellow due to jaundice caused by the rapid breakdown of red blood cells. Blindness may result from sickle-cell blockage of the retina. Arthritis is a common source of chronic pain in older patients.

NEW HOPE FOR TREATMENT

In January 1995, the drug hydroxyurea was deemed "the first effective treatment for sickle-cell disease," according to Dr. Samuel

Charache of Johns Hopkins University Medical School. A five-year nationwide trial of the drug was so successful that it was halted early, and results of the research were rushed in a "clinical alert" to thousands of doctors nationwide.

Researchers and doctors are extremely optimistic that this new treatment will greatly improve the quality of life for SCD patients. The drug trial consisted of a blind test of 299 adults with severe sickle-cell disease. Half of the patients received hydroxyurea and the other half received a placebo. The results were so dramatically positive that the National Institutes of Health, sponsors of the trial, stopped the study early in order to switch the placebo patients to hydroxyurea and to alert doctors of the drug's benefits.

During the trial, hydroxyurea proved effective both in decreasing the number of sickle-cell crises and in limiting their severity. One of the participants, a forty-year-old secretary who had endured frequent hospitalizations in the past, experienced fewer than half her usual number of episodes, and she was able to treat all of these at home, using prescription pain medicine. Similarly positive results were achieved studywide. Hydroxyurea reduced by 50 percent the number of crises, hospitalizations, and blood transfusions needed, along with incidents of life-threatening "acute chest syndrome," which is characterized by fever and severe chest pain.

Hydroxyurea is the first treatment for sickle-cell anemia that attacks the cause of the disease rather than simply combating its symptoms. Hydroxyurea caused the body to produce a different kind of hemoglobin, called fetal hemoglobin, which does not sickle. Fetal hemoglobin is produced by babies before and shortly after birth, although adults normally have less than 1 percent of this type of hemoglobin. In patients who took hydroxyurea, the level of fetal hemoglobin rose to as high as 20 percent.

Unfortunately, hydroxyurea is not yet recommended for children, nor for women who plan to have children. A two-year study aimed at developing the proper dose for children will begin soon, however.

Hydroxyurea is a treatment, not a cure. Its long-term use has potential adverse effects, including an increased risk in some people for one type of leukemia. High doses of hydroxyurea can also cause the suppression of bone marrow, which manufactures red blood cells; this was the only adverse effect observed during the drug trial itself. All of the long-term effects have yet to be determined.

Hydroxyurea must be taken daily for the rest of a patient's life (once a day in pill form in low, nontoxic doses). Blood counts must be monitored every two weeks until a safely effective dose can be determined.

Yet another difficulty is purely economic: Use of hydroxyurea costs about one hundred dollars a month, and, while the drug is pending FDA approval, the treatment is not covered by most insurance plans.

Still, it's impossible to overstate the bright hope that hydroxyurea brings. The enthusiasm created by the successful hydroxyurea trial bodes well for efforts to perfect and broaden its use now that it has burst upon the scene.

For now, SCD continues to be a devastating illness in children and adults. However, there are some ways that parents can manage the disease and, in some cases, modulate its worst effects.

TESTING

If you are thinking of having children, you should know whether you or your partner carry the sickle-cell trait. Testing and counseling can take place before pregnancy, and also during it.

The goal of genetic counseling is to *provide information* so that parents can make decisions that are right for them, in an environment free of judgment.

- Before pregnancy, testing tells whether you or your spouse carries the sickle-cell trait. If so, your odds of passing the trait or the disease to your child can be determined. The decision on whether or not to become pregnant is up to you.

- During pregnancy, the fetus can be tested at about nine weeks through a procedure called chorionic villus sampling. (A bit of tissue is extracted from the membrane surrounding the fetus and analyzed.) This is the earliest available diagnostic procedure. Later diagnosis can be made at about fifteen weeks through amniocentesis.

  The advantage of fetal testing is to give parents options and to prepare for the outcome if the fetus has SCD. Parents who choose abortion should be able to do so without criticism from health-care professionals. Likewise, those who decide to continue their pregnancies, knowing that their infant will be born with SCD, and later have a child who experiences a great deal of pain and suffering should not be humiliated by health-care providers who believe that early abortion would have been a more merciful choice.

- At birth: If either parent carries the sickle-cell trait and the fetus was not tested before birth, it's *crucial* that the newborn be screened immediately following delivery. An infant born with SCD can receive antibiotics to protect against life-threatening infection. And parents can receive counseling that will help prepare them to manage the baby's health.

Forty states now require routine infant screening for SCD to protect newborns from the earliest possible date; however, not all provide the money to implement the testing programs effectively. If you know, or suspect, that you carry the trait, insist that your newborn be tested.

A baby who tests positive for SCD is immediately retested. The baby should also be tested again when he is several months old. A complete blood analysis will be done to see what kind of hemoglobin, and how much, he produces and to distinguish between sickle-cell disease and the sickle-cell trait.

WHAT PARENTS CAN DO

Newborns known to have SCD should immediately be enrolled in a pediatric health-care program, which mobilizes doctors, nurses, and family members into a team. (See pages 403–404 for a list of regional sickle-cell treatment centers.)

Any illness in a sickle-cell child is a potential medical emergency, and most doctors try to head off this danger with heavy use of antibiotics. Babies who receive daily penicillin have a dramatically increased chance of staying healthy. For the first five years of a child's life, management of SCD requires daily doses of penicillin and frequent visits to the doctor. It's not unusual for doctors to continue penicillin treatment up to age ten or through adolescence.

Immunization is crucial for SCD babies. In addition to the usual immunization schedule (see chapter 6), most doctors recommend that SCD kids receive pneumovax when they are two years old.

This vaccine reduces the chance of pneumococcal infections, to which sickle-cell children are especially vulnerable.

Parents will learn how to take their child's temperature and be alert for symptoms. Symptoms that the blood count is falling include tiredness, fever, pallor or yellow cast to the skin, loss of appetite, yellow eyes, and dark urine. Other symptoms to watch for include respiratory distress, unexplained irritability, diarrhea, and vomiting. An extremely low red blood cell count may require a blood transfusion. (You will need advice on blood banking options in your area, since transfusions may be a vital part of your child's health care.)

Parents will also learn how to examine their child's spleen in order to monitor its size and report changes to the doctor. (Spleen enlargement is common in children with sickle-cell anemia, and it can lead to severe anemia.)

Your child's doctor will monitor her growth and development closely. As a child grows, joint pain in the spine and hips becomes a chronic problem. It is extremely difficult for parents to stand by and watch a child suffer. Episodes of acute pain lead to a buildup of toxic substances that can further injure cells, causing more pain and inflammation.

The onset of pain cannot be predicted, and its intensity varies from person to person. When your child experiences pain, the first approach is a medical exam to rule out any underlying complications.

If the pain is a sickle-cell episode, you may be able to relieve it with home therapy, which includes over-the-counter painkillers, warm baths, heating pads, fluids, and massage. If home treatment does not bring relief, your child's doctor must intervene with stronger analgesics, even narcotics. The American medical community is slowly coming to terms with our chronic undertreatment of pain from all diseases.

Doctors are also experimenting with antiinflammatory steroid drugs as well as epidural injections of anesthesia. So far, in limited studies, children with SCD appear to respond better to epidural injections, rather than steroids.

Like any chronic illness, SCD brings with it a number of emotional and financial stressors affecting each member of the family. It's important to establish good working relationships with your child's schoolteachers, principal, and school medical staff. You will also need a backup plan for homework in case your child misses school. Look for a tutoring program or other at-home study programs your child can join if necessary.

As your child grows up, discuss sexual development with him. Explain that puberty may come a little later than it does for most kids, but he (or she) will catch up. At the same time, you should know that some teenagers with SCD are identical to their peers when it comes to their sexual development. You will want to discuss contraception and prevention of sexually transmitted diseases with your child, just as you would with any other youngster of the same age.

If your daughter has SCD, be certain she understands that pregnancy could have life-threatening consequences for her. Be absolutely up front about sex and birth control. If you are uncomfortable talking to your preteen about sexual activity, or are uncertain yourself about birth-control options, ask a member of your child's health-care team to have this discussion with her. Even if you do explain the facts of life, it's a good idea for your teen to hear it from her doctor, too. Reinforcement and repetition of information is effective.

NUTRITION

Nutrition plays an important part in managing sickle-cell disease. Folic acid, zinc, vitamin E, and cyanate are the nutrients that play an especially important role in SCD management. Folic acid boosts the immune system. Zinc is critical to normal growth and sexual development. Vitamin E, a powerful antioxidant, enables the body to use oxygen more efficiently. And cyanate, a nontoxic relative of the poisonous chemical cyanide, has been found to inhibit the sickling process in red blood cells.

All of these critical vitamins and minerals are readily available in foods (see table on page 330). Every SCD child should eat a well-balanced and varied diet, with particular emphasis on foods high in these nutrients. During crises, when it's common for a child to have little or no appetite, try giving him small meals throughout the day. It's interesting that several foods commonly eaten in Africa contain rich sources of cyanate, particularly yams and cassavas. The true African yam is seldom grown in the United States, but it is sometimes imported. African yams and cassavas can usually be found in specialty stores in cities with large populations of West Indians and Africans.

Foods High in Specific Nutrients

Folic Acid	Zinc	Vitamin E	Cyanate
Raw spinach	Eggs	Egg yolk	African yams
Dark green leafy vegetables	Pumpkin and sunflower seeds	Whole grains	Cassavas
		Wheat germ	Radishes
	Red meat	Wheat-germ oil	Carrots
Whole grains	Seafood	Polyunsaturated vegetable oils	Millet
Pumpkin and sunflower seeds			Kidney beans
		Nuts	Lentils and other legumes
Nuts		Dark green leafy vegetables	
Chickpeas			
Pinto beans			

VITAMIN/MINERAL SUPPLEMENTS

Your child may benefit from specific vitamin/mineral supplements. At about one year of age, some children are given 1 mg per day of folic acid. Some benefit from supplements of zinc, iron, and vitamin E. However, don't self-prescribe; discuss supplements with your child's physician or nutritionist.

WATER

Children with sickle-cell disease need more fluids than other children, and they usually get thirsty more often. Keep enough fluids on hand so that your child can have as much as he wants. Plain water and fruit juices are the best choices. The following circumstances require even more fluids than usual.

- If your child has a fever or is experiencing pain
- In very hot weather
- When your child is very active
- While traveling

An infant needs extra fluids only during the special circumstances mentioned above. At these times, encourage your baby to take all of his breast milk or formula, unless he is vomiting.

PRECAUTIONS

- Avoid any situation where the oxygen supply may be compromised, including flying in small, unpressurized airplanes. (Almost all commercial planes are pressurized.)
- Drink plenty of fluids when traveling—flying in an airplane, riding in a car, riding or walking at high altitudes, visiting in a dry climate.
- Let your doctor know if you plan to take your child on a trip and ask for a letter describing your child's condition so that you can give it to a local physician should your child become ill during the trip.
- Be certain your teenage daughter discusses the risks of pregnancy with a physician.
- Teach your child to avoid cuts and injuries (especially to the arms, legs, toes, and fingers) and to seek immediate help if he or she is injured.
- Get a doctor's okay before any sports and other physical activities.

YOUR CHILD'S LIFE

Children with SCD can participate in a wide range of activities, but let your child set her own pace. Taking care of herself means resting when she feels tired, drinking extra fluids when she is active, and dressing warmly during cold weather. Beyond these precautions, encourage your child to find her own level of activity and enjoy it. Try to foster an attitude of self-sufficiency, which will help your child maintain her self-esteem and live life fully.

Encourage your child to develop a wide range of interests and to get a good education, even if this means home tutoring. Your goal is to make your child independent and well educated, with a positive attitude about life, work, and the future.

Having a chronic illness is stressful, and stress creates its own set of physical and emotional problems, which can exacerbate the disease. Help your child explore relaxation techniques—from yoga to biofeedback—that can help alleviate tension.

Little research has been done concerning the impact of SCD on the family, but the stress load associated with medical costs, impact on family relationships, and parents missing days at work can be enormous. Any guidance or counseling you can get will be useful. If possible, join a support group. Look for advice about educational scholarships and vocational rehabilitation.

It's not unusual for SCD children to grow up to become unemployed adults either because they have fallen behind in school or because they think of themselves as sickly and unable to compete in the workplace. The problem is compounded by the biases of employers who are reluctant to hire people who may have a high rate of absenteeism. Although it's true that people with SCD are at risk for unpredictable pain attacks, most do not have crises frequently enough to disqualify them for employment.

LOOKING TOWARD THE FUTURE

Since red blood cells are manufactured in the bone marrow, modern research toward a cure has focused on bone marrow transplantation. This process is still in the experimental stage and has been tried only in a limited number of people. It's a difficult procedure at best, because the donor must be a perfect match.

Gene therapy is another area of new research, in which the gene for sickle hemoglobin is replaced with a gene for normal hemoglobin. This technique is still highly experimental and has not yet been successfully achieved. In the long run, the prospects for a cure using bone-marrow transplantation or gene therapy are excellent, because the same research can be applied to many other diseases besides SCD, which means that funding is more generally available.

30

COMMON CHILDHOOD AILMENTS

PROTECTING AGAINST INFECTIONS

All children are vulnerable to infections, but African-American kids have a greater incidence of serious infections—*not because they're black, but because they are more likely to have poor housing and less access to regular medical care.*

Viruses and bacteria are spread through human contact—from kissing, sharing eating utensils, and simply being around someone who's sneezing and coughing. All children touch things that cross their path, then inevitably put miscellaneous objects, along with their fingers, into their mouths.

Enrollment at day-care facilities is another way infection commonly occurs, especially among infants and toddlers who require a lot of physical attention during feedings and diaperings. (The risk of your child coming down with something appears to be highest during his first month in day care. The risk tapers off the longer a child is enrolled, undoubtedly because his immune system gets stronger.)

Maintaining a clean home, teaching children to wash their hands frequently, providing sound nutrition, helping children to cope with stress, and encouraging exercise are all ways to minimize the spread of infection and keep children resilient and healthy.

When choosing a day-care center for your child, look for a staff that maintains high levels of cleanliness and hygiene. They should wash their hands frequently and thoroughly, and the facility should look clean. (By the way, there are some built-in protections. The American Academy of Pediatrics and the American

WHEN TO CALL THE DOCTOR

Good judgment is your best ally, but here are some guidelines.

Infants:

- *Unexplained illness of more than twelve hours*
- *Unexplained constant crying (more than one hour) or crying that sounds unusual*
- *Vomiting lasting over twelve hours*
- *Bloody diarrhea*
- *If your baby feels floppier than normal*
- *If the soft spot (fontanel) on your baby's head becomes sunken (possible dehydration) or bulged out (possible meningitis)*
- *If your baby holds her head back or won't let you move her head*
- *If your baby shows signs of dehydration (sunken eyes, infrequent or dark urine, sticky saliva, and loss of skin elasticity)*
- *If your baby stops eating or drinking a bottle*
- *Difficulty breathing or rapid breathing*
- *Face and lips look blue*
- *Skin has a yellowish cast (jaundice)*

Toddlers:

- *Any of the above symptoms*
- *Confusion or delirium*
- *Child can't stay awake, seems dazed*
- *Unexplained head, chest, or stomach pains that worsen*
- *Unusually high temperature*
- *Stiff, painful neck (can't touch chin to chest)*
- *Rash of small, flat purple blotches*
- *Swelling around the eyes and mouth*

Public Health Association have recommended guidelines for day-care centers to minimize the spread of disease, and each state also has individual standards.)

Your part of the bargain is to keep sick children home, especially if a child is seriously ill, has a known contagious disease, or is so uncomfortable that he cannot participate in normal activities.

Fever, aches, rashes, and minor infections are a normal part of childhood. Let's look at some of the most common ailments children are vulnerable to, and some of the ways you can at least reduce transmission of germs.

CANKER SORES

It's quite common for kids to develop lesions in and around their mouths. Some are caused by biting the inside of the mouth, and others appear for unknown reasons. Most disappear on their own.

If a canker sore makes eating painful for your child, be certain that she at least drinks plenty of fluids to avoid dehydration. Offer her cold liquids and ice pops. Sores just inside the lip and on the gums may be helped by a preparation called Orabase, which is sold over the counter. Sores on the outside of the mouth and lips respond to phenol and camphor preparations such as Blistex or Campho-phenique. If your child develops a fever, you can give her acetaminophen. If the sore doesn't disappear within three weeks, take your child to the doctor.

COLDS

Every cold is caused by a distinct and separate virus. Children encounter so many new strains that it's not uncommon for youngsters to have between four and six colds every year. Coming down with one cold creates antibodies for that particular virus, and the child will be immune to that virus the next time around. Eventually, the number of colds a child gets every year decreases.

Contrary to old wives' tales, colds are not caused by getting wet, standing in a draft, or skipping a hot breakfast. More children get sick during the winter because bad weather keeps them indoors, where the air isn't well circulated and where they are exposed to more germs.

HOME TREATMENT

Colds are characterized by sneezing, runny nose, cough, sore throat, tiredness, and headache. Unless there are complications, the best remedy is to let your child rest and drink fluids. You can give your child acetaminophen for fever or aches, and use a cool mist vaporizer for the cough. If your child is too young to blow his nose, you can remove mucus with a nasal aspirator.

Drugs are not very effective against colds. A 1990 study reported in *The Journal of Pediatrics* showed that the most commonly prescribed cough suppressants, codeine and dextromethorphan, were ineffectual. Children who received placebos bounced back from the illness just as quickly as those on medication. Since all drugs have some side effects, it may actually be better to withhold medication. However, antibiotics may be needed if a secondary infection has occurred due to a prolonged cold.

It's also not recommended to megadose children with vitamin C, since that can cause diarrhea, which in turn causes dehydration.

WHEN TO CALL THE DOCTOR ABOUT A COLD

- If your child is under eight weeks old
- If the cough interferes with his or her breathing
- If the cough is painful, persistent, and accompanied by a whooping noise on inspiration
- If your child is vomiting or turns blue
- If the cough persists longer than a week, especially if accompanied by a fever

CONSTIPATION

"Regular" is not the same for every person, particularly *normal* younger children and infants. Many children experience hard, painful stools or no bowel movement at all. Sometimes children with diaper rash withhold their bowel movements by sheer force of will in order to avoid pain. (Treat the diaper rash, and the constipation will take care of itself naturally.) Children in the throes of toilet training may also refuse to have bowel movements as part of the power struggle with their parents.

HOME TREATMENT

If your child becomes constipated, try increasing his liquid intake with diluted apple juice and other clear liquids. Prune juice really works. Older children can eat more vegetables and fruits. A mild children's laxative may be required, but don't give infants mineral oil (which can travel to the lungs, causing pneumonia). Nor should children receive enemas.

WHEN TO CALL THE DOCTOR ABOUT CONSTIPATION

- If there's no bowel movement after three days
- If constipation is accompanied by a fever that doesn't respond to acetaminophen
- If stools smell bad when they do appear
- If stools are bloody
- If your child has stomach pain
- If your child's bowel movements are very painful, or if a crack or fissure appears around the anus

DIARRHEA

Children's normal bowel movements vary considerably. For example, some infants produce stools several times daily, others once every other day. You can only observe your baby's general pattern and extrapolate differences from there.

Generally, diarrhea is characterized by loose, watery stools. Children taking antibiotics may have diarrhea. Diarrhea may also be caused by infection, contaminated food or water, or a change in diet.

HOME TREATMENT

Foods suitable for infants and toddlers with diarrhea are soy milk and rice soup, and bland, nonallergenic foods are the order of the day. For older children, fluids such as soup, diluted juice, water, electrolyte solutions, and flat soda help prevent dehydration. Avoid solid foods and avoid fats. Try bananas, rice, toast, and applesauce.

WHEN TO CALL THE DOCTOR ABOUT DIARRHEA

- If your child is under one year
- If stools smell particularly bad or shows signs of blood or mucus

- If your child has a fever, stomach pain, seems especially lethargic, or exhibits behavioral changes
- If diarrhea persists longer than two to three days

EARACHES

Earaches are usually caused by fluid building up in the middle ear due to cold or infection. The ear can become infected by bacteria trapped there. Symptoms include pain in the ear, fever, irritability, sleep disturbance, and a temporary decrease in hearing. Be especially concerned if the ear is leaking fluid, if your baby is extremely fussy or irritable, and if she cries more than normal.

HOME TREATMENT

Call the doctor. You can safely use over-the-counter acetaminophen (Tylenol) to ease the discomfort until the child can be seen by her physician. Your physician may even feel comfortable enough to call in a topical anesthetic to be used until the child can be seen.

Never put nonprescribed treatments in your child's ears without first consulting her physician, including Q-Tips, sweet oils, warmed mineral oil, or peroxide.

MEDICAL TREATMENT

Your child's physician will prescribe medication to resolve the infection. Antibiotics may or may not be prescribed; the majority of ear infections (called otitis media) are nonbacterial and will resolve spontaneously.

If a child has a history of acute ear infections (three or more within six months), a doctor may put her on a low daily dose of an antibiotic during the cold-weather months, when ear infections are most prevalent.

Some persistent earaches are not caused by infection, however. These are called serous otitis media and are treated by a minor operation in which drainage tubes are placed within the middle ear.

FEVER

Fevers in children are common signals that the body is fighting off infection. Even minor infections can trigger high fevers in children.

As long as your child is eating and drinking fluids, and smiles and plays, there is probably no cause for concern.

HOME TREATMENT

Children should be encouraged to eat when feverish. The body needs more calories to replace those used up by the higher internal temperature. Fluid is even more important than food, however, to avoid dehydration. Keep your child lightly dressed and give him plenty of fluids (water, uncarbonated drinks, diluted fruit or vegetable juice). A sponge bath with tepid water is another method for reducing high fevers.

Acetaminophen effectively lowers fever in children. Follow package directions, or speak to a doctor or pharmacist about the correct dosage. However, never give oral medications to children who are having a seizure or unconscious (see below).

You can use a rectal or oral thermometer to take a child's temperature. Insert a lubricated rectal thermometer just one inch (be sure your child is comfortable and lying still). Leave the thermometer in place for about three minutes, until the mercury stops rising and remains at the same temperature for one or two minutes.

Individual temperatures vary throughout the day. Also remember that some healthy children do not have the classic 98.6 temperature. You should establish your child's typical temperature when he is healthy and feeling well, so you have a point of comparison. Here are some guidelines.

WHEN TO CALL THE DOCTOR ABOUT A FEVER

- If fever is over 101° F (birth to one year)
- If fever is 106° F or higher, no matter what the child's age
- If child is especially weak and lacking energy, won't take liquids, vomits, or is extremely uncomfortable

FEVER WITH SEIZURE

Febrile convulsions are not uncommon even for healthy kids, and are not in themselves dangerous. Seizures occur when the brain overheats and sends scrambled messages throughout the body, causing muscles to spasm or stiffen. Seizures end quickly for most children; it's imperative to call a doctor, especially if a seizure lasts longer than five minutes. Afterward, children tend to be groggy or weak. Luckily, most children rarely have more than one experience of febrile seizures. You should do the following during a seizure.

- Protect your child's head.
- Put him into bed.
- Do not force anything into the mouth.
- Clear the mouth/nose of any obstructions and pull the child's head back slightly to elongate the neck and facilitate breathing.
- Sponge off the child's body with tepid water.
- Call the doctor.

HICCUPS

Everyone has a favorite remedy for hiccups. Some people swallow nine gulps of water without taking a breath; others drink out of the "wrong" side of the glass. Some people believe a good scare stops hiccups, and some recommend breathing into a brown paper bag. A study recently published in *The New England Journal of Medicine* delivered the news that swallowing a teaspoonful of table sugar cures hiccups immediately.

Hiccups result from a rhythmic contraction of the diaphragm which is usually transient. Hiccups can be dangerous if they are prolonged and if related to underlying disease. For example, prolonged hiccups can be associated with some brain tumors and brain injuries. In the vast majority of instances, however, hiccups are benign and the cause unknown. As far as home cures go, pediatricians say never try anything scary.

NOSEBLEEDS

Nosebleeds may be caused by colds, dry heat, picking the nose, blowing the nose, and injury; nosebleeds do not signal high blood pressure or the advent of a stroke. Most stop on their own within ten minutes.

To prevent nosebleeds, keep the air at home moist by using a vaporizer or humidifier. Teach children not to pick their noses. At bedtime, thinly coat the inside of your child's nostrils with Vaseline to keep the tissues lubricated.

HOME TREATMENT

Keep your child sitting up, without tipping his head back. Try to calm the child, since crying aggravates bleeding. Do not pack the nose with gauze or tissues. Instead, pinch the *middle* of the nose (not the tip and not close to the eyes) for about five minutes, and tell your child to breathe through his mouth. If bleeding persists, repeat this process for another five minutes. Sometimes a cold compress or even an ice pack on the bridge of the nose stops the bleeding.

WHEN TO CALL THE DOCTOR ABOUT A NOSEBLEED

- If bleeding persists
- If your child's nose hurts or appears to have something shoved into it
- If nosebleeds occur frequently

SKIN PROBLEMS

PRICKLY HEAT

This is characterized by slightly raised white or red dots surrounded by red skin on the trunk, neck, and the skin folds on the arms and legs, and by itching.

Home Treatment. Keep infant lightly dressed in hot weather to avoid excessive perspiration. Emollient lotions (Nutraderm) and clear calamine lotion can be applied to the rash to make the baby feel more comfortable.

POISON IVY AND OAK

Raised blisters that are red and intensely itchy may be a symptom of poison ivy or poison oak. The rash begins twelve to forty-eight hours after exposure and lasts roughly two weeks. The blisters may swell and ooze. By scratching, one can spread the blisters to different areas of the body. Towels can spread the infection and people can infect one another. One can even contract poison ivy internally from breathing smoke from areas where leaves have been burned.

Home Treatment. Cleanse your child's skin thoroughly. Compresses of Burrow's solution, oatmeal baths, and aspirin help relieve itching. Calamine lotion may help, but may also spread the rash. Do not use Caladryl or Zyradryl, since many children are allergic to them.

The best thing you can do is to teach your kids to recognize poison ivy and poison oak plants so they can stay away from them in the future.

ACNE

Acne may include red pimples and cysts along the face, back, and chest as well as blackheads and whiteheads. Acne is almost inevitable in adolescence because a new flood of hormones increases oil production, which clogs pores. Although dirt and oil promote and aggravate acne, excessive cleaning doesn't eliminate it. Benzoyl peroxide and tretinoin are two of the current and most effective preparations available. Encourage your adolescent to clean the skin gently and to avoid coarse, gritty soaps. If acne is very severe or persists for more than a few years, consult a dermatologist. Sometimes long-term antibiotics in low dosages or steroids are prescribed to control severe acne and prevent permanent scarring.

ATHLETE'S FOOT

The symptoms of athlete's foot are cracks, scaly patches, or blisters on the skin between toes. Athlete's foot also itches—a lot.

Home Treatment. Teach your child to wash frequently with soap and water and to dry carefully between the toes. He should change his socks every morning (twice a day is better) and wear shoes that allow feet to breathe (no plastic- or rubber-lined shoes). Dry shoes and medicated over-the-counter foot powder will help. These same methods will also prevent athlete's foot.

WARTS

Warts are caused by viruses, and they tend to recur. You can try removing the warts by applying over-the-counter remedies, including salicylic acid plasters or compounds featuring salicylic and lactic acid, Compound W, or Vergo.

If the warts don't disappear, take your child to the doctor. Warts can be frozen with liquid nitrogen, then removed with an electric needle. They can also be burned off with chemicals.

VOMITING

Nausea and vomiting may be caused by any number of problems—bad food, too much food, viral and bacterial infection, or riding in cars, boats, trains, and planes. The greatest immediate danger is dehydration.

HOME TREATMENT

Vomiting can usually be treated at home by giving a child small amounts of clear liquids every ten to fifteen minutes. A child who can't keep anything down can suck on ice chips, followed by sips of water, sweetened tea (without milk), or bouillon every fifteen minutes. Bland food can join the menu once your child has spent from twelve to twenty-four hours without vomiting. However, do not offer fatty foods, dairy products, or spicy foods. Stick to gelatin, cooked cereal, rice, and applesauce.

WHEN TO CALL THE DOCTOR ABOUT VOMITING

- If vomiting is frequent and violent
- If vomiting is accompanied by severe stomach pain
- If vomit is bloody (bright red or dark coffee colored) or yellow or green in color

31

CHILDHOOD DISEASES

COMMON CHILDHOOD ILLNESSES

CHICKEN POX

Symptoms. Initially, these are fatigue and mild fever; twenty-four hours later, a rash appears, beginning as flat red splotches that look like pimples and turn into small clusters of blisters. The rash starts on the scalp or trunk. Within hours, blisters form a crust, and the tops scratch off easily. Itching can be severe. Fever subsides as the crust forms. Crusts fall off around days nine to thirteen.

Incubation. This takes from fourteen to seventeen days. This disease is highly contagious from twenty-four hours before rash to six days after.

Treatment. The FDA has approved an antiviral prescription drug called acyclovir for the treatment of chicken pox in children over two years of age. Given within twenty-four hours of the rash's appearance, the drug tends to reduce symptoms and the length of the illness. This new drug therapy is most useful for adolescents, who tend to have more severe symptoms than younger children, and children with chronic health problems such as respiratory illness or skin diseases.

Itching can also be helped by warm baths of baking soda (half a cup in a tub of water); calamine lotion; occasionally antihistamines by prescription. Wash your child's hands frequently to prevent possibility of infecting a lesion. For sore throat: Have a child suck on throat lozenges; encourage cold, soft foods and fluids (avoid hot or spicy foods). For fever: Give acetaminophen. (Children with viral diseases should not be given aspirin because they risk coming down with Reye's syndrome, a rare but potentially fatal side effect.)

Complications. The same virus causes shingles, which may develop later in life. Rare complications include encephalitis, pneumonia, and severe bacterial infection of lesions. This disease can be serious for children with cancer or those taking steroids and drugs affecting the immune system.

When to see a doctor. See a doctor *immediately* if your child has convulsions, a stiff neck, severe lethargy, or a severe headache. See a doctor *as soon as possible* if lesions appear infected. Make a *phone call* to your child's doctor if your child is breathing rapidly.

Note: There has been recent (1995) FDA approval of a chicken pox vaccine. The recommended age of immunization for otherwise healthy children is between twelve and eighteen months of age.

CONJUNCTIVITIS (PINKEYE)

Symptoms. Inflamed membrane lining of the front inner lid and some puss discharge are the symptoms. Conjunctivitis may be caused by a bacterial or a viral infection, or by an allergic reaction. If the infection is bacterial, the discharge is heavy and the eye may be crusted over when the child wakes up; a child may complain of grit or pain in his eyes.

Transmission. Both bacterial and viral conjunctivitis are highly contagious, and run through schools and day-care centers like water under a bridge.

Treatment. For allergic conjunctivitis, avoid the irritant, if known, and wash the eye gently. A doctor usually recommends antihistamines to reduce itching and swelling and prescribes antibiotic ointment. Avoid over-the-counter eyedrops.

Complications. The herpes virus can cause ulceration of the cornea; iritis or uveitis can affect the deep layers of the eye, causing irregularity of pupil and/or pain.

When to see a doctor. Always consult with a physician to determine the cause of the conjunctivitis and receive advice on appropriate treatment.

IMPETIGO

Symptoms. Multiple infected sores, some red and others blisterlike; most common on unclothed parts of the child's body (head, face, lower arms, and legs).

Transmission. Contagious through close physical contact.

Treatment. Clean sores vigorously with antibacterial soaps and apply antibacterial ointments two to three times a day. If there are multiple lesions or large areas of the limb affected or sores are blisterlike (which suggests a staph infection) oral and injected antibiotics are important to resolve the problem and prevent complications. Your physician will prescribe the appropriate therapy.

Complications. Commonly, highly pigmented scars and keloids. Rarely glomerulonephritis, an acute form of kidney failure, manifested by reduced urine output, swelling in the lower legs, headaches from brain swelling, bloody urine, and high blood pressure. Though rare, impetigo is the most common cause of childhood glomerulonephritis in the Deep South and the second-most common cause nationwide (after strep throat).

When to see a doctor. See a doctor *immediately* if your child is running a fever or if anyone in your family or neighborhood has had glomerulonephritis recently. See or call a doctor *as soon as possible* if the lesions do not show prompt improvement and are spreading.

MONONUCLEOSIS

Symptoms. The symptoms are severe sore throat accompanied by a fever for over seven days, weakness, swollen lymph nodes.

Transmission. The incubation period is from thirty to fifty days. It is infectious from the onset of the fever until the fever is gone (seven days).

Treatment. Get rest. Symptoms last from one to four weeks.

Complications. A person will experience prolonged tiredness and weakness. Enlarged spleen commonly occurs, so physicians advise against contact sports for about six months after the illness.

When to see a doctor. See a doctor *immediately* if your child has severe difficulty swallowing or breathing; excessive drooling. See a doctor *as soon as possible* when symptoms first appear, for accurate diagnosis.

PINWORMS

Pinworms are the most common parasite infecting the intestines of children in the United States. (Thirty percent of all children around the world are estimated to have pinworms.)

Symptoms. The most common symptoms are intense itching around the anus that is worse at night. At night, female pinworms emerge from the intestines through the rectum, deposit their eggs around the anal opening, then die. Worms resemble white threads about a quarter of an inch long. Your doctor may request samples; collect them on transparent tape. Even if you can't see any worms, the eggs will be visible under a microscope.

Transmission. Pinworms are highly contagious. Children become infected after coming in contact with contaminated objects— garden dirt, bedding, furniture, toys—then placing their fingers in their mouths. Pinworm eggs can be transmitted in food or by any contaminated object that a child puts in his mouth. Once infected, children easily transfer pinworms or pinworm eggs to others.

Treatment. Avoid home remedies such as tincture of turpentine with peppermint, which can be toxic. For itching, your physician may recommend Benadryl or topical creams such as clear Caladryl or Itch-X. Your physician may also prescribe a single dose of Vermox (mendazole), a chewable tablet, for your child and also for each person with whom your child is in intimate contact. The medication may be repeated in two weeks.

Keep your child's hands and body clean (cut fingernails short; stress the importance of washing hands after using the bathroom). The doctor may prescribe medication; the entire family may need treatment.

Complications. In girls, worms can move to the vagina, causing infection there.

When to see a doctor. See a doctor *as soon as possible* if your child is symptomatic. Call the doctor *immediately* if your newborn has bloody stool.

PNEUMONIA

Symptoms. Any signs of difficulty in breathing, pain in the chest with concomitant fever and/or cough or pain on breathing suggests an infectious inflammatory disease of the lungs (pneumonia, bronchitis, pleurisy).

Pneumonia can follow a cold if the fever does not abate after several days; it can also be a complication of measles and other viral diseases such as flu, as well as secondary to inhaled substances such as talcum/baby powder or perfumes.

Treatment. Cough medicine/expectorants (remember that cod liver oil and honey your parents used to make you take); lots of fluids. Your doctor may prescribe antibiotics depending on the cause of the pneumonia and the age of your child, as well as her general condition.

Hospitalization is rarely required (thus the well-known phrase "walking pneumonia"), but can be lifesaving, especially in very young children and immune-compromised children. Your doctor may perform a chest X ray and will prescribe antibiotics.

When to see a doctor. See a doctor *immediately* if your child has a fever; drools, breathing with his chin jutting out and his mouth open; is hoarse; has difficulty breathing in; wheezes.

ROSEOLA

Symptoms. Days of recurring fever are symptomatic. As the fever wanes, the rash appears. The rash looks like pink patches on the trunk (turns white when pressure is applied); can be bumpy; spreads to arms and neck (rarely face or legs); lasts less than twenty-four hours. Your child may have a runny nose, a red throat, or swollen glands in the neck.

Contagious. Roseola is contagious from the onset of the fever until the rash disappears.

Treatment. For fever, give acetaminophen.

When to see a doctor. Since roseola is almost over by the time the rash appears, contact your physician if any unusual problems occur during the feverish stage (see Fever in previous chapter), or if the illness lasts more than five days. Roseola is essentially a self-limited, mild viral disease that in itself should not produce any significant problems.

SCARLET FEVER

Scarlet fever is essentially a complication of the untreated Group A strep tonsillitis.

Symptoms. Initially, there is fever and weakness accompanied by a headache, stomachache, vomiting, and a sore throat. A fine sandpapery red rash appears from twelve to forty-eight hours later—first on the face, trunk, and arms; it then covers the body in twenty-four hours. The skin around the mouth will be pale, but skin creases will be more deeply red.

Incubation. This period is from three to six days. Scarlet fever is highly contagious from the onset of the fever or rash until twenty-four hours after an antibiotic is begun.

Treatment. For infection, your doctor will prescribe antibiotics. For fever, give acetaminophen and plenty of fluids.

Complications. Rheumatic fever is a rare complication.

When to see a doctor. See a doctor *immediately* for antibiotics and to rule out other illnesses.

TONSILLITIS

Symptoms. Inflamed tonsils, difficulty swallowing, a scratchy, sore throat, and a fever are symptomatic; tonsils look red and inflamed and are flecked with pus.

Treatment. Your doctor will prescribe antibiotics if the infection is caused by bacteria. If an infection is viral, antibiotics are not effective. Cold, soft foods and fluids are recommended. Surgery to remove tonsils is usually recommended only when a child has chronic tonsillitis.

Complications. Permanently enlarged tonsils, which can interfere with breathing and swallowing, are a complication. Chronic respiratory problems are also a complication. Symptoms include loud snoring, breathing through the mouth, restless sleep, and poor growth. Surgery is usually recommended for children who experience four or more episodes of tonsillitis a year and those whose tonsils are permanently enlarged.

When to see a doctor. Call the doctor *immediately* and describe the symptoms. The doctor will make an appointment to examine your child and prescribe appropriate treatment.

WARNING: TUBERCULOSIS ALERT

Since 1985, the incidence of tuberculosis in the United States has risen dramatically, particularly among poor inner-city families and individuals with HIV infection. Tuberculosis is caused by a specific type of bacterium (mycobacterium) that usually affects the lungs. TB destroys lung tissue and severely impairs breathing, but it may also affect other parts of the body, including the brain, heart, kidneys, and gastrointestinal tract. Left untreated, TB may be fatal.

We know that TB is infectious, but to become infected requires repeated prolonged exposure to airborne particles from an infected person's coughing or sneezing. Poor living conditions make this much more likely. Overcrowding, poor nutrition, inadequate hygiene, and stress all contribute to the spread of disease. TB spreads more quickly in confined, poorly ventilated spaces, including tenements, homeless shelters, jails, and even hospitals.

Beyond this, the most significant factor responsible for the rise in TB cases is that the treatment is lengthy and many people stop when they start feeling better, even though the disease is not yet cured. A combination of three to four antibiotics must be taken daily for six months or longer. These drugs kill the weakest bacteria first, and symptoms subside after a few weeks. Many people stop taking the drugs at this point. Yet stronger, more resistant bacteria have survived the initial drug assault. Stopping the medication encourages their growth, and they will be even stronger and more resistant than before.

According to a study of more than 25,000 residents of an integrated nursing home in Arkansas, blacks are twice as likely to be infected with tuberculosis, despite identical living conditions. This suggests that we are naturally more susceptible, though no reasons for this have been found.

A majority of children around the world have been inoculated with BCG, a vaccine designed to lessen the severity of TB if the child is stricken. However, this vaccine has not been recommended in the United States. While the inoculation may help children temporarily, no one knows for how long. This inoculation also leads to a positive tuberculosis test, which means it may negate the screening test for TB. BCG cannot be given to HIV-infected people—who presently account for most new cases of tuberculosis.

WHEN TO SEE THE DOCTOR

There is a screening test for TB that's suitable for children. The American Academy of Pediatrics recommends routine, yearly screening of children who live in areas where TB is known to be prevalent or who live with an HIV-positive person, who is more susceptible to developing TB.

Adults who screen positive for TB have a 10 percent chance of contracting the disease. Of those who get sick, the death rate from drug-resistant strains is about 50 percent. Children have an even greater risk of developing the disease once they become infected. As many as 40 percent of infants in their first year of life may develop TB once they become infected.

Symptoms of TB:

> *Persistent cough, possibly with bloody sputum*
> *Chest pain*
> *Shortness of breath*
> *Night sweats*
> *Fever*
> *Fatigue*
> *Loss of appetite; weight loss*

In addition to the long course of antibiotics, children should get plenty of rest until symptoms subside. Children should be taught to sneeze or cough into disposable tissues to prevent the spread of infection. In some cases, particularly if the TB is resistant to standard treatment, a child may have to be hospitalized in an isolation room to receive additional treatment and prevent spread of the drug-resistant strain.

To fight TB effectively, and to prevent the growth of drug-resistant strains of the bacteria, requires regular screening of high-risk individuals, as well as full courses of treatment.

DISEASES CHILDREN MAY BE IMMUNIZED AGAINST

PERTUSSIS (WHOOPING COUGH)

Stage one is similar to an upper respiratory infection for from one to seven days—nasal congestion, runny nose, sneezing, coughing.

Stage two consists of two weeks of intense periods of coughing lasting several minutes each; a child gasps between coughs; inspiration makes the sound that gives this disease the nickname "whooping cough."

Stage three is the convalescent period of from three to four weeks, notable for chronic cough.

Complications most commonly occur in infants under six months of age: pneumonia; aspiration; pneumothorax; atelectasis; sinusitis; failure to thrive; seizures; encephalopathy; and death.

DPT vaccine. The diphtheria immunization is given in combination with pertussis vaccine and tetanus toxoid (DPT), or in combination with tetanus toxoid alone (DT, or Td, which is an adult tetanus and diphtheria immunization). This vaccine is contraindicated for children who are over seven years of age, or who may have a progressive neurological disorder. It is also contraindicated in children who have a current fever or a history of prior DPT reaction. DPT is not a live viral vaccine. Thus, it is not contraindicated in children who are receiving immunosuppressive therapy. But it may not be given to such patients because they may not make antibodies to the vaccine as long as they are immune-suppressed.

Vaccine reactions: Roughly half of the children receiving DPT shots develop fever. About one-third become drowsy; some children feel pain and anxiety; others temporarily lose their appetite. Some have swelling at the injection site.

More severe side effects include high fever, collapse, or shock. By far the most serious reaction affects a child's central nervous system. Episodes of high-pitched screaming, persistent crying jags, and even seizures are followed by a period of exhaustion or sleep, but they begin again when the child awakens. Severe reactions are rare. If your child develops any of these symptoms after DPT vaccination, call the doctor immediately.

Most children who have reactions recover completely. If your child has any extreme reaction to DPT, let your physician know. It's possible that your child will be able to tolerate diphtheria-tetanus immunization without the pertussis.

DIPHTHERIA

Diphtheria attacks the throat, nose, and skin. It is highly infectious.

Complications include paralysis in 20 percent of patients; heart damage in 50 percent; it is fatal in approximately 10 percent of patients.

The diphtheria immunization is given in combination with pertussis vaccine and tetanus toxoid (DPT), or in combination with tetanus toxoid alone (DT, or Td, which is an adult tetanus and diphtheria vaccine). For DPT reactions, see the entry for pertussis.

MUMPS

Initial symptoms include headache or earache; weakness. After several days, salivary glands around the ears may swell, causing painful chewing and swallowing; sour tastes exacerbate pain. Glands under the jaw and tongue may become inflamed and the inside of the mouth may become red and puffy.

The virus is most contagious two days before symptoms begin until the swelling is completely gone. Susceptible individuals (those who have never had mumps or never been exposed to them) will develop symptoms from sixteen to eighteen days after exposure.

Treatment is acetaminophen and fluids. Avoid sour or acidic foods and citric juice such as orange juice.

Complications include (rarely) encephalitis; pancreatitis; kidney disease; deafness; inflammation of testes/ovaries.

Call the doctor or clinic immediately if your child is lethargic; has convulsions or a stiff neck; if testicles hurt or swell; abdominal pain or vomiting occurs; child experiences dizziness or difficulty in hearing.

The mumps vaccine: Mumps vaccine is given in combination with measles and rubella vaccine (MMR). Reactions to the vaccine may not occur until several days after the shots.

Some children who receive the MMR vaccine experience a lowering of blood platelets. Roughly one out of every one hundred develops swollen glands under one or both ears. Some children develop a mild rash all over. The child will not be contagious, and side effects will disappear without treatment. Children experiencing joint pains after an MMR shot usually respond to acetaminophen.

The vaccine should not be given to children who are known to have serious allergic reactions to eggs (hives, difficulty breathing, low blood pressure, throat swelling, or shock). MMR is also contraindicated in children who have fever; those who are hypersensitive to the antibiotic neomycin; those who have immunodeficiency (except HIV infection). Any female who is pregnant or is planning to become pregnant within three months should not receive MMR vaccine.

MEASLES

When measles swept Chicago in the late 1960s, most of the stricken came from the poorest neighborhoods. When it erupted again in 1989, children from the inner city were hardest hit. In these outbreaks, even some who had been vaccinated for measles contracted the disease. There's an obvious connection between measles and poor nutrition, inadequate health care, and substandard living conditions.

Between birth and four months of age, most infants are naturally protected against measles by antibodies inherited through their mother's blood, if she had measles as a child.

Symptoms of measles do not begin until eight to twelve days after the initial infection. Early symptoms include fever; weakness; dry cough; inflamed eyes—red, itchy, light-sensitive; white spots on a red base inside the mouth.

About five days later, the rash appears around the hairline, face, neck, and ears. It is first pink, blotchy, and flat; the spots may fade if touched, but eventually they darken, merging into large red patches;

the rash spreads to the body and lasts from four to seven days; it is itchy; lesions can turn light brown.

The incubation period is from eight to twelve days. The period of contagion is from three to six days before the rash appears and about seven days afterward.

Treatment is limited to acetaminophen for fever; vaporizer for cough. If eyes are photosensitive, draw the shades and dim the lights.

Common complications requiring additional treatment are sore throat, ear infection, and pneumonia. Rarely, encephalitis and seizures are complications.

If severe lethargy, headache, vomiting, or convulsion occurs, call a doctor or clinic immediately for an emergency appointment; wrap your child up and *go!* If the child is having a convulsion, or is too sick to move, call 911 for an ambulance. (See Fever with Seizure, previous chapter.)

Somewhat less urgent complications also require a visit to the doctor: bleeding from nose, mouth, rectum, or into the skin; difficulty breathing; earache; rapid breathing; or a sore throat.

Measles vaccine is the same as recommended for rubella (below).

RUBELLA (GERMAN MEASLES)

Rubella is a mild disease that poses little threat to children. However, rubella is extremely dangerous to a developing fetus whose mother contracts the disease during pregnancy, especially in the first trimester, when the baby's systems are initially developing. In a developing fetus, rubella can cause heart defects, blindness, deafness, and mental deficiency. The risks decrease as pregnancy advances.

Initial symptoms include mild fatigue and enlarged and tender lymph nodes at the base of the neck. The rash begins on the face as flat or slightly raised red spots, then spreads to the body in large patches. But often no rash appears, and even when it does many parents and doctors don't recognize it. There is some brief low fever. Between 10 and 15 percent of older children and teens experience joint pains that begin around the third day.

Rubella is not as contagious as measles and chicken pox; it incubates for twelve to twenty-one days (average sixteen) and is contagious from four days before the rash develops until the rash disappears about seven days later.

Treatment is limited to acetaminophen for fever.

Child should see a doctor immediately if lethargy or convulsions occur, or if there is any bleeding into the skin.

Rubella vaccine: The vaccine may be given separately or in combination with measles and mumps vaccine (MMR).

Rubella vaccine or MMR should not be given if a child has an active infection accompanied by fever or has a respiratory illness. It is also contraindicated if a child is being treated with immunosuppressive therapy. (Any female who is pregnant or is planning to become pregnant within three months should not receive rubella vaccine alone or MMR vaccine.)

TETANUS

Since 1976, there have been fewer than one hundred cases of tetanus (lockjaw) annually in the United States, almost none of them occurring in children.

Tetanus is caused by bacterial spores that exist all around us in dirt and human and animal waste. These spores grow in the absence of air, and therefore tetanus thrives in puncture wounds (from stepping on a nail, being bitten by a cat or dog, or being stabbed with a narrow sharp object). If these or any similar injuries occur, it's imperative to cleanse the wounds thoroughly and get an immediate tetanus shot, either from the emergency room or from your doctor. Tetanus causes severe muscle spasms, predominantly in the neck and jaw. Though treatable, it still claims the lives of 40 percent of its victims.

Tetanus toxoid: Tetanus (and also diphtheria) infection is caused by toxins produced by bacteria. Therefore, the immunizations for these diseases use toxoids (a weakened form of toxin) to stimulate antibody production. Toxoids are not truly "vaccines" (which are composed of weakened bacteria or viruses). The tetanus immunization can be given alone or in combination (see DPT for pertussis on page 352). It protects a child for roughly twelve years.

Severe allergic reactions to the tetanus vaccine are extremely rare. Such a reaction immediately after immunization contradicates any further dose.

POLIO

Polio is an infectious and often deadly viral disease that can crip-
ple, as well as cause meningitis or respiratory infections. There has
been no polio epidemic in the United States since the mid-1950s,
when the famous Salk vaccine was invented. Salk's original vaccine was an injectable form made from killed polio virus. It is still
approved for use by the American Academy of Pediatrics, but
because the injectable form requires repeated boosters, it is primarily used as an alternative for children whose immune systems
are compromised.

Oral polio vaccine: The oral vaccine (OPV) is made from a live
polio virus. This is the popular favorite today because it works in
the infant's upper respiratory tract, where the disease grabs hold.
This vaccine also lasts longer because it creates both intestinal and
circulating antibodies.

Reactions to vaccine: Very rarely (1 or 2 per 10 million), a child
develops paralytic polio, either by receiving the oral vaccine or by
coming in contact with someone who did. Since 1961, approximately 260 cases of paralytic polio have occurred among youngsters
receiving the oral vaccine and people who have come into contact
with these children.

OPV should not be given to children who have a family history
of immunodeficiency disease (unless they are tested first) or who
are known to be immune-deficient. However, immune-deficient
children may receive *inactivated* polio vaccine (IPV), which is given
by intramuscular injection. Children who are taking drugs that
lower resistance—corticosteroids, alkalating drugs, radiation, or
antimetabolites—should not receive OPV. Any child who has
received OPV should not come in contact with household members who are immune-deficient.

The vaccine is also contraindicated in children who are acutely
sick or who have persistent vomiting or diarrhea. Pregnant women
should not receive OPV.

HEMOPHILUS INFLUENZA B (HIB)

Hemophilus influenza B is the most common cause of bacterial
meningitis in children, and it is also responsible for several other

deadly illnesses. It also causes inflammation of the epiglottis and arthritis, generally before the age of four.

The risk for Hib is greatest for children under two, and the incidence is higher among blacks than among whites. Hib is sometimes fatal and can cause permanent disability.

Hib vaccine: The current Hib vaccines have been very successful in boosting children's immune systems and preventing additional infections of Hib. They can be used in infants under eighteen months of age.

The Hib vaccine should not be given to children who are known to be sensitive to the materials in the vaccine, including thimerosal (a preservative) and diphtheria toxoid. The vaccine should not be given to those with illness accompanied by fever.

Part Five

———

TROUBLESHOOTING

32

CHILDREN AND LEAD EXPOSURE

Exposure to environmental hazards—including pollution, toxic waste, and secondhand smoke—can lead to a variety of health problems for children. Poor children especially are more likely to live in areas where they are exposed to industrial wastes and pollution, putting them at risk for respiratory infections, skin ailments, and some cancers. The most common and most serious environmental hazard affecting African-American children is lead. African-American children are more likely than any other group to suffer damages from lead exposure.

Symptoms of lead exposure include delayed mental development and reduced IQ, behavioral problems, and anemia. Very severe exposure, which is rare, may cause convulsions, coma, and death.

About 75 percent of the lead children take in comes from paint dust in their homes. Another 20 percent comes from drinking water. And the rest comes from air, soil, and food.

WHICH CHILDREN ARE VULNERABLE?

New studies show conclusively that all children are vulnerable to lead exposure. However, the lower the family income, the higher the risk. Any child living in poverty is more likely to live in an old building where lead paint peels from the ceilings and walls. Children living in inner cities tend to be even more exposed, because they are also more likely to live in areas where lead contamination from industry and vehicles is high.

However, the percentage of poor black children who get lead

poisoning is significantly higher than the percentage of poor white children living in the same circumstances (33⅓ percent versus 6 percent). The reason for this startling difference is not known, but it might reflect how lead is absorbed and stored in the body.

Lead is more easily absorbed by children who suffer from nutritional iron deficiency. Studies in both humans and animals have proved that a diet low in iron and calcium (and possibly protein) increases the body's absorption and retention of lead, while a diet rich in these nutrients protects against lead buildup. Therefore, nutritional differences may partly account for varying lead levels among poor children.

Obviously, researchers must start looking into these and other possible factors present in an African-American child's life that might account for the serious discrepancy.

LEAD LEVELS: HOW LOW IS LOW ENOUGH?

Recent findings show that even though efforts to reduce lead exposure have drastically cut cases of obvious lead poisoning, current exposure limits are still not low enough to prevent brain damage in millions of American children.

For the past five years, syndicated *New York Times* science writer Jane E. Brody has been diligently following the story of "silent" lead poisoning among children. Her reports on three large ongoing studies in Australia and the United States support the opinion of federal health officials who describe lead poisoning as the number-one environmental problem facing American children. These findings contradict assertions by the lead industry that genetic and economic factors are mainly responsible for lowered intelligence and behavioral problems.

In 1991, the federal Centers for Disease Control and Prevention found that earlier definitions of lead poisoning were too high and reduced the poison level to 10 mcg per dl of blood. That's where it still stands. Today, this amount can be found in 3 million children under age six, or 10 to 15 percent of the nation's preschoolers. And the new studies show that even low levels of lead, under 10 mcg/dl, are linked to diminished IQ.

The studies found lasting losses in children's intelligence, even when children had no obvious physical symptoms of lead poisoning. They also showed that lead damage to a child's brain can start even before birth if the pregnant mother has elevated levels of lead in her own body. The brain is most vulnerable to toxic substances from the seventh month in utero through the first two years of life, when most of the connections between brain cells are formed.

These new findings have led many public health experts to conclude that there is no such thing as a "safe" level of lead in young children.

EFFECTS OF LEAD EXPOSURE

The Australian study found that lead exposure had a particularly harmful impact on a child's *visual-motor abilities*. These are deficits that can hamper a child's ability to read, write, and solve math problems by interfering with the brain mechanisms involved in recognizing and copying shapes, visualizing objects in space, and forming nonverbal concepts. Similar findings have come out of ongoing studies in Cincinnati and Boston.

Even in families that are financially secure, where lead levels are generally lowest and children are best able to compensate for small declines in cognitive abilities, the effects of lead are notable.

In the continuing study of 170 children from middle- and upper-middle-income families in Boston, Dr. David Bellinger and his colleagues found significant signs of lasting brain damage from lead exposure. The children in the study had lead levels of up to 25 mcg. For every 10 mcg of lead above the danger zone (10 mcg/dl), first measured when the children were two years old, there was a decline of 5.8 in overall IQ and a decline of 8.9 in achievement-test scores by age ten.

Dr. Bellinger, a psychologist and epidemiologist at Children's Hospital and an associate professor of neurology at Harvard Medical School, said that the findings strongly suggest that the cognitive losses are permanent.

The Cincinnati study was conducted among low-income families. Here, researchers found that IQ points fell as the average lifetime blood-lead concentrations increased from 10 to 35 mcg per dl. The average loss was 8 IQ points—from 91 to 83.

In children with above-average IQs, these losses may not make a significant impact on achievement. But for children whose IQ is on the low end of normal, even a small drop can make the difference between success and failure in school.

Despite the evidence that even low levels of lead can harm the brains of young children, further reducing amounts of lead in the environment remains a controversial issue. Special interests, most notably the lead industry, argue that reducing lead exposure would cost millions, with virtually no benefit. In an editorial in *The American Journal of Diseases of Children,* Dr. Claire B. Ernhart, of Case Western Reserve School of Medicine in Cleveland, and Dr. James W. Sayre, of Family Health Associates of St. Mary's Hospital in Rochester, New York, stated that resources would be better put to use on other factors known to affect child development, such as prenatal care, vaccinations, and Head Start.

Yet the CDC conservatively estimates that the costs of removing lead from children's homes would ultimately bring a net savings of $28 billion, through reduced medical and special-education costs, as well as the increased wages that typically accompany higher IQ and better education. (Not included in the estimate were the potential savings from a reduction in juvenile delinquency, along with the costs of treating high blood pressure and heart disease in adults, which can result from long-term exposure to low levels of lead.)

Thus, although the science is becoming clearer, politics and budget cuts govern solutions. Right now, precious little money is going toward lead abatement, universal prenatal care, or Head Start. It's a lose-lose situation.

LEAD DANGERS: WHERE THEY ARE

Lead is everywhere: in air, water, soil, food, dust. It gets into the air from industrial and vehicular emissions, from tobacco smoke and paint dust, and from the burning of solid wastes that contain lead. Airborne lead levels dropped sharply after the nation began phasing out leaded gasoline, but many vehicles still use fuel containing lead.

Lead occurs naturally in soil, which also collects lead from the air and other sources. When crops are grown in soil containing lead, the poison can enter the food chain. Other sources of lead include foods stored or served in lead-glazed pottery or lead crystal, as well as processed foods sold in cans soldered with lead. Despite a federal ban on using these cans for food, many imported foods are still sold in lead-soldered cans.

Lead is also a natural constituent of surface and ground waters that provide drinking water to many millions of Americans. Although the use of lead in plumbing is now banned, many homes still have old water pipes that can transfer lead to drinking water.

The use of indoor paints containing lead was banned in 1977, but about 57 million older homes still contain lead paints. Of these, 14 million are believed to contain lead paint in unsound condition and 3.8 million of these deteriorated units are occupied by at least one young child. The highest concentration of lead paint is in homes built before 1960. The same goes for day-care centers and nursery schools. When this lead paint flakes off or is disturbed during even minor renovations, the area becomes filled with lead-containing dust. Sweeping or vacuuming spreads the dust to furniture, toys, and food, from which it readily goes into the hands and mouths of infants and toddlers. In this way, young children absorb far more lead than adults living under the same conditions.

WHAT PARENTS CAN DO

Let's look at some solutions that parents can put into effect in their own homes to help protect children from lead exposure. It's important to use caution, as those who are concerned about lead can sometimes make the problem worse by trying to remove it in ways that introduce even further hazards.

REMOVING OLD PAINT

A new federal law will soon require that potential occupants of housing units built before 1980 be notified of known or possible lead hazards in them. However, the mere presence of lead paint doesn't mean an active lead hazard exists. Trying to remove all lead paint from a home can be costly, dangerous, and perhaps impossible.

Lead paint that is not flaking does not necessarily have to be removed. The old paint can be covered with an impervious material like wallboard, plywood, ceramic tile, or vinyl-coated fabric. Regular wallpaper or painting the wall over with a lead-free paint are quick fixes, not permanent solutions, according to the New York Public Interest Research Group's booklet *Get the Lead Out.*

Before considering removing old paint, lead levels should be tested in household dust. The most comprehensive guidelines for lead testing and control are described in the HUD Guidelines for the Evaluation and Control of Lead-Based Paint Hazards (see pages 411–412).

Lead paint should be removed only by a licensed abatement contractor, an individual who has been trained and certified by the Environmental Protection Agency. Lead-based paint should be removed with a chemical stripper, not torched, sanded, or scraped off. Pregnant women and small children should stay out of the home until the job is completed. Professional lead removal includes a thorough cleanup with an industrial HEPA (high-efficiency particle accumulator), filtered vacuum, and a wet mop dipped in a hot-water solution of a phosphate polymer such as powdered dishwasher detergent.

Thirty states do not license or certify paint-removal contractors. Anyone can claim to be a lead abatement contractor. As a result, parents with the best of intentions may unwittingly subject young children to lead poisoning through the work of incompetent and sometimes unscrupulous contractors.

DRINKING WATER AND LEAD

Never use water from the hot-water tap for cooking or for mixing drinks or infant formula. In general, it is wise to let even the cold water run for a few minutes before using it for cooking or drinking.

If you are concerned about lead levels in your water, call your area EPA or have it tested. The EPA Safe Drinking Water Hot Line is available to answer consumer questions about water (see page 398). If you use a well, check with your public health department.

If you have concerns about the safety of the water supply in your area, the best way to find out what's in it is to have it tested. Costs range from twenty dollars to two hundred dollars, depending on how many tests are performed. Be sure to consult a reputable state-certified independent laboratory, which can be found in the Yellow Pages under "Laboratories—Testing." (Companies that sell home water-treatment devices are not objective testers.)

If lead levels in your water are high, either a reverse osmosis filter or a distiller can be used to remove the lead. There are also inexpensive countertop units with replaceable filters that remove most of the lead from drinking water.

STORING AND COOKING FOOD

Never store food or drinks in decorative ceramic containers or lead crystal decanters. Unless you are sure the glaze is free of lead, avoid cooking in ceramic ware, and do not routinely use ceramic dishes or old china with a damaged glaze to serve hot or acidic foods and beverages, including coffee and tea. Imported pottery is best checked for lead content before it is used for food. Avoid imported canned foods; the cans may contain lead. Look for canned food products with "lead free" on the label.

NUTRITION

Make sure children consume adequate amounts of iron, calcium, and protein, as deficiencies in these nutrients increase a child's absorption of lead.

SOIL

If the soil surrounding your home contains a lot of lead, it should be removed and replaced. If this is not possible, it should be covered with grass or a layer of mulch, or planted with shrubbery to discourage children from playing in the area.

TESTING CHILDREN

The American Academy of Pediatrics recommends that all children be routinely screened for lead. However, most young children, including those most heavily exposed to lead, have not been tested even once to see if their bodies are harboring dangerous amounts.

Testing should start at about six months of age, with repeat tests at twelve and twenty-four months and every year afterward until the child is six years old. Waiting to test when a child is ready to start school is a little late; serious damage may already have occurred, since the developing brain is most vulnerable to lead damage between birth and age three.

If your child's lead levels are found to be high on an initial test and a confirming second test, there is no need to panic. Rather, a systematic approach to identifying and eliminating sources of lead is what's called for. When lead levels exceed 25 mcg, most lead experts recommend chelation therapy (the use of oral or intravenous drugs that carry lead out of the body), in addition to environmental cleansing.

33

CHILDHOOD SAFETY

Accidents are the leading cause of death in children, and African-American children are particularly at risk. Automobile accidents are the most common cause of death; in about half of the accidents, children are hit by cars, and in the other half, they are passengers in cars involved in accidents. Drownings and fires account for most other injury-related deaths among children.

Household fires are a special risk to children, because they have more difficulty escaping than adults and are less likely to survive fire-related injuries. Fire-related deaths are often due to asphyxiation and traumatic injuries, as well as burns. Children under the age of five who live in substandard housing without smoke detectors are most at risk.

Falls and poisonings cause many nonfatal injuries. Playground equipment and upper-story windows are frequently implicated in fall-related injuries in children.

Many injuries can be and are being prevented. But safety remains a serious problem in some neighborhoods. Low income is the single most important predictor of injury. Children living in poverty are more than twice as likely to receive injuries from all causes, and four and one half times as likely to be assaulted. Poor neighborhoods have fewer safe play areas, and more children are likely to play in the streets, abandoned buildings, and other hazardous areas. Broken playground equipment, broken glass, poor housing, drug activity, violence, and a high prevalence of firearms in the hands of children, adolescents, and young adults are all contributing factors.

The Safe Kids/Healthy Neighborhoods Injury Prevention Program has shown that neighborhood intervention can make a difference in these statistics. The program involved children in central Harlem and Washington Heights, two contiguous neighborhoods in Manhattan with large numbers of residents living below the poverty line.

Parents and teachers in Harlem requested a program in playground safety from health professionals. Intervention was planned for central Harlem, with Washington Heights serving as the control group.

A community coalition involving twenty-six separate organizations, both voluntary and city agencies, planned and executed the program. The plan was to renovate central Harlem's playgrounds, involve children and adolescents in safe, supervised activities that would teach them useful skills, provide injury- and violence-prevention education, and provide safety equipment such as bicycle helmets at reasonable costs. Over the first three years, the program saw a 44 percent reduction in accidents among school-aged children. The positive effects appeared to spill over into Washington Heights, for that neighborhood also reduced the number of accidents among children, although not as much.

Clearly there are things we as communities and as individuals can do to improve the circumstances of the huge number of American children who live in dangerous environments.

SAFEGUARDING YOUR CHILD

INFANTS

Inspect carefully all the small environments in which your baby spends his day: the crib, the changing table, the car, the high chair, and the bathtub. Check for anything that could cause strangulation (window blind cords or strings on crib toys, for example), or suffocation (gaps between a baby's mattress and bumpers, or plastic bags), and put away all small objects he could choke on. Close supervision is the main thing. Just because your infant hasn't turned over yet doesn't mean that today won't be the day he learns.

Car safety. Babies must be strapped into their car seats, which in turn must be securely fastened to the car. Babies need rear-facing car seats until they weigh at least twenty pounds. Follow the manufacturer's directions for using your car seat. It is never safe to travel in the car with your baby on your lap or in your arms. He needs a car seat beginning with his very first trip—home from the hospital.

Crib safety. To prevent strangulation, crib slats should be no wider than 2⅜ inches apart. The mattress should be the same size as the crib, with no gaps. New cribs, or those manufactured after 1974, will meet these strict safety standards. Remember to check all cribs that your baby sleeps in—at the baby-sitter's and grandparents' homes, too—to be sure they're safe. Always keep the rails up when your baby is in the crib.

Falls. Never leave your baby alone on your bed or on other high places. Always keep one hand on your baby during diaper changing. Have everything out and ready before you begin in order to prevent awkward reaching or the need to leave your child unattended.

Fire. To keep your whole family safe, install smoke detectors on each floor of your home and near sleeping areas. If you smoke, never do so while holding your baby or child. Keep ashtrays, matches, and lighters out of a baby's reach.

Burns. Be careful when warming infant formula, and do not heat bottles in a microwave oven—the formula becomes too hot too quickly. A bowl of warm water is all that's needed to warm a bottle. Always test the formula's temperature on your wrist before feeding it to your baby.

Turn down your water heater to 120–130° F to prevent scalds. Always check bathwater with your forearm first, and never let go of your baby during a bath. To avoid serious burns, put your baby down when you're having a cup of coffee. Cups can be very fascinating, and your baby will be at the perfect height for grabbing hold and spilling the hot contents all over both of you.

BABIES ON THE MOVE: CREEPERS, CRAWLERS, AND TODDLERS

Once a baby becomes mobile, usually around six or seven months, full-scale childproofing of your home and other environments is vital. The best advice from safety experts is, "Think like a toddler, act like an adult."

Car safety. When your baby weighs twenty pounds, you can change your car seat from rear-facing to front-facing. The center seat in the back is the safest place to put it in your car.

When children weigh forty pounds, they no longer need a car seat, but they still need to buckle up. A car booster seat will let your growing boy or girl watch the scenery go by.

A child over sixty pounds can use the regular car seat without a booster seat and with a lap belt low on the hips. When your child is over four and a half feet tall, you can add the shoulder strap. In children under four and a half feet tall, the shoulder harness can cause neck injuries. If the strap runs across the neck (rather than the shoulder), put it behind your child. Never put the shoulder belt under both arms.

Crib toys. Once a baby can pull up to stand, remove toys hung across the crib rails and decorative crib bumper pads.

High places. Block all stairways with safety gates that fit snugly. Never leave your baby unattended in a high chair, infant seat, swing, or walker. Grocery carts, high chairs, changing tables, and beds are common sites for babies' tumbles. Use all restraints provided and never turn your back on your child.

As children begin climbing and jumping, they can slip and fall. Keep chairs away from counters. Install guards on windows above the first floor.

Walkers. Walkers are a leading cause of accidents. The American Academy of Pediatrics recommends against using them; if you choose to have one, be sure to avoid the situations in which the most accidents occur. These include spills down steps, tipping over on uneven surfaces, and dangerous access to hot radiators, plants, and other hanging objects a baby can pull down or ingest. Never be out of range of a quick rescue.

Small objects. Watch for hidden dangers. Once babies discover their mouths, it seems everything they touch goes into them. Keep all small objects out of reach. Older kids' toys, buttons, paper clips, safety pins, insect traps, and candy are just some of the things your baby will find tempting. Keeping an older child's toys from getting into a baby's hands can be a special problem. Experts on child safety caution that preschoolers should never be left unsupervised with a baby.

Never feed your baby hard pieces of food, like peanuts. And beware of another source of dangerous objects that mothers frequently overlook: their open pocketbooks.

Choking. Ask your pediatrician to show you how to perform first aid on a choking baby—just in case.

Choking is always a potential threat with infants and toddlers. If the baby is obviously coughing and making noise, the best thing to do is nothing—coughing is the most effective way to clear the air passages.

If the baby can't cough or move air and her face is turning blue, emergency measures are mandatory. Quickly place the baby face-down on your knee, with her body tilted downward (the head lower) at a thirty-degree angle. Administer four sharp blows between the baby's shoulder blades.

Burns. During cold winter months, block your baby's path to heat registers, ducts, and portable heaters. It's okay to warm toddler food in the microwave *if you follow the directions on the label carefully. Always check the food's temperature by tasting it yourself first.*

Electrical outlets and cords. Electrical outlets in every room should have guards to protect against electrical shock, as children are often fascinated with these openings and like to poke objects into them. There are several types of outlet protection, including simple plastic caps that fit directly into the socket; outlet plates that prevent access to the outlet; and outlet guards that completely cover the outlet, plugs and all. Your choice should depend on how persistent your child is about outlets. Never leave an extension cord plugged into an outlet with the other end open, such as for Christmas tree lights.

Electrical cords are another irresistible temptation to some children. A cord shortener helps get extra cord up and away from your crawler. Also available are clamps that attach to furniture and prevent a lamp from toppling, even if the cord is pulled.

Doors. A squeaky door can be intriguing to a creeping child. Doorstops can keep little fingers from being pinched.

Shoelaces. In a recent study of three thousand children treated at the Children's Hospital of Philadelphia emergency room, more than a third of the injuries treated were related to loss of footing—and 67 percent of these were associated with dangling laces. Untied shoelaces can be a serious threat. Teach your kids how to double-tie their laces.

Kitchen. Knives and scissors should be locked securely away. Childproof latches on drawers and cabinets within a child's ever-lengthening reach will keep harmful substances secure. Keep all corrosives and poisons in high cabinets. Install appliance latches to prevent a child from opening the oven, refrigerator, dishwasher, and microwave doors. You can also purchase range knob covers and a plastic range guard to safeguard your stove. Remember to keep all pot handles turned toward the back of the stove and hot pans out of reach. If possible, use back burners when cooking.

Never use a knife or fork to remove toast from the toaster in front of your child—even if the toaster is unplugged. Use wooden toast tongs instead.

Bathroom. Place medicines and other potentially harmful substances, including mouthwash and cleaning solutions, in child-proofed cabinets. A toilet seat lock is a helpful product, as a toddler who's attracted to the water in the toilet bowl could drown from toppling into it. Unplug and coil the cords of hair dryers, curling irons, electric shavers, and other bathroom appliances when they're not in use. Store them out of sight so there is no possibility that they might fall into the tub with your young bather.

To avoid slips and falls in the bathtub, apply nonskid appliqués or use a rubber bath mat. A cushioned spout guard helps prevent the possibility of banged heads and burns from a faucet that may remain hot after filling the tub.

Bath safety. Don't let your child turn on hot faucets alone. Even tap water can cause a serious burn. Double-check your water heater's temperature to make sure it's not set too high. And get into the habit of turning the cold water off last. This will help prevent scalding and keep the metal faucet cool.

Never leave your baby or child alone in the tub. If the phone rings, don't answer it. (They will call back.) It only takes a few seconds and a few inches of water for a child to drown.

Living room. Evaluate your furniture in light of your child's constantly improving ability to climb. Can it be pulled over? Bolt bookshelves and other pieces of furniture that could topple to the wall with L-braces. Keep drawers that could pull chests off balance fully closed.

If you have a fireplace, a glass screen will keep a child away from the fire, ashes, and soot. However, remember that a glass screen gets hot when the fireplace is in use.

Apply cushioned corner guards to tables and other pieces of furniture with sharp corners. If your VCR is accessible, you might want a VCR lock that inserts in the front (like a tape) and prevents a child from reaching inside. (This also protects your VCR from being damaged by your child.)

TOYS

Do not let your toddler play with balloons or plastic bags. Check to see that lids of toy boxes and other cabinets your child has access to do *not* shut tight—curious children can get trapped inside.

Choose toys that are safe for your child. Watch for sharp edges and small pieces that could come off. When consulting guidelines on toy packages, consider your own child's ability to play safely with the toy, not just the toy's "safety age."

Art supplies. Believe it or not, a recent survey of crayons imported from China turned up twelve brands that contained lead. These have been recalled and banned by the Consumer Product Safety Commission. Most crayons in the United States are made here and are safe: Check labels of all children's art supplies to make sure they conform to ASTM D-4236 or similar codes. This label shows that the material has been okayed by a toxicologist. Even better, look for a seal on the label from the Art and Craft Materials Institute (ACMI) certifying that the product is nontoxic.

PLAYING OUTSIDE

Children can be risk-takers and may not be afraid of many things that can cause them harm. Fence in play areas. Teach your child where it is safe to play in your yard. Check for poisonous plants and other hazards. Just in case—learn CPR and first aid. These informative, useful courses are often offered by the local YMCA and various community organizations.

Never leave your child alone near water—whether it's a wading pool, stream, birdbath, bathtub, or puddle. Of all drowning victims, 75 percent are between one and three years old.

If you have a swimming pool, put a fence around it, and always keep the pool gate locked, as well as any doors that access your pool from inside the house. This protects your child, as well as any other children in the neighborhood who may wander into your yard.

Teach your child how to cross streets safely and about traffic dangers. Set and enforce rules for riding trikes and bikes. Be sure your child wears a helmet and rides on the sidewalk or a path, never in the street.

Watch your child carefully on the playground. Kids don't realize how dangerous some of their play can be.

See that your child learns to swim. Even knowing how to tread water can prevent panic if he accidentally falls in the water. Instruct your child not to run around water, not to push or dunk others, and never to depend on inflatable toys as life preservers. Never let your child swim alone. Even children who are comfortable in water can find themselves in life-threatening situations. (This is true for adults, too.)

Personal safety. Teach your children to be cautious around people they don't know and to stick close when you go shopping together. Teach them what to do if they get separated from you in the mall or store.

BIKE HELMETS

Several states now have bicycle helmet laws, but even if yours does not, insist that your child wear a safety helmet when riding her bike. As many as one thousand bike riders, six hundred of them under the age of fourteen, die each year, and thousands of others suffer brain damage from head injuries. Helmets worn by cyclists have been shown to reduce the risk of serious, permanent, and sometimes fatal head injuries by 85 percent. Choose a helmet that meets accepted safety standards of the American National Standards Institute or the Snell Memorial Foundation. (These will be clearly stated on the label.) New, all-purpose helmets that can be worn by children while riding bikes, roller skating, and participating in a variety of sports are also available.

POISON CONTROL

Each year, 2 million children under five come into contact with household poisons, leading to frightening emergency room visits.

Many accidental poisonings occur while adults are using such products. Don't use medicines or cleaners when your baby is in the room.

Safeguard your child's environment from the following dangerous household poisons.

Air fresheners
Alcohol (rubbing alcohol, liquor, etc.)
Ammonia
Batteries
Bleaches
Bug killers
Cleaners
Cosmetics (including nail-polish removers and hair products)
Detergents
Drain and toilet cleaners
Fertilizers
Furniture polish
Gasoline
Kerosene
Lighter fluid
Lye
Medicines
Paints
Paint removers and thinners
Pesticides
Plants, indoor and outdoor
Rat poisons
Weed killers

Store all cleaning products, insecticides, and medicines *in their original containers* in places where your child can't reach them.

Keep medicines in child-resistant packaging. Check to be sure grandparents and baby-sitters also buy their medicines in child-proof containers. Never refer to any medicine as candy.

If a child accidentally swallows a poisonous substance, seconds count. Keep the phone number of your local poison-control center (PCC) near your phone. (There is also a place in the back of this book to write in the PCC numbers and other emergency phone numbers. Use it as a backup to the list you keep by your phone.)

PCCs are staffed by medical professionals who can help you quickly. If you suspect your child has ingested something poisonous, find out immediately what was swallowed, when, and how much. Be ready to give this information to the PCC. Always call first, before taking action, as different substances require different treatment.

The PCC may instruct you to induce vomiting by giving your child syrup of ipecac. (You should have this ready in your first-aid kit, but do not administer ipecac unless told to do so by a poison expert.) Afterward, you may be instructed to give your child an activated-charcoal tablet, which will counteract the remaining poison in the body.

However, not every situation benefits from vomiting. If a child is unconscious, is having a seizure, or has ingested any corrosive or petroleum substance (acid, alkali, gasoline) or is known to have a heart condition, the PCC will give you special instructions.

Take your child (and the poison he swallowed) to the telephone when you call for help, so you will be ready to describe the poison and your child's condition when you are given instructions.

FOOD POISONING

Ninety percent of all food poisoning is the result of undercooked meat, fish, and eggs. Dangerous salmonella bacteria can be killed only by thorough cooking.

Ground beef should be cooked until it is well done inside and out. Chicken juices should not be pink. Pork should have absolutely no pink in it when it is eaten. Soft-boiled eggs can contain salmonella, as can anything with raw eggs—even cookie dough, which in the past we all loved to sample from the bowl.

In addition to thorough cooking, the way you handle and prepare food can also prevent food poisoning. For example, after cutting raw chicken or meat, wash the cutting surface and knife in warm soapy water before using for other foods.

Your sense of smell is your first defense against food poison. If food smells bad, throw it out. However, not every contaminated food smells bad. Other precautions are also important:

Refrigerate anything made with mayonnaise, which contains raw eggs. Thaw frozen foods in the refrigerator. Once food is completely thawed, use within two to three days. Use fish within three days of purchase, and always refrigerate.

Don't buy food in dented or swollen cans; they may contain botulism.

Symptoms of food poisoning. Symptoms are similar to flu or viral infection and include severe diarrhea, nausea, and vomiting, usually two to three hours after ingesting contaminated food. If symptoms do not subside within twenty-four hours, call a doctor.

TEENAGERS AND SAFETY

Accidents are the number-one cause of death in adolescents, and the single-most-important category is that of motor vehicle crashes. Drinking is usually involved. Many community organizations are working to reduce the accident rate among teens.

Homicide and suicide are also high. African-American teens have a greater risk of dying in a homicide; white teens have a higher risk of suicide. But both homicide and suicide occur among both groups.

Read chapters 19 and 22 carefully. Think about getting involved in community activities aimed at risk prevention. If your teen is drinking, using drugs, or appears depressed, seek professional help. Resources on pages 398–416 provide names and addresses of mental-health organizations and community-empowerment organizations.

34

FIRST AID

BROKEN BONES

The nature of the injury can help you determine whether a bone is broken. For example, a car accident is more likely to produce bone fractures than simple roughhousing. If you suspect your child has broken a bone, apply ice to the site immediately to minimize swelling. Keep the limb still by immobilizing the joint above and below the suspected break. You can use cardboard or newspapers to stabilize the limb, but don't move your child. Be careful not to wrap the limb too tightly, thereby cutting off circulation. Call the doctor.

Go to the emergency room or doctor's office immediately if:

- The skin is punctured and bone is sticking out.
- The limb appears unnaturally bent or crooked.
- The limb is cold, blue, or numb.
- Your child is in so much pain that he cannot or will not use the limb.
- The injury is to the pelvis or thighs. It's almost impossible to detect fractures in these areas.
- Your child appears to be in shock (pale, sweating, dizzy, and thirsty).

The doctor will x-ray the injury. Fractured bones will have to be properly set and placed in a cast; injuries to joints may be held together with surgical pins.

BURNS

Burns can be first-, second-, or third-degree, escalating in severity as the numbers rise. First-degree burns are akin to mild sunburn. Though painful, they rarely require medical attention. Second-degree burns split the skin, creating blisters and causing fluid loss.

To treat first- and second-degree burns, immediately apply an ice bag, a cloth soaked in ice water, or a cloth containing ice. If the burn is on the hand, plunge it in and out of a bowl of ice water several times. Keep up the treatment for from five minutes to one hour (depending on the severity of the burn)—long enough to lessen the pain but not to cause numbness.

Do not break blisters or disturb blisters that break on their own. Don't use Vaseline or butter! Do not use anesthetic or antibiotic creams or sprays, unless your doctor makes a specific recommendation.

You can give children acetaminophen for the pain.

If a second-degree burn is larger than the palm of your hand, if it occurs on your child's face or hands, and if pain persists after forty-eight hours, take your child to the doctor.

Third-degree burns require immediate medical intervention, no matter what. These burns damage every layer of skin and can harm deeper tissues, as well. They are prone to infection, cause fluid loss, and create pronounced scars. The doctor may prescribe antibiotics to guard against infection. Very severe burns may require skin grafts.

BEE STINGS AND INSECT BITES

Most stings and bites are trivial, but they can be painful on tender young skin. Apply a cold pack or a few ice cubes wrapped in a washcloth to the spot, which will prevent swelling. Applying a tea bag soaked in cold water directly to the skin will also work wonders to relieve swelling.

Occasionally, insect stings and bites cause more severe, widespread reactions. Wheezing, difficulty breathing (asthma), hives or skin rashes, or fainting following a bite or sting indicate a severe allergic reaction. Call the doctor immediately. Antihistamines can help somewhat, but in the case of severe allergic reaction, injections may be required. Once an allergic reaction has occurred in response to an insect bite or sting, it is likely to recur if the child is bitten or stung again.

Abdominal pain, nausea, vomiting, headaches, and shaking are signs that a child may have been bitten by a poisonous spider. These are rare events, and most are traced to the female black widow. Call the doctor immediately.

TICK BITES

In some localities, ticks may carry Rocky Mountain spotted fever or Lyme disease. Ticks bites are usually easy to see because the insect buries its head and pincers in the skin, but the body and legs stick out. It stays there until you remove it, or it simply lets go or "festers" out.

The idea is to get the tick to relax its pincers before removal so you can remove the whole body at once. Heat causes the tick to wiggle its legs and begin to withdraw. Try applying a warm paper clip or warm oil to the bump. Grasp the tick with your fingers or a tissue and remove it quickly with a twisting motion. If the whole body and head doesn't come out, soak the skin gently with warm water twice a day until the bite heals itself. If your child develops symptoms—fever, rash, red or swollen eyes, or headache—within three weeks of a tick bite, call the doctor.

CAT AND DOG BITES AND SCRATCHES

The main concern from pet bites and scratches is infection. Teeth and/or claw wounds often go deep and immediately seal over (puncture wounds), trapping bacteria inside; infection can travel quickly through the bloodstream. It's almost impossible to wash out the wound successfully. Puncture wounds are serious, particularly cat punctures on the hand, and require prompt medical attention. First, wash the area with liquid soap and running water for ten minutes to flush out the wound; then take your child to your physician's office or the emergency room.

Because tetanus bacteria can be introduced by an animal bite, most doctors give a tetanus shot if a child has not had an inoculation within the recommended time period.

Dog and cat scratches that don't penetrate the skin can be

washed with lots of water and liquid soap for five minutes. Leave the scratch exposed to air, unless it's in a spot that can easily get dirty. If the area begins to look infected or if the pain and redness increases after the second day, call your child's physician.

Generally, minor wounds from other indoor pets such as gerbils, hamsters, guinea pigs, and white mice can be treated in the same way.

Rabies. Humans seldom contract rabies, but the incidence is rising. Rabies almost always comes from wild animals, particularly squirrels, mice, skunks, foxes, bats, raccoons, and possums. If your child is bitten by a wild animal, try to get your child to tell you if the animal attacked without provocation or behaved in an otherwise strange manner—such as a nighttime animal (raccoon) appearing in the daylight. A rabid animal may also foam at the mouth. Take your child to the doctor, and ask your child to repeat the description. If you saw the animal yourself, give the doctor a careful report.

The doctor won't want to give your child a series of rabies shots unless absolutely necessary. Rabies vaccine must be administered in five injections over twenty-eight days. The vaccine can cause skin reactions, as well as fever, chills, aches, and pains. However, reactions are uncommon in children.

YOUR HOME FIRST-AID KIT

Every home with children needs a first-aid kit that is always handy and always in order. It should include the following products, which are available at your local drugstore:

- *Ipecac syrup*
- *Activated charcoal*
- *Band-Aids of varying sizes*
- *Gauze*
- *Antiseptic solution (hydrogen peroxide)*
- *Citrate of magnesia*
- *Antibiotic cream/ointment (Neosporin). (Do not keep or use red-colored antiseptics such as Mercurochrome or methiolate.)*
- *Antibacterial cleaner (Phisoderm, or even Safeguard, Dial, or Lever 2000)*

EMERGENCY ALERT

Call a doctor immediately if your baby or child has trouble breathing. Labored breathing that involves a grunting sound with every breath means your baby could be in serious trouble.

If your child is bitten or scratched by someone else's pet, ask the owners if the animal has been immunized against rabies; also ask them to observe their pet for the next two weeks to make sure it shows no sign of rabies infection.

One of the most important early skills parents should teach young children is how to behave around animals. This is particularly true—and most likely to be overlooked—when you have no pets of your own around the house. Even the most tolerant house pet can lose its composure and flash a claw or a tooth when confronted with a gleeful toddler trying to hold and squeeze it. The animal who scratches or bites in these circumstances isn't mean; it's simply terrified.

Teach your child to treat domestic pets with respect and gentleness, *never* to try to pick up a cat or dog, and never to scream at it, bang on it, or pull its hair. Children do not realize that animals are not toys unless you teach them that. Teach your child not to go near a dog that's eating and never to try to take away a bone or other food from a dog's mouth. Always ask people the child knows whether it is okay to pet their animal. Also, show your child how to extend a hand, never approaching a pet from above its head. Children under five or six years old should never be left alone around dogs or cats.

If you have pets, make sure they are well trained, too. Animals trained to attack do not belong in the same house, or even the same neighborhood, with children. Teach your child not to touch strange animals, strays, or wild animals of any kind—not even to reach out with a friendly pat.

HUMAN BITES

Human bites are more likely than any other animal bite to become infected. If your child receives a bite from another child during play or roughhousing, wash the wound thoroughly with soap and running water; then take your child to the doctor or the emergency room. If the bite is a superficial scrape, wash the area with lots of soap and water for at least five minutes and leave it exposed to the air. If the wound starts to look infected, or if pain increases after the second day, take your child to the doctor.

CUTS

Clean cuts with soap and water or 3 percent solution of hydrogen peroxide. Apply a butterfly bandage or strips of sterile paper tape to pull the edges of the cut together and speed healing.

A wound that won't close may require stitches; this should occur within eight hours in order to prevent infection.

Injuries to the face, chest, stomach, and back are potentially the most serious, so have a doctor look at these wounds unless they are extremely small or shallow.

Call or see the doctor immediately if:

- Your child feels numbness, bleeds uncontrollably, or feels tingling and weakness near the cut.
- You suspect a major blood vessel or nerve has been cut.
- Fever, pus, or extensive redness and swelling is present.

SCRAPES

Scrapes may look terrifying, but most are shallow and not nearly as serious as they appear. However, they usually hurt a lot more than cuts because so many nerve endings are damaged.

Clean the scrape thoroughly. Then apply an ice pack to the wound to lessen pain, or try giving your child acetaminophen. The scab that forms over the scrape will provide a natural protection to the area. Try to keep your child from picking at it.

Call the doctor if:

- Foreign matter is stuck in the wound and you are unable to remove it.
- You notice signs of infection such as pus, a lump, or a bad odor.

EMERGENCY PHONE NUMBERS

Keep these numbers by your telephone.

> *Life-threatening emergencies: 911*
>
> *Non-life-threatening emergencies: Call your child's physician or the nearest emergency room.*
>
> *Doctor:*
>
> *Hospital Emergency Room:*
>
> *Poison-Control Center:*
>
> *Fire Department:*
>
> *Police:*
>
> *Gas Emergency:*
>
> *Electric or Steam Emergency:*
>
> *Crime Victims Hot Line:*
>
> *Missing Child Hot Line:*
>
> *Child Abuse Hot Line:*

With recent budget cutbacks at the city, state, and federal levels many child health and nutrition agencies are in the process of reducing and sometimes eliminating services.

You will find the most current listings of available child health information and services to the public in your telephone book. Local help lines are listed in the White Pages (first few pages); Yellow Pages (under "Social and Human Services Organizations"); Blue Pages (under city, state, and federal health departments).

PUBLICATIONS

The National Center for Education in Maternal and Child Health distributes a wide variety of books and pamphlets on maternal, child, and adolescent nutrition and health. You can call or write the following for the full catalog of publications.

American Dietetic Association
216 West Jackson Boulevard, Suite 800
Chicago, IL 60606-6995
(800) 877-1600
(312) 899-0040

Food and Drug Administration
Office of Consumer Affairs
5600 Fishers Lane (HFE-88)
Rockville, MD 20857
(301) 443-3070

National Maternal and Child Health Clearinghouse
8201 Greensboro Drive, Suite 600
McLean, VA 22102
(703) 821-8955, ext. 254 or 265
Fax: (703) 821-2098

USDA Human Nutrition Information Service
6505 Belcrest Road
Hyattsville, MD 20782
(301) 436-8498

HELP FOR SPECIFIC PROBLEMS

AIDS

Many local African-American organizations and churches around the country offer help and information to AIDS patients. The AIDS Project at Glide Memorial Church in San Francisco is one of the oldest and best-known help groups in the country. Almost every local chapter of the Urban League also offers some kind of AIDS program.

Many other African-American organizations, such as People of Color Against AIDS Network in Seattle, have been created especially to serve AIDS patients. Others focus on all minorities. The Multicultural AIDS Coalition (United South End Settlement) in Boston and the Minority AIDS Project in Los Angeles are examples.

You will find these and many more AIDS help groups listed in the Yellow Pages under "AIDS—Testing and Counseling Services."

On the national level, the following institutions provide important HIV/AIDS information to everyone.

The AIDS Clinical Trials Information Service
(800) TRIALS-A
> Information on federally funded clinical trials for patients with AIDS or HIV, including eligibility requirements and locations of study centers.

AMFAR
American Foundation for AIDS Research
Box AIDS, Dept. P
New York, NY 10016
(800) 521-8110
> AMFAR publishes a compendium called *Learning AIDS,* which reviews seventeen hundred books, pamphlets, videotapes, and other educational materials available to the public— $24.95 (softcover).

The CDC National AIDS Clearinghouse
PO Box 6003
Rockville, MD 20849-6003
(800) 458-5231
(301) 217-0023
Fax: (301) 738-6616
> Free educational materials on HIV and AIDS; names,
> addresses, and phone numbers of local African-American
> organizations working with AIDS.

Centers for Disease Control and Prevention
CDC National AIDS Hot Line
(800) 342-2437
(800) 344-7432 (Spanish-speaking)
> Free national hot line for anyone with questions about AIDS.
> Confidential and anonymous referrals to local health organiza-
> tions, counselors, and support groups. Open twenty-four
> hours a day.

Gay Men's Health Crisis (GMHC)
Pediatrics Program
129 West 20th Street
New York, NY 10001
Hot Line: (212) 807-6655
Hot Line-TDD (hearing-impaired): (212) 645-7470

National Pediatric HIV Resource Center
15 South 9th Street
Newark, NJ 07107
(800) 362-0071
(201) 268-8251

ALCOHOL AND DRUGS

Treatment Programs

RADAR—The Regional Alcohol and Drug Awareness Resources is
a network of state information centers. The RADAR office in your
state should be able to get a list of all the treatment and counseling
programs available in your area. You can also call your local health
department for information, or the state Office of Minority Health.

Al-Anon/Alateen Family Group Headquarters, Inc.
PO Box 862
Midtown Station
New York, NY 10018-0862
(800) 356-9996 or 344-2666
(212) 302-7240

Alcoholics Anonymous
PO Box 459
Grand Central Station
New York, NY 10163
(800) 344-2666
(212) 870-3400
AA has special meetings for teenagers.

Cocaine Anonymous (CA)
6125 Washington Boulevard, Suite 202
Los Angeles, CA 90230
Hot Line: 1-800-COCAINE (262-2463)

Cocaine Baby Help Line
(800) 638-2229

Narcotics Anonymous (NA)
World Service Office
PO Box 9999
Van Nuys, CA 91409-9999
(818) 780-3951
     NA has special meetings for teens—(800) 662-4357 for a
     referral in your area.

Northeast Drug/Alcohol Referral Station
1809 N. Broadway, Suite C
Wichita, KS 67214
(316) 265-8511

Partnership for a Drug-Free America
National Help Line: (800) 662-HELP (4357)

     For a free copy of *A Parent's Guide to Prevention,* call (800)
     624-0100.

Information and Publications

The U.S. Department of Health and Human Services offers a variety of publications for parents and children concerning the prevention of alcohol and drug abuse. Write or call:

ACTION
Drug Prevention Program
1100 Vernon Avenue, NW, Suite 8200
Washington, DC 20525
(202) 634-9759

National Association of Alcoholism and Drug Abuse Counselors
3717 Columbia Pike, Suite 300
Arlington, VA 22204
(703) 920-4644

National Clearinghouse for Alcohol and Drug Information
PO Box 2345
Rockville, MD 20852
(800) 729-6686
(301) 468-2600

National Council on Alcoholism
12 West 21st Street
New York, NY 10010
(212) 206-6770

National Institute on Alcoholism and Drug Abuse (NIDA)
5600 Fishers Lane
Rockville, MD 20857
(800) 662-4357
(301) 443-4373

National Urban League, Inc. (Yellow Pages for local listings)
500 East 62nd Street
New York, NY 10021
(212) 310-9000

Office of Minority Health Resource Center
PO Box 37337
Washington, DC 20013-7337
(800) 444-6472

ASTHMA AND ALLERGIES

American Academy of Allergy and Immunology
611 East Wells Street
Milwaukee, WI 53202
(800) 822-ASMA (2762)

American Lung Association (White Pages for local listings)
1740 Broadway
New York, NY 10019-4374
(800) LUNG-USA (5864-872)
    The American Lung Association publishes a pamphlet called
    Let's Talk About Asthma: A Guide for Teens. For a free copy, con-
    tact your local chapter, or call (800) LUNG-USA.

Asthma and Allergy Foundation of America
1717 Massachusetts Avenue, NW, Suite 305
Washington, DC 20036
(202) 385-4403

Asthma Today (newsletter)
412 State Street
Bangor, ME 04401

Mothers of Asthmatics, Inc.
10875 Main Street, Suite 210
Fairfax, VA 22030
(703) 385-4403

DENTAL CARE

Look for child dental clinics in the Blue Pages under city and/or
state health departments. (Professional associations are listed under
"Community Empowerment" on pages 405–407.)

DIABETES

American Diabetes Association
Diabetes Information Service Center
1660 Duke Street
Alexandria, VA 22314
(800) ADA-DISC (232-3472)
(703) 549-1500

American Dietetic Association
216 West Jackson Boulevard, Suite 700
Chicago, IL 60606
(312) 899-0040

Juvenile Diabetes Foundation
432 Park Avenue South, Sixteenth Floor
New York, NY 10016
(212) 889-7575

National Diabetes Information Clearinghouse
Box NDIC
9000 Rockville Pike
Bethesda, MD 20892
(301) 468-2162

EATING DISORDERS

American Anorexia/Bulimia Association
418 East 76th Street
New York, NY 10021
(212) 734-1114

National Anorectic Aid Society
1925 East Dublin Granville Road
Columbus, OH 43229
(614) 436-1112

National Association of Anorexia Nervosa and Associated
Disorders (ANAD)
PO Box 7
Highland Park, IL 60035
(708) 831-3438

National Food Addiction Hot Line
(800) 872-0088

FITNESS

National 4-H Council
Public Affairs, Fitness Leadership Program
7100 Connecticut Avenue
Chevy Chase, MD 20815
(301) 961-2800

President's Council on Physical Fitness and Sports
Market Square East Building, Suite 250
701 Pennsylvania Avenue, NW
Washington, DC 20004
(202) 272-3430
Fax: (202) 504-2064

HEALTH CARE/PEDIATRIC PHYSICIANS

To locate child health clinics in your area, look in the Blue Pages of
your telephone book under city and state health department
services.

Various child and youth organizations also offer assistance and
information about health-care options in local communities. For
example, the local Boys' Club and Girls' Club often have health
programs (check your White Pages). Their national headquarters are
in New York City (212) 351-5900.

In addition, the following organizations can supply the names of
physicians who treat children in your area:

American Academy of Family Physicians
Committee on Minority Health Affairs
8880 Ward Parkway
Kansas City, MO 64114-2797
(800) 274-2237
> Provides voluntary information on race and ethnicity of
> members so they may be identified as advocates and role
> models.

American Academy of Pediatrics
141 Northwest Point Boulevard
PO Box 927
Elk Grove Village, IL 60009-0927
(708) 981-7384

Black Women's Physicians Project
3300 Henry Avenue
Philadelphia, PA 19129
(215) 842-7124

National Medical Association (professional association for
    African-American doctors)
1012 Tenth Street, NW
Washington, DC 20001
(202) 347-1895

HEALTH STATISTICS

Centers for Disease Control and Prevention
Office of Public Inquiry
1600 Clifton Road, NE
Atlanta, GA 30333
(404) 639-3534
Fax: (404) 639-1623

Children's Defense Fund
122 C Street, NW
Washington, DC 20001
(202) 628-8787

National Health Information Center (ONHIC)
PO Box 1133
Washington, DC 20013-1133
(No telephone number listed.)

HEART DISEASE

American Heart Association
National Center
7272 Greenville Avenue
Dallas, TX 75231
(214) 373-6300

American Heart Association Schoolsite Programs
7272 Greenville Avenue
Dallas, TX 75231
(214) 373-6300

National Cholesterol Education Program
NHLBI Information Center
PO Box 30105
Bethesda, MD 20824-0105
(301) 251-1222

National Heart, Lung, and Blood Institute
Education Programs Information Center
PO Box 30105
Bethesda, MD 20814-0105
(301) 251-1222

HERBALISTS

Herbalists use natural plants or plant-based substances to treat illnesses and to promote optimal health. They often use iridology (examining the iris of the eye) as a diagnostic tool.

American Herbalism Guild
PO Box 1683
Soquel, CA 95073
(408) 464-2241

The Herb Research Foundation
1007 Pearl Street, Suite 200
Boulder, CO 80302
(303) 449-2265

HOLISTIC AND HOMEOPATHIC PRACTITIONERS

Holistic health treatments seek to strengthen the connection between body and mind. Homeopathic practitioners may combine traditional medicine with alternative approaches to health, including acupuncture, ethnic diets, and herbs.

The American Holistic Medical Association
4101 Lake Boone Trail, Suite 201
Raleigh, NC 27606
(919) 787-5181

National Center for Homeopathy
801 N. Fairfax Street, Suite 306
Alexandria, VA 22314
(703) 548-7790

HYPERTENSION

National High Blood Pressure Education Program
Information Center
PO Box 30105
Bethesda, MD 20814-0105
(301) 251-1222

INFANT HEALTH AND NUTRITION

WIC (Women's, Infants', and Children's Supplement Nutrition Program): For WIC programs, look in the Blue Pages of your phone book under city and/or state health departments.

LaLeche League International
PO Box 1209
Franklin Park, IL 60131-8209
(708) 455-8317

National Association of Pediatric Nurse Associates and
    Practitioners
1101 Kings Highway North, Suite 206
Cherry Hill, NJ 08034
(609) 667-1773

The Organization for Obstetric, Gynecologic, and Neonatal
    Nurses
409 12th Street, SW
Washington, DC 20024-2191
(No telephone number given.)
    Consumer education brochures on questions to ask when
    your baby is in a special-care nursery.

LEAD EXPOSURE

Environmental Protection Agency
Public Information Center
401 M Street, SW
Mail Code PM 3404
Washington, DC 20460

Lead Hot Line: (800) 424–LEAD (5323)
  Will mail information about the dangers of lead and how to
  remove it safely.

Learning Disabilities Association of America
3115 North 17th Street
Arlington, VA 22201
(703) 243-2614

New York Public Interest Research Group Publications
9 Murray Street, Third Floor
New York, NY 10007-2272
(212) 349-6460
  Distributes *Get the Lead Out,* a fifty-four-page handbook for
  preventing lead poisoning—$7 each.

Safe Drinking Water Hot Line:
(800) 426-4791

Toxic Substance Control Act
Assistance Information Service Hot Line
East Tower, Garage Level
401 M Street, SW
Washington, DC 20024
(202) 554-1404
Fax: (202) 554-5603

MENTAL HEALTH

Association of Black Psychologists
PO Box 55999
Washington, DC 20040-5999
or
821 Kennedy Street, NW
Washington, DC 20011
(202) 722-0808

Learning Disabilities Association of America
3115 North 17th Street
Arlington, VA 22201
(703) 243-2614

National Clearinghouse on Child Abuse and Neglect and Family
   Violence Information
3998 Fairridge Drive, Suite 350
Fairfax, VA 22033
(800) 394-3366
(703) 385-7565
Fax: (703) 385-3206

National 4-H Council
Cooperative Extension System
7100 Connecticut Avenue
Chevy Chase, MD 20815
(301) 961-2800

National Institute of Mental Health
Depression Awareness/Treatment Program
5600 Fishers Lane, Room 10A-85
Rockville, MD 20857
(800) 421-4211 (free brochures on depression)
(301) 443-4140 (information)

National Institute of Mental Health
Public Information
Parklawn Building, Room 7C-02
5600 Fishers Lane
Rockville, MD 20857
(301) 443-4513 (many publications on mental health)

NUTRITION

American Dietetic Association
216 West Jackson Boulevard, Suite 700
Chicago, IL 60606
(312) 899-0040

Food and Nutrition Information Center
National Agricultural Library, Room 304
10301 Baltimore Boulevard
Beltsville, MD 20705-2351
(301) 504-5719

National 4-H Council
Expanded Food and Nutrition Education Program
7100 Connecticut Avenue
Chevy Chase, MD 20815
(301) 961-2800

National Health Information Center
PO Box 1133
Washington, DC 20013-1133
(800) 336-4797

PREGNANCY AND CHILDBIRTH

African-American Women for Wellness
PO Box 52378
St. Louis, MO 63136
(314) 385-2784

American College of Nurse Midwives
1522 K Street, NW, Suite 1000
Washington, DC 20005
(202) 728-9860

Maternity Center Association
48 East 92nd Street
New York, NY 10128
(212) 369-7300
> Promotes safe and affordable family-centered maternity care.
> Operates an out-of-hospital birth center and publishes educa-
> tional material used by parents and professionals in fifty states
> and eighty-two countries.

National Association of Childbearing Centers
3123 Gottschall Road
Perkiomenville, PA 18074-9546
(215) 234-8068
Fax: (215) 234-0564

National Black Women's Health Project
1237 Abernathy Boulevard, SW
Atlanta, GA 30310
(404) 758-9590

National Dairy Council (publication: *Great Beginnings*)
6300 North River Road
Rosemont, IL 60018-4289
(708) 696-1020

National Maternal and Child Health Clearinghouse
8201 Greensboro Drive, Suite 600
McLean, VA 22102
(703) 821-8955, ext. 254 or 255
Fax: (703) 821-2098

The Organization for Obstetric, Gynecologic, and Neonatal
  Nurses
409 12th Street, SW
Washington, DC 20024-2191
(No telephone number given.)
  Offers brochures on planning for pregnancy prior to
  conception.

Planned Parenthood Federation of America
810 Seventh Avenue
New York, NY 10019
(800) 230-PLAN (7526)
(212) 603-4600
  Planned Parenthood publishes a variety of reliable books and
  pamphlets for parents on teenage sexuality, reproductive
  health, pregnancy nutrition, contraception, AIDS, and STDs.
  Write or call for their catalog of publications. They also have
  many clinics serving women. Call the 800 number for
  appointments.

Women's Health Network
1325 G Street, NW
Washington, DC 20005
(202) 347-1140

SAFETY

Mothers Against Drunk Driving (MADD)
511 East John Carpenter Freeway, Suite 700
Irving, TX 75062
(800) 438-6233
> MADD has developed community, youth, and public affairs
> and volunteer programs offering victim services in an all-out
> effort to reduce the numbers of drunk drivers, including teens,
> on the street. Drunk drivers kill some 22,000 people each year.

Students Against Drunk Driving (SADD)
PO Box 800
Marlboro, MA 01752
(508) 481-3568

SEX EDUCATION

Family Planning Publications
Seattle-King County Department of Public Health
110 Prefontaine Avenue South, Suite 300
Seattle, WA 98104
(206) 296-4672

Planned Parenthood Federation of America
810 Seventh Avenue
New York, NY 10019
(800) 230-PLAN (7526)
(212) 603-4600

SICKLE-CELL DISEASE

National Association for Sickle Cell Disease, Inc.
3345 Wilshire Boulevard, Suite 1106
Los Angeles, CA 90010-1880
(800) 421-8453
(213) 736-5445

National Center for Education in Maternal and Child Health
38th and R Streets, NW
Washington, DC 20057
(202) 625-8400

Sickle-Cell Disease
AHCPR Publications Clearinghouse
PO Box 8547
Silver Spring, MD 20907
(800) 358-9295

Sickle-Cell Disease Branch
National Heart, Lung, and Blood Institute
Federal Building
7550 Wisconsin Avenue
Bethesda, MD 20205
(301) 251-1222

Sickle-Cell Treatment Centers

Ten regional comprehensive sickle-cell centers have been established to conduct basic and clinical research, as well as to provide educational information and testing.

Boston City Hospital
818 Harrison Avenue
Boston, MA 02118
(617) 424-5727

Children's Hospital Medical Center
Elland and Bethesda Avenues
Cincinnati, OH 45229
(513) 559-4534

Children's Hospital of Michigan
3901 Beaubien Boulevard
Detroit, MI 48201
(313) 494-5611

Howard University
2121 Georgia Avenue, NW
Washington, DC 20059
(202) 636-7930

Medical College of Georgia
1435 Lancy Walker Boulevard
Augusta, GA 30912
(404) 828-3091

St. Luke's Hospital Center
419 West 114th Street, Room 403
New York, NY 10025
(212) 870-1756

San Francisco General Hospital
1001 Potrero Avenue
San Francisco, CA 94110
(415) 821-5169

University of Chicago
950 East 59th Street
Chicago, IL 60637
(312) 947-5501

University of Illinois
1959 West Taylor Street
Chicago, IL 60612
(312) 996-7013

University of Southern California
1129 North State Street, Trailer 12
Los Angeles, CA 90033
(213) 226-3853

SMOKING

American Cancer Society
   See Yellow Pages for local listings.

American Lung Association
1740 Broadway
New York, NY 10019-4374
(800) LUNG-USA (5864-872)

Stop Teenage Addiction to Tobacco (STAT)
PO Box 60658
Longmeadow, MA 01116
(413) 567-2070

SUDDEN INFANT DEATH SYNDROME

National SIDS Alliance
6065 Roswell Road, Suite 876
Atlanta, GA 30328
(800) 232-7437
(800) 847-7437 (in Georgia)

National SIDS Resource Center
8201 Greensboro Drive, Suite 600
McLean, VA 22102-3810
(703) 821-8955 or -2098

Southwest SIDS Research Institute
Brazosport Memorial Hospital
100 Medical Drive
Lake Jackson, TX 77566
(800) 245-7437

Sudden Infant Death Syndrome Alliance
10500 Little Patuxent Parkway, Suite 420
Columbia, MD 21044
(800) 221-7437

COMMUNITY EMPOWERMENT PROFESSIONAL ASSOCIATIONS AND INSTITUTIONS

With cutbacks in government funding of health-care projects, community empowerment daily becomes more urgent. Many private professional associations and several federal institutions continue to provide educational workshops and conferences and to print information to support community action. If you are already involved, or if you or your club or organization wishes to develop a new program in your community, here are some people who can help you.

GENERAL RESOURCES

Advocacy Institute
1730 Rhode Island Avenue, NW, Suite 600
Washington, DC 20036
(202) 659-8475

> The Advocacy Institute teaches low-cost, high-impact lobbying and public relations techniques to nonprofit grassroots organizations. You can also write for publications on developing strategies and publicizing your community's efforts.

Center for Science in the Public Interest
1875 Connecticut Avenue, NW
Washington, DC 20009-5728
(202) 332-9110

> CSPI is a nonprofit independent consumer advocacy group specializing in health issues. They offer several handbooks providing strategies to challenge companies marketing and advertising alcohol and tobacco in our communities.

Join Together
441 Stuart Street, Sixth Floor
Boston, MA 02116
(617) 437-1500

> Join Together is a national program to help communities fight substance abuse. Join Together offers a national computer network to share information and ideas; a communication and technical assistance program to help coalitions develop and implement strategies; and a National Fellows Program to train community leaders.

Special Minority Health Agencies

Twenty-eight states have established official minority health entities (such as an office, commission, council, center, branch, project, or other unit). Other states may designate minority health contacts for various purposes. Look in the Blue Pages under "State Government Offices, Health Department."

Here are the names and addresses of major agencies dedicated to improving the health of all children, with special attention to African Americans.

Child and Adolescent Branch
Maternal and Child Health Bureau
U.S. Department of Health and Human Services
Parklawn Building, Room 6-37
5600 Fishers Lane
Rockville, MD 20857
(301) 443-6600

Children's Defense Fund
122 C Street, NW
Washington, DC 20001
(202) 628-8787
> CDF is a nonprofit research and advocacy organization that works to provide a strong and effective voice for all American children. They promote child health, child care and development, child welfare, teen pregnancy prevention, and many other topics related to the welfare of children.

National Health Information Center (ONHIC)
PO Box 1133
Washington, DC 20013-1133
(800) 336-4797

National Minority Health Association
PO Box 11876
Harrisburg, PA 17108-1876
(717) 761-1323

Office of Minority Health Resource Center
PO Box 37337
Washington, DC 20013-7337
(800) 444-6472,
(301) 587-1938

CHILDREN'S HEALTH ISSUES

AIDS

CDC National AIDS Clearinghouse
PO Box 6003
Rockville, MD 20850-6003
(800) 458-5231/(301) 217-0023
Fax: (301) 738-6616

ALCOHOL AND DRUGS

Center for Substance Abuse Prevention
820 First Street, NE, Suite 510
Washington, DC 20002
(800) 937-6727
(202) 408-5556

Institute on Black Chemical Abuse
2616 Nicollet Avenue South
Minneapolis, MN 55408
(612) 871-7878

> The Institute on Black Chemical Abuse will provide guide-
> lines for starting community-based alcohol and drug abuse
> prevention strategies and show you or your organization how
> to get involved.

The Links, Inc.
National Headquarters
1522 K Street, NW
Washington, DC 20005
(202) 783-3888

> Two hundred local chapters are working to prevent and treat
> substance abuse among black youth. The Services to Youth
> division will provide their expertise and time to help commu-
> nities develop alcohol-abuse programs.

National Black Alcoholism Council
School of Social Welfare
Health Sciences Center, Level 2, Room 093
State University of New York
Stonybrook, NY 11794
(No telephone number given.)

> NBAC's one thousand members and twenty chapters
> throughout the United States work to raise the consciousness
> of the black community about the impact of alcoholism. It
> publishes a semiannual newsletter, sponsors workshops and
> conferences, and supervises a national speakers' bureau.

National Clearinghouse for Alcohol and Drug Information
PO Box 2345
Rockville, MD 20847-2345
(800) 729-6686
(301) 468-2600

> NCADI is the information service for the Center for Substance Abuse Prevention. It offers extensive resources, bibliographies, free computer searches, treatment referral, alcohol- and drug-education materials, and prevention and education services.

National Council on Alcoholism and Other Drug Dependencies
12 West 21st Street, Seventh Floor
New York, NY 10010
(212) 206-6770

> A voluntary health agency with over two hundred state and local affiliates, whose purposes include promoting effective and accessible prevention and treatment programs and representing local programs before government groups. Publishes and distributes an extensive collection of books and pamphlets on alcohol-related topics, including materials for African Americans and other minorities.

National Federation of Parents for Drug-Free Youth
1820 Franwell Avenue, Suite 16
Silver Spring, MD 20902
Help Line for Parents: (800) 554-5437
(301) 649-7100

> This is a national network of parents working to combat drug and alcohol abuse in their communities. The federation publishes newsletters and brochures for parents and children, as well as manuals for organizers and speakers.

Drug-Free Schools

The following regional centers assist schools and communities to develop alcohol- and drug-prevention and early-intervention programs.

Midwest Regional Center
1900 Spring Road
Oak Brook, IL 60521
(708) 571-4710

Northeast Regional Center
12 Overton Avenue
Sayville, NY 11782
(516) 589-7022

Southeast Regional Center
Spencerian Office Plaza
University of Louisville
Louisville, KY 40292
(502) 588-0052

Southwest Regional Center
University of Oklahoma
555 Constitution, Suite 138
Norman, OK 73037-0005
(800) 234-7972

Western Regional Center
101 SW Main Street, Suite 500
Portland, OR 97204
(503) 275-9480

Asthma and Allergies

National Institute for Allergy and Infectious Diseases
Building 31, Room 7A32
9000 Rockville Pike
Bethesda, MD 20892
(301) 496-5717
Fax: (301) 402-0120

Dental Care

American Academy of Pediatric Dentistry (AAPD)
211 East Chicago Avenue
Chicago, IL 60611
(312) 337-2169

Healthy Mothers, Healthy Babies Coalition
409 12th Street, SW
Washington, DC 20024-2188
(202) 863-2458

Provides educational material on dental care and access. This is
an informal association of more than 104 national and 100
state and local professional, voluntary, and governmental health
organizations, including several professional dental associations.

National Dental Association
5506 Connecticut Avenue, NW, Suite 24-25
Washington, DC 20015
(202) 244-7555

National Institute of Dental Research
Public Information Office
Building 31, Room 2C35
9000 Rockville Pike
Bethesda, MD 20892
(301) 496-4261
Fax: (301) 496-9988

Infant Nutrition

WIC (Women's, Infants', and Children's Supplement Nutrition
Program): To locate WIC programs in your area, look in the Blue
Pages of your phone book under city and state health departments.

LaLeche League International
PO Box 1209
Franklin Park, IL 60131-8209
(708) 455-8317

Lead Hazards

American Board of Industrial Hygiene
(517) 321-2638
     Will verify if a contractor is licensed for lead paint removal.

National Center for Lead-Safe Housing
(410) 992-0712
     Distributes HUD guidelines.

New York Public Interest Research Group Publications
9 Murray Street, Third Floor
New York, NY 10007-2272
(212) 349-6460
> Distributes *Get the Lead Out,* a fifty-four-page handbook for
> preventing lead poisoning—$7 each.

Toxic Substance Control Act
Assistance Information Service Hot Line
East Tower, Garage Level
401 M Street, SW
Washington, DC 20024
(202) 554-1404
Fax: (202) 554-5603

Mental Health

National Association of Black Social Workers, Inc.
15231 West McNichols
Detroit, MI 48235
(313) 862-6700

Nursing Associations

National Association of Pediatric Nurse Associates and
    Practitioners
1101 Kings Highway North, Suite 206
Cherry Hill, NJ 08034
(609) 667-1773

National Black Nurses' Association, Inc.
PO Box 1823
Washington, DC 20013-1823
(202) 393-6870

The Organization for Obstetric, Gynecologic, and Neonatal
    Nurses
409 12th Street, SW
Washington, DC 20024-2191
(No telephone number given.)

Nutrition

The American Dietetic Association, often in conjunction with the Department of Health and Human Services (NIH), publishes many valuable brochures and booklets for the public. You may order publications from:

American Dietetic Association
216 West Jackson Boulevard
Chicago, IL 60606-6995
(800) 745-0775

National Center for Nutrition and Dietetics
Consumer Nutrition Hot Line
(800) 366-1655

National 4-H Council
Expanded Food and Nutrition Education Program
7100 Connecticut Avenue
Chevy Chase, MD 20815
(301) 961-2800

Pediatric Physicians

American Academy of Family Physicians
Committee on Minority Health Affairs
8880 Ward Parkway
Kansas City, MO 64114-2797
(800) 274-2237
> Provides voluntary information on race and ethnicity of members so they may be identified as advocates and role models.

American Academy of Pediatrics
141 Northwest Point Boulevard
PO Box 927
Elk Grove Village, IL 60009-0927
(708) 981-7384

National Black Child Development Institute, Inc.
1023 Fifteenth Street, NW
Washington, DC 20005
(202) 387-1281

National Medical Association
1012 Tenth Street, NW
Washington, DC 20001
(202) 347-1895

Pregnancy/Childbirth

American College of Nurse Midwives
1522 K Street, NW, Suite 1000
Washington, DC 20005
(202) 289-0171

Healthy Mothers, Healthy Babies Coalition
409 12th Street, SW
Washington, DC 20024-2188
(202) 863-2458

> This is an informal association of more than 104 national and
> 100 state and local professional, voluntary, and governmental
> organizations with a common interest in maternal and infant
> health. Offers public and professional education materials on
> topics related to improving maternal and child health.

National Association of Childbearing Centers
3123 Gottschall Road
Perkiomenville, PA 18074-9546
(215) 234-8068
Fax: (215) 234-0564

National Center for Education in Maternal and Child Health
2000 North Fifteenth Street, Suite 701
Arlington, VA 22201-2617
(703) 524-7802

National Maternal and Child Health Clearinghouse
8201 Greensboro Drive, Suite 600
McLean, VA 22102
(703) 821-8955, ext. 254 or 255
Fax: (703) 821-2098

National Resource Center for Prevention of Perinatal Substance
  Abuse (CSAP)
9302 Lee Highway
Fairfax, VA 22031
(703) 218-5700

Safety

Advocates for Highway and Auto Safety
777 North Capital Street, NE, Suite 410
Washington, DC 20002
(202) 408-1711
> This is a nonprofit lobbying organization that works on high-
> way safety issues. At no cost they provide technical assistance
> in coalition building, lobbying legislators, and working with
> the media.

Mothers Against Drunk Driving (MADD)
511 East John Carpenter Freeway, Suite 700
Irving, TX 75062
(800) 438-6233
> MADD has developed community, youth, and public affairs
> and volunteer programs offering victim services in an all-out
> effort to reduce the numbers of drunk drivers, including teens,
> on the street. Drunk drivers kill some 22,000 people each
> year.

National Highway Traffic Safety Administration
400 Seventh Street, SW
Washington, DC 20590
(202) 366-2588
> NHTSA will provide copies of *Community Assessment Tool,*
> which is part of Tools for Community Action: Youth Traffic
> Safety Program.

National Injury Information Clearinghouse
USCPSC
Washington, DC 20207
(301) 504-0424
Fax: (301) 505-0124

Students Against Drunk Driving (SADD)
PO Box 800
Marlboro, MA 01752
(508) 481-3568
> SADD provides students with prevention and intervention
> strategies to help them deal with the issues of underage drink-
> ing, impaired driving, and substance abuse.

Sickle-Cell Disease

March of Dimes
National Foundation
Box 2000
White Plains, NY 10602
(800) 326-2229

Sickle Cell Disease Branch
National Heart, Lung, and Blood Institute
Federal Building
7550 Wisconsin Avenue
Bethesda, MD 20205
(301) 251-1222

Sudden Infant Death Syndrome

U.S. Public Health Service
American Academy of Pediatrics, SIDS Alliance and Association of
    SIDS Program Professionals
PO Box 29111
Washington, DC 10040
(800) 505-CRIB (2742)

INDEX

AA (Alcoholics Anonymous), 264–67
Abortion, 282–83
Accidents, 5, 71
Acetaminophen, 345
Acne, 342
Acyclovir, 345
Addiction counselors, 266–67
Adolescents, *see* Teenagers
After-school snacks, 167
Agriculture, U.S. Department of (USDA), 105, 163, 165
    Dietary Guidelines for Americans, 112, 166
    Food Guide Pyramid, 109
AIDS, *see* HIV/AIDS
Alateen, 265
Alcoholics Anonymous (AA), 264–67
Alcohol use and abuse, 252–53, 257–58
    diabetes and, 309
    hypertension and, 321
    pregnancy and, 13
    resources, 389–91, 408–10
    treatment programs for, 264–69
    talking about, 263–64
Allergies
    food, *see* Food allergies
    resources, 392, 410
Allergists, 191–92
Almond cookies, 211
American Academy of Pediatrics, 31, 69, 76, 125, 333–34, 367, 372
American Academy of Psychiatrists in Alcoholism and Addiction (AAPAA), 266
American Anorexia/Bulimia Association, 240
American College of Nurse Midwives, 32
American Dental Association, 82
American Dietetic Association, 125, 181, 238
American Health Foundation, 162
American Heart Association, 4, 312
American Journal of Diseases of Children, The, 364
American Medical Association Council on Ethical and Judicial Affairs, 84
American Public Health Association, 334
American School Food Service Association, 166
American Society of Addiction Medicine (ASAM), 266
Amniocentesis, 24–25
Angel dust, 261
Ankles, swollen, 40
Anorexia, 239
Antiretroviral medications, 297
Art and Craft Materials Institute (ACMI), 375
Art supplies, safety and, 375
Aspirin, 345
Asthma, 300–304
    preventing attacks, 302–4
    resources, 392, 410
    treatment of, 301–302

Athlete's foot, 342
Athletic programs, low-cost, 246–47
Attention deficit-hyperactivity disorder (ADHD), 61–62
AZT, 295, 297

Babies
    bottle-feeding, 129–33
    breast-feeding, 124–29, 131–33
    caloric needs of, 138
    checkups for, 67–69
    emergencies and, 71
    health resources for, 397, 411
    HIV/AIDS and, 294–96
    premature and low-birth-weight, 141–48
    safety and, 370–75
    sickle-cell disease and, 327
    solid foods for, 134–39
    teething, 79
    vegetarian, 138
    weaning to regular milk, 139–40
    when to call doctor, 70, 334
    see also Newborns
Baby food, homemade, 140
Bailey, Eric J., 86
Bathroom safety, 374
B-complex vitamins, pregnancy and, 16–17
Beef sloppy joes, 203
Bee stings, 381–82
Behavioral problems, 61–62
    food allergies and, 190
Bellinger, David, 363
Berenson, Gerald S., 314
Beta-carotene, 117–18
Bike helmets, 376–77
Birthing centers, 31–32
Bites
    insect, 381–82
    cat and dog, 382–84
    human, 384–85
Blistex, 335
Blood in diaper, 70
Body image, 60
    eating disorders and, 237–40
Bogalusa Heart Study, 149, 311–14, 316
Bones, broken, 380
Bottle-feeding, 129–31
Boys
    nutritional needs of, 176
    preparing for puberty, 275–76
Boys' Club, 246
Boy Scouts, 247
Breads, 158
Breakfast, importance of, 105–7, 165
Breast-feeding, 124–29
    premature and low-birth weight babies, 144
Breathing problems, 70, 71
Broccoli-stuffed potatoes, 205–6